Pediatric Endoscopic Surgery

Edited by
George W. Holcomb III, MD
Assistant Professor of Surgery and Pediatrics
Children's Hospital, Vanderbilt University Medical Center
Nashville, Tennessee

Foreword by
Judson G. Randolph, MD
Former Professor of Surgery
George Washington University
Former Surgeon-in-Chief
Children's Hospital National Medical Center
Washington, DC

Illustrations by
Paul Gross

APPLETON & LANGE
Norwalk, Connecticut

94 95 96 97 98 / 10 9 8 7 6 5 4 3 2 1

Prentice Hall International (UK) Limited, *London*
Prentice Hall of Australia Pty. Limited, *Sydney*
Prentice Hall Canada, Inc., *Toronto*
Prentice Hall Hispanoamericana, S.A., *Mexico*
Prentice Hall of India Private Limited, *New Delhi*
Prentice Hall of Japan, Inc., *Tokyo*
Simon & Schuster Asia Pte. Ltd., *Singapore*
Editora Prentice Hall do Brasil Ltda., *Rio de Janeiro*
Prentice Hall, *Englewood Cliffs, New Jersey*

Library of Congress Cataloging-in-Publication Data
Pediatric endoscopic surgery / edited by George W. Holcomb III.
p. cm.
ISBN 0-8385-8047-5
1. Endoscopic surgery. 2. Children—Surgery. I. Holcomb, George W. III
[DNLM: 1. Endoscopy—in infancy & childhood. 2. Endoscopy—methods. 3. Surgery, Operative—in infancy & childhood. WO 500 P3712 1994]
RD137.P39 1994
617'.05–dc20
DNLM/DLC
for Library of Congress 93-13799

ISBN 0-8385-8047-5
90000
9 780838 580479

Acquisitions Editor: Edward H. Wickland, Jr.
Designer: Penny Kindzierski

PRINTED IN THE UNITED STATES OF AMERICA

This book is dedicated to
George W. Holcomb, Jr, MD
Father, Teacher, Friend

Contributors

N. Scott Adzick, MD
Associate Professor of Surgery and Pediatrics
University of California at San Francisco School of Medicine
San Francisco, California
Fetoscopic Surgery

Richard G. Azizkhan, MD
Professor of Surgery and Head, Section of Pediatric Surgery
University of Buffalo, State University of New York
Surgeon-in-Chief, The Children's Hospital of Buffalo
Buffalo, New York
Bronchoscopy and Endobronchial Procedures

David A. Bloom, MD
Associate Professor, Department of Surgery
Chief, Pediatric Urology
Mott Children's Hospital
University of Michigan Medical Center
Ann Arbor, Michigan
Laparoscopy for the Nonpalpable Testis

John W. Brock III, MD
Associate Professor of Urology
Director, Division of Pediatric Urology
Children's Hospital, Vanderbilt University Medical Center
Nashville, Tennessee
Endourology

Ralph V. Clayman, MD
Professor of Urological Surgery and Radiology
Washington University Medical Center
St. Louis, Missouri
Laparoscopic Nephrectomy

James M. Estes, MD
Postdoctoral Research Scholar
University of California at San Francisco School of Medicine
San Francisco, California
Fetoscopic Surgery

Stephen L. Gans, MD
Clinical Professor of Pediatric Surgery
University of California, Los Angeles, College of Medicine
Senior Attending, Division of Pediatric Surgery
Children's Hospital, Los Angeles
Chairman, Subdivision of Pediatric Surgery
Cedars-Sinai Medical Center
Los Angeles, California
Historical Development of Endoscopic Surgery

Michael W.L. Gauderer, MD
Professor of Pediatric Surgery and Pediatrics
Case Western Reserve University School of Medicine
Director of Surgical Services
Rainbow Babies and Children's Hospital
Cleveland, Ohio
Percutaneous Endoscopic Gastrostomy

Keith E. Georgeson, MD
Professor of Surgery and Director, Division of Pediatric Surgery
University of Alabama at Birmingham
Surgeon-in-Chief, Children's Hospital of Alabama
Birmingham, Alabama
Laparoscopic Gastrostomy

Michael R. Harrison, MD
Professor of Surgery and Pediatrics
University of California at San Francisco School of Medicine
Chief, Division of Pediatric Surgery, and Director, The Fetal Treatment Center
The Medical Center at the University of California
San Francisco, California
Fetoscopic Surgery

George W. Holcomb III, MD
Assistant Professor of Surgery and Pediatrics
Children's Hospital, Vanderbilt University Medical Center
Nashville, Tennessee
Diagnostic Laparoscopy: Equipment, Technique, and Special Concerns in Children
Laparoscopic Cholecystectomy
Percutaneous Endoscopic Gastrostomy
Future Applications in Children

Louis R. Kavoussi, MD
Assistant Professor of Urology
Harvard Medical School
Boston, Massachusetts
Laparoscopic Nephrectomy

Kurt Kerbl, MD
Research Fellow, Division of Urology
Washington University Medical Center
St. Louis, Missouri
Laparoscopic Nephrectomy

Thom E Lobe, MD
Chairman, Section of Pediatric Surgery
LeBonheur Children's Medical Center and St. Jude's Children's Research Hospital
Memphis, Tennessee
Laparoscopic Appendectomy
Laparoscopic Management for Inguinal and Hiatal Hernia (Nissen Fundoplication)

Giantonio Manzoni, MD
Specialist in Pediatric Urology
Ospedale di Circolo e Fondazionne Macchi
Varesse, Italy
Laparoscopy for the Nonpalpable Testis

Christopher R. Moir, MD
Assistant Professor of Surgery
Mayo Medical School
Consultant in Surgery, Mayo Foundation
Rochester, Minnesota
Laparoscopy for the Female Patient

Kurt D. Newman, MD
Associate Professor of Surgery and Pediatrics
George Washington University School of Medicine
Attending Surgeon, Children's Hospital National Medical Center
Washington, DC
Laparoscopy for Intersex Anomalies

James A. O'Neill, Jr, MD
C.E. Koop Professor of Pediatric Surgery
University of Pennsylvania School of Medicine
Surgeon-in-Chief, Children's Hospital of Philadelphia
Philadelphia, Pennsylvania
Rigid Esophagoscopy

David M. Powell, MD
Senior Fellow, Department of Surgery
Children's Hospital National Medical Center
Washington, DC
Laparoscopy for Intersex Anomalies

Michael L. Ritchey, MD
Assistant Professor, Department of Surgery
University of Michigan Medical Center
Ann Arbor, Michigan
Laparoscopy for the Nonpalpable Testis

Bradley M. Rodgers, MD
Professor of Surgery and Pediatrics
Chief, Division of Pediatric Surgery
Children's Medical Center
University of Virginia Health Sciences Center
Charlottesville, Virginia
Thoracoscopy

David A. Rogers, MD
Senior Fellow, Department of Pediatric Surgery
LeBonheur Children's Medical Center
Memphis, Tennessee
Laparoscopic Management for Inguinal and Hiatal Hernia (Nissen Fundoplication)

Arthur J. Ross III, MD
Associate Professor of Pediatric Surgery
University of Pennsylvania School of Medicine
Senior Attending Surgeon, Children's Hospital of Philadelphia
Philadelphia, Pennsylvania
Rigid Esophagoscopy

Felix Schier, MD
Associate Professor of Pediatric Surgery
University Medical Center Steglitz
Berlin, Germany
Laparoscopic Procedures in Neonates and Infants

Kurt P. Schropp, MD
Assistant Professor of Surgery and Pediatrics
LeBonheur Children's Medical Center and St. Jude's Children's Research Hospital
Memphis, Tennessee
Laparoscopic Appendectomy
Laparoscopic Management for Inguinal and Hiatal Hernia (Nissen Fundoplication)

Joseph D. Tobias, MD
Associate Director, Division of Pediatric Anesthesia/Critical Care Medicine
Associate Professor of Anesthesiology and Pediatrics
Children's Hospital, Vanderbilt University Medical Center
Nashville, Tennessee
Anesthetic Management for Endoscopic Procedures

Jürgen Waldschmidt, MD
Professor and Chairman, Department of Pediatric Surgery
University Medical Center Steglitz
Berlin, Germany
Laparoscopic Procedures in Neonates and Infants

Robert E. Wood, PhD, MD
Professor of Pediatrics and Chief, Division of Pulmonary Medicine, Department of Pediatrics
University of North Carolina at Chapel Hill School of Medicine
Chapel Hill, North Carolina
Bronchoscopy and Endobronchial Procedures

Contents

Preface

The advent of laparoscopic and thoracoscopic surgery has changed the way in which surgery is practiced today. Five years ago, very few surgeons knew about these minimally invasive techniques and even fewer surgeons were practicing them. In the last 5 years, there has been an explosion of new laparoscopic and thoracoscopic techniques with progressive refinement of previously used endoscopic techniques.

This book is intended to provide an introduction to the basic principles of laparoscopy, thoracoscopy, and endoscopy in the care of the infant and child. The authors have been carefully selected because of their expertise in the areas about which they write. In addition, the primary emphasis of the book is on the newer modalities of laparoscopy and thoracoscopy, but it should be remembered that these are merely another form of endoscopic surgery.

It is my hope that this text will provide information and guidance to those practicing minimally invasive surgery and will stimulate others to apply these techniques when it is in the patient's best interest.

This book could not have been completed without the help of three people. My secretary, Nancy Hanna, has provided more than secretarial assistance in the completion of this book. She has been of immense help in the organization and completion of the entire project. In addition, Paul Gross has provided superb graphics to demonstrate the various procedures described in the chapters. The final person, without whose help I could not have completed this book, is my father, who has served as a reviewer, mentor, and friend during the time it has taken to complete this effort. All three people deserve special recognition for their time and attention to this book.

George W. Holcomb III

Foreword

Over time, a series of intersecting events, sharply focused by chance or by The Grand Design, can produce an extraordinary work. Witness the confluence of interlocking coincidences that has led to this important book. In the late 1940s, Dr. George Whitfield Holcomb, a Nashville physician, watched with pride as his son, George W. Holcomb, Jr, MD, traveled to Boston to study with Dr. Robert E. Gross in the nascent specialty of pediatric surgery. Returning to his boyhood home in Tennessee, Dr. Holcomb, Jr, established one of the early practices of pediatric surgery in this country and began service on the clinical faculty of Vanderbilt University Medical Center.

In the early 1960s, a bright young physician named James A. O'Neill, Jr, arrived at Vanderbilt as a resident in general surgery. There, Dr. O'Neill was captivated by the challenges of pediatric surgery and secured a position in Columbus, Ohio, to learn children's surgery in the well-known training program directed by Dr. William Clatworthy. In 1970, Dr. O'Neill returned to Vanderbilt to develop a full-time department of pediatric surgery. Subsequently, he and Dr. Holcomb created a unique academic and clinical partnership which thrived thereafter. A decade passed with increasing strength and productivity of the growing pediatric surgery service at Vanderbilt. Another significant note in this narrative is Dr. Holcomb's ongoing interest in and contributions to the body of knowledge of biliary tract disease in infants and children. In 1980, Dr. O'Neill left Nashville and Vanderbilt to head one of the nation's premier programs in pediatric surgery at the Children's Hospital of Philadelphia. Concomitantly, Dr. Holcomb's son, Dr. George W. Holcomb III, began his career as an intern on the Vanderbilt surgical service. Perhaps by genetic leanings and by environmental stimuli, the younger Dr. Holcomb became enamored with the surgical problems of infants and children. Accepted for the training program at Children's Hospital of Philadelphia under Dr. O'Neill, he spent two highly productive years, then returned in 1988 to Nashville to join the faculty at Children's Hospital, Vanderbilt University Medical Center.

As these connecting events unfurled, the creation of this textbook received a boost from a startling development close at hand. After appropriate literature search and laboratory work, two Nashville surgeons, Dr. Reddick and Dr. Olsen, successfully introduced clinical laparoscopic cholecystectomy. From their educational seminars, endoscopic cholecystectomy rapidly spread across the country. With the advice and instruction of Dr. Olsen immediately available, Dr. George W. Holcomb III was in the vanguard of pediatric surgeons who adapted the technique of laparoscopic cholecystectomy to small subjects.

Members of my generation remember three or four decades ago when we struggled with long alligator forceps passed down a brass No. 3 bronchoscope. The tiny light showed a peephole 18 inches away with a wisp of foreign body waving maddeningly at the operator. It was difficult to acquire the necessary touch with that outmoded equipment, and we challenged all principles of experiential education to teach it to residents. Fiberoptics and modern lens systems have eliminated those indelible agonies. Similarly, even the most hidebound skeptics, who long for a generous incision and finger control of anatomic structures, must lay aside their reluctance and realize, yea marvel at, the results innovative pediatric surgeons are obtaining with this remarkable miniaturized equipment.

It is not, however, simply a fortuitous series of events that led to the construction of this book. A blend of curiosity, skill, industry, and surgical insight led Editor Holcomb to master the techniques, then marshal this new body of knowledge. As so ably detailed by the work of experts gathered in this timely volume, a new highway in children's surgery has been charted. On the basis of these principles, ever-widening applications of the endoscope for investigation and therapy in pediatric patients will be realized.

The new methodology described here demands old-fashioned attention to anatomy and pathology and the deft touch that every surgical house officer throughout history has sought to acquire. Among his many other attributes, Dr. Robert E. Gross, pioneer pediatric surgeon and teacher, was a master mechanic. Without hesitation, he would have seized on this new technology. Dr. Gross would have thrilled to the delicate techniques described in this book and would have recognized the splendid contribution that this text makes to the science, the art, and the triumphs of pediatric surgery.

Judson G. Randolph

CHAPTER 1

Historical Development of Pediatric Endoscopic Surgery

STEPHEN L. GANS

The appearance and workings of the tissues of the living human body underneath its dermal covering have always been a matter of great curiosity and importance to scientists and particularly to practitioners of the medical arts. Studies of the body fluids moved from speculation to present-day sophistication and unimaginable complexity. Imaging methods proceeded along similar pathways to their present, almost artistic, state.

Creative but crude attempts to directly examine body cavities began to be made in the early nineteenth century. Bozzinni recognized the need to provide a direct light for these purposes and devised a wax candle with a mirror reflection to illuminate shallow orifices for examination and manipulation.[1]

In Paris in 1867, Desormeaux designed an open-tube endoscope for use in examining the urethra and bladder. For illumination he used the light of a small flame of a mixture of alcohol and turpentine. He found that a lens, appropriately placed, could condense the light to a narrower and brighter spot. In Freiburg, Kussmaul, hearing about this instrument, was intrigued with its possibilities and sent one of his assistants to visit Desormeaux to learn about this endoscope. He was interested primarily in using it for esophagoscopy.

Hitherto it had been assumed that a tube had to be fitted with some sort of mirror, prism, or reflector to overcome the angle made by the horizontal axis of the mouth and the vertical axis of the pharynx and esophagus. As one more demonstration that all of the solutions to technical problems do not emanate from the laboratory, this problem was solved by chance at an inn in Freiburg called the Wolfschlucht, much frequented by students and clinical assistants at the nearby medical school. Here, a professional sword swallower performed his act, and one of the assistants, fascinated by the feat, persuaded the performer to visit the clinic for observation by Kussmaul. Noting that the previously mentioned angle could be overcome by proper positioning of the head and neck (Figure 1–1), Kussmaul had a local instrument maker fashion tubes of the Desormeaux type and introduced them into the gullet of his willing subjects in 1868. The view was hindered by poor lighting, fluid collection, and reflux, but it was a notable accomplishment and the start of a new art.[2] Because of this pioneering work of Desormeaux and Kussmaul, urethrocystoscopy and primitive esophagoscopy could be accomplished.

Others were also inspired by the sword swallowers[3,4] and, concurrent with and following these events, numerous tubes of several varieties were devised, and methods of use were developed in singular ways.[5,6] These efforts were punctuated by attempts to improve illumination. These ranged from the use of Bozzinni's reflected candle light, to the use of the flame lamps of Desormeaux, Kussmaul, and others condensed with lenses, and platinum wires heated by batteries to provide light, and finally to the electric filament globe developed by Nitze and based on Edison's concept.[7]

As the result of the preceding investigations, endoscopy has evolved around the use of an open tube with a light source, applied either distally at the end of a light holder (Figure 1–2) or at the proximal (eye) end, sometimes aided by a reflector or lens. Although quite acceptable in adults for many years for a variety of examinations and procedures, the field of view became very small and the image dim and less than satisfactory when reduced in size for pediatric use. For example, if a tube with a small diameter is used, such as that used for infant bronchoscopy with an inside diameter of 3.0 mm and a 200-mm length, the visual field is determined by the diameter of the small tube: 3.0 mm at one end is 3.0 mm at the other end (Figures

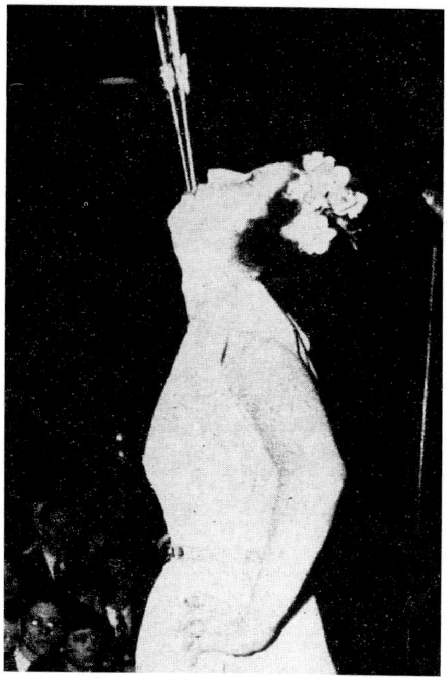

Figure 1–1. This is not "Kussmaul's patient" but a professional sword swallower demonstrating how to overcome the oropharyngoesophageal angle.

1–2 and 1–3A). The addition of a magnifying loupe at the proximal end does not change the size of the visual field. Because of the tiny view and the long focal distance through the tube, only a very small part of the organ is visible. For this reason, orientation is difficult and illumination is inadequate.[8,9] Recognizing that the use of a telescope could transmit an image from a deep hole to the examiner's eye, Nitze developed such a lens system and introduced the first cystoscope in 1879 (Figures 1–3B and 1–4).[10] This system became a standard over the years. Although the viewing angle was increased, it remained small. A greater drawback, however, was the enormous light absorption by the lens system. Again, this telescope was reasonably satisfactory for adults, but when the diameter was decreased for pediatric use, the light absorption became even more significant and the image quite dim as compared with that obtainable in adults.

Therefore, to this point, the limiting factor in pediatric endoscopy had been the size of the instrument. With the open-tube bronchoscopes and esophagoscopes, and with the conventional telescopes used in urethrocystoscopy and laparoscopy, the field of view was too small and too dim, making orientation difficult and the image less than satisfactory. As a result a large number of endoscopic procedures in infants and children were unduly prolonged, repeated, or abandoned even in skillful and experienced hands. For these and other technical reasons, pediatric laparoscopy was not possible at this time. In addition, the teaching of endoscopic techniques and principles was difficult and lengthy.

Miniaturization of endoscopes for all purposes in infants and children was made possible by two significant advances: fiberoptic illumination, and the Hopkins rod-lens telescope. In 1930 Lamm described successful experiments in transmitting light through small fiberglass threads held together in a flexible bundle.[11] If a bundle of these threads is sorted with great care, fiber A next to B next to C at each end, in exactly the same relationship, an image can be transmitted even if the bundle is in a bent position (a coherent bundle) (Figure 1–5A). If the individual fiber threads are not assorted in such an orderly manner but run haphazardly, each individual thread will not transmit its respective part of the image in position and the image is distorted (incoherent bundle), but it will still *transmit light* (Figure 1–5B). In the *rigid telescopes*, brilliant light is furnished by such incoherent threads placed along the lenses, but the *image* is transmitted by the *lens system*. In the *flexible endoscopic instruments*, both incoherent and coherent fibers are used, one for light and the other for image.

The invention by Hopkins of a rod-lens telescopic system provided the other move into miniaturization of endoscopes.[12] Instead of the traditional set of lenses spaced in air channels (Figure 1–3B), this telescope used rod lenses with small intervening air spaces (Figure 1–3C). As a result, the viewing angle was significantly enlarged, which provided a wider field of view and made orientation much easier. It also provided an important increase in light transmission, thereby making a much brighter image. Optical resolution was excellent. The previously mentioned light-transmitting fibers were wrapped along the telescope for brilliant illumination and the system was now complete. With this ingenious system, miniaturization became possible with exceptional performance.

Karl Storz undertook the development of such

Figure 1–2. Open-tube endoscope with distal illumination provided by a tiny globe at the end of a wire filament holder.

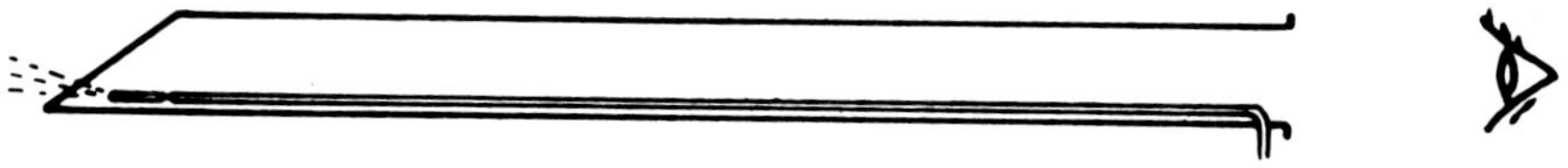

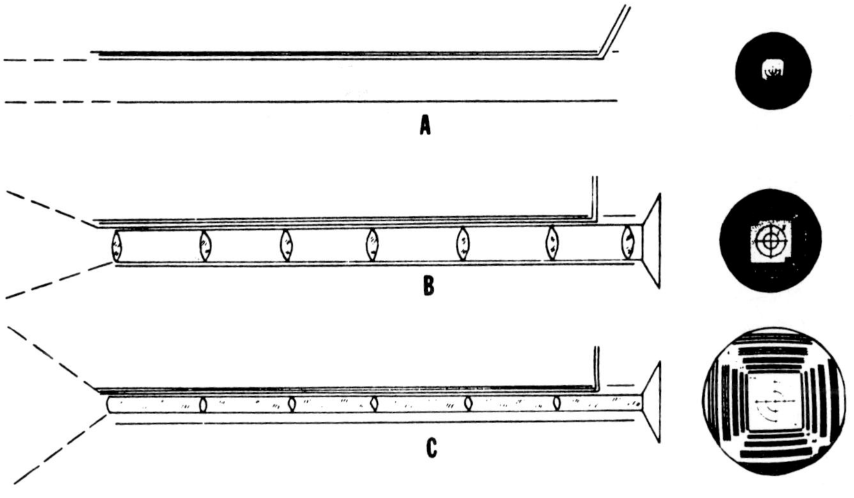

Figure 1–3. **A.** Open-tube endoscope with 3.0-mm lumen partially occupied by light carrier. The field of view is somewhat less than 3.0 mm and is quite dim and poorly delineated. **B.** Endoscope with conventional telescope. Although the field of view is somewhat increased, much light is lost in transmission, which makes the image relatively dim and resolution poor. **C.** Endoscope with Hopkins rod-lens telescope. Rod lenses are shaded. Compare lens arrangement with that in B. As a result, light transmission is greatly increased and the field of view is expanded and sharp. (*Reprinted, with permission, from Gans and Berci.*[8])

instruments, appropriate for the smallest of infants, at his plant in Germany (Karl Storz GmbH & Company, Tuttlingen). Provided only with charts and drawings, we planned a program of study and clinical trial. Prototype instruments were supplied to us by Mr. Storz in 1969. With these miniaturized instruments, the first few endoscopies were among the most rewarding and thrilling events of my professional career. The difference from precariously peering through dimly lit "straws" was a sensational turn of affairs. Subsequently, we visually explored all body tubes and cavities and developed new sets of indications and parameters for pediatric endoscopy. Sufficient light was transmitted so that split-lens teaching attachments could be used and photograph and television documentations were possible.

I made several visits to Mr. Storz and his brilliant crew of optical and mechanical engineers in Tuttlin-

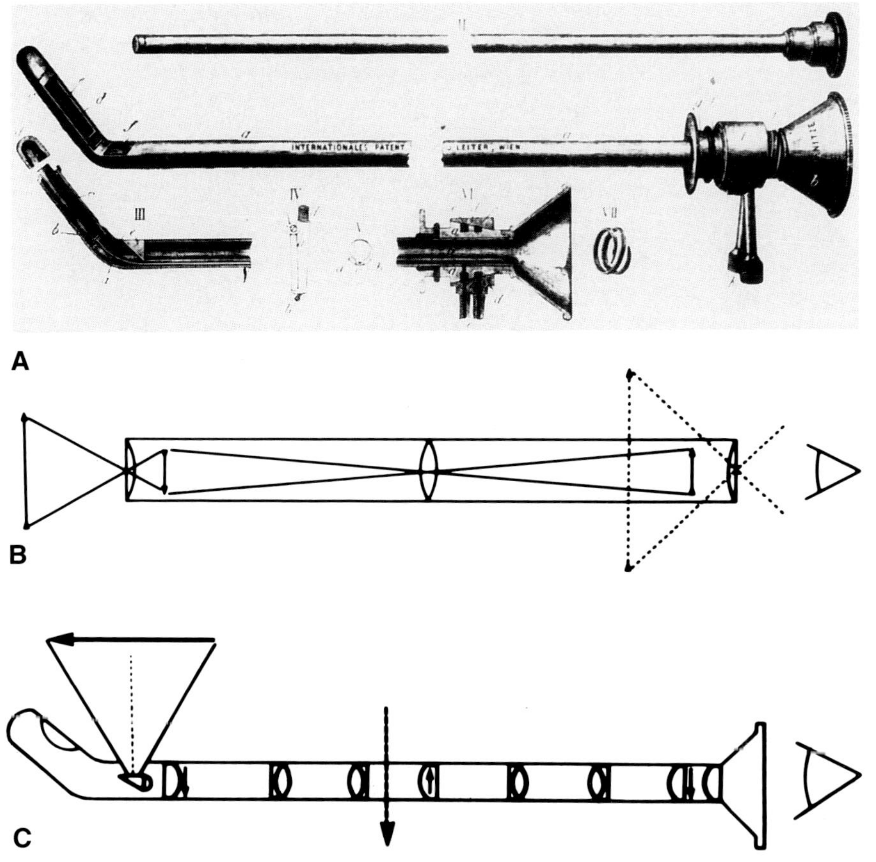

Figure 1–4. **A.** Nitze's first cystoscope employing an image-transmitting lens system. **B.** A schematic drawing illustrating the wider view obtained by his traditional telescope, although considerable light transmission is lost and the view is quite dim. (***A**, reprinted, with permission, from Nitze.*[10])

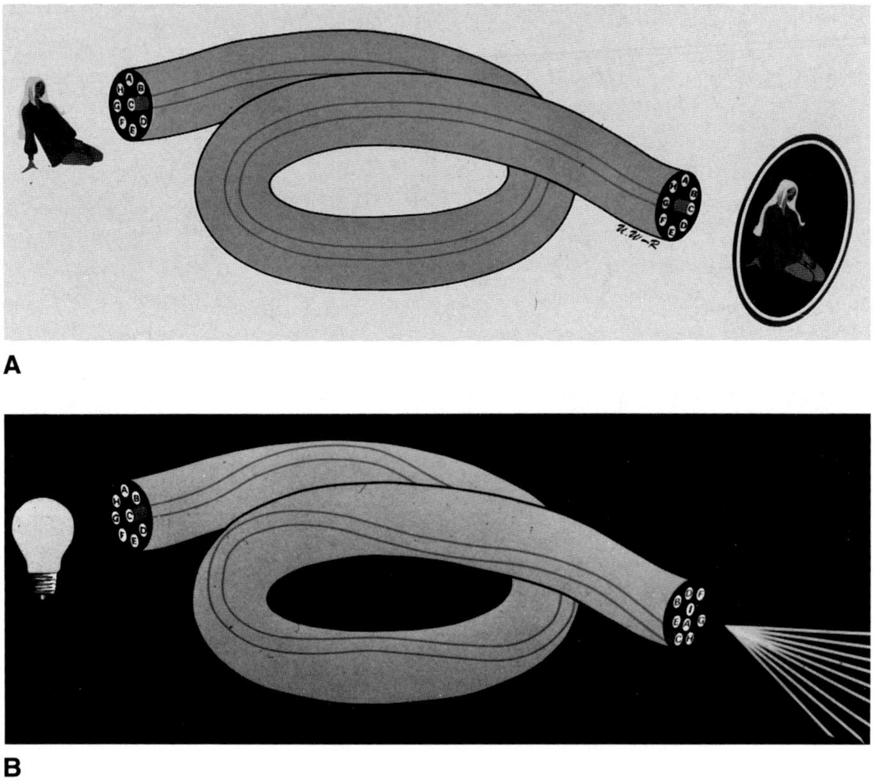

Figure 1–5. **A.** Coherent bundle: the glass fibers are in the same relationship to each other at both ends and thus transmit an image. **B.** Incoherent bundle: glass fibers are haphazardly arranged and will transmit light only. (*Reprinted, with permission, from Gans et al.*[35])

gen, which provided reasonable exchange of experiences and ideas for improvements. Initial results from these new endoscopic improvements were reported in 1971.[13] Pediatric endoscopy had now emerged from its "dark ages."

BRONCHOESOPHAGOSCOPY

These miniature bronchoscopes not only provided a sharp, magnified, and wide-angle view, but at the same time had sufficient space within the sheath for adequate ventilation and/or anesthesia and for the use of a number of manipulating instruments. With the same telescope, esophagoscopy was now possible with additional space for manipulation, injection, electrocautery (now laser), and safer dilation. For these reasons it became possible for surgeons with reasonable dexterity and surgical and anatomic experience with the involved organs to become proficient in related bronchoesophagoscopic procedures. Yet, some of the already proficient bronchoesophagoscopists who could see so much through the traditional open-tube instrument were not as convinced of the superiority of these new improvements. I can best illustrate this with the following story:

> A young pastor prepared a beautiful sermon describing the plight of the poor and how it was the charitable duty of the rich to share their wealth with the poor. After the service a friend asked how it went.
>
> "Well," said the young minister, "it was partially successful. I convinced the poor."

The "poor" were convinced, and these telescopic endoscopes became the standard for use throughout the world.

URETHROCYSTOSCOPY

In urethrocystoscopy the Hopkins telescope again provided a superior view and manipulative/operative possibilities. In 1971 Dr. Hardy Hendren visited our institution and we invited him to try our new instruments. After his initial shock in comparing the traditional view with the new view, we proceeded to endoscopically incise large urethral valves using a specially made television camera, with our black and white television monitor as the viewing field. This was probably the first endoscopic pediatric operation performed in this way, long before the era of microvideo cameras and high-resolution color monitors.

LAPAROSCOPY

Laparoscopy was first described by Kelling in 1902 using an optical instrument in dogs.[14] In 1910, Jacobaeus was the first to describe laparoscopy in the human, using a trocar and cystoscope.[15] Kalk and Bruhl advocated it in Europe and produced a series of 2000 cases without fatality.[16] Even in adults, however, acceptance for the procedure was slow and it was practiced by only a few hepatologists and gynecologists. As a result of the availability of improved telescopic instruments, laparoscopy became more popular with gynecologists.

The use of laparoscopy in the *pediatric* age group was virtually unknown until we obtained the first prototype instruments in 1969. We developed and tested our own method of laparoscopy suitable for infants and children, and this is still the method accepted and practiced on most pediatric surgical services today. We reported our results first in 1971 and later in 1973.[13,17] At that time we referred to the procedure as *peritoneoscopy*, and the use of this name resulted in future difficulties in searching the literature for *laparoscopy*.

Our first case was the successful verification of a hernia on the opposite side by an endoscope introduced through the contralateral known hernia sac. This was followed by a succession of cases using a pneumoperitoneum established by our conventional method for liver and pelvic problems. This series also included a 2-kg 1-day-old with severe neonatal ascites, the youngest and smallest reported, and a case of the removal of a foreign body (a piece of Raimondi tube broken off and lying free in the pelvis).

Although our initial efforts were widely reported,[17–25] and presentations and demonstrations were provided at many major centers in many countries (Figure 1–6), laparoscopy failed to achieve wide acceptance in pediatric surgery. Notable exceptions were individuals who not only followed our initial efforts, but broadened the indications and parameters of the field. In Zurich, Stauffer gained considerable experience, particularly in hepatobiliary conditions.[26] From Boston, Leape reported the use of laparoscopy in pediatric gynecologic disorders and in the investigation of abdominal pain.[27,28] Rodgers and colleagues were the first to describe treatment of malfunctioning ventriculoperitoneal shunts in pediatric patients.[29] Rodgers was also the first to report on thoracoscopy in children.[30] In addition, we reported the advantages of laparoscopy in the management of abdominal trauma.[31]

Aided by the availability of the computer-chip television camera and high-resolution color monitors, creative general surgeons "discovered" laparoscopy and started the widespread performance of major procedures with this method. With the experience gained, the development of better and smaller instruments has brought the pediatric surgeon into the field. These events are chronicled in the following chapters of this book.

PEDIATRIC ENDOSCOPY WITH FLEXIBLE FIBERSCOPES

Although the problem of the oropharyngoesophageal angle had been solved by sword swallowers so that rigid endoscopes could be used, the more distal angles of the gastrointestinal tract still remained a problem. Several flexible scopes were made using lenses and reflectors in jointed tubes, but all provided insufficient

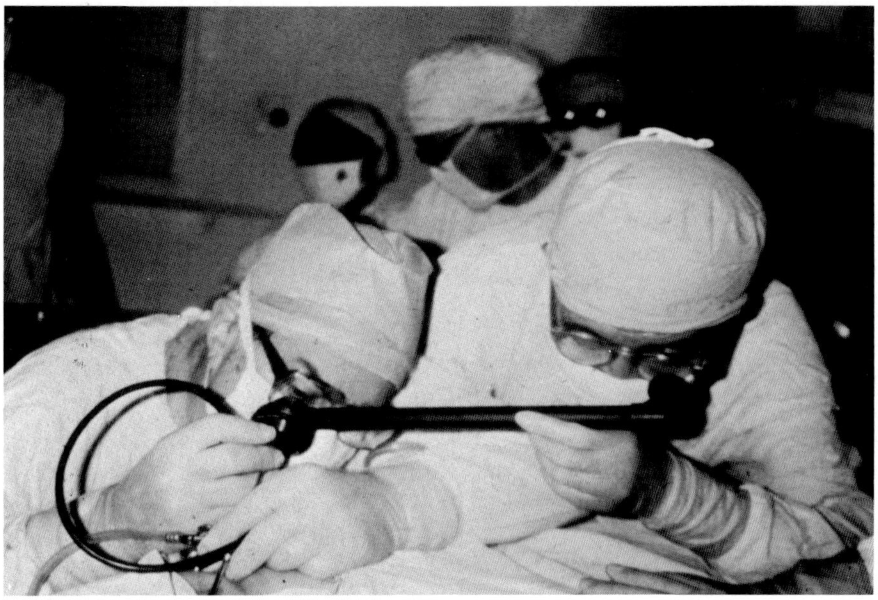

Figure 1–6. Demonstration of the techniques of laparoscopy to Professor Zhang Jin-Zhe (pictured on the right of the photograph) in Beijing in 1981.

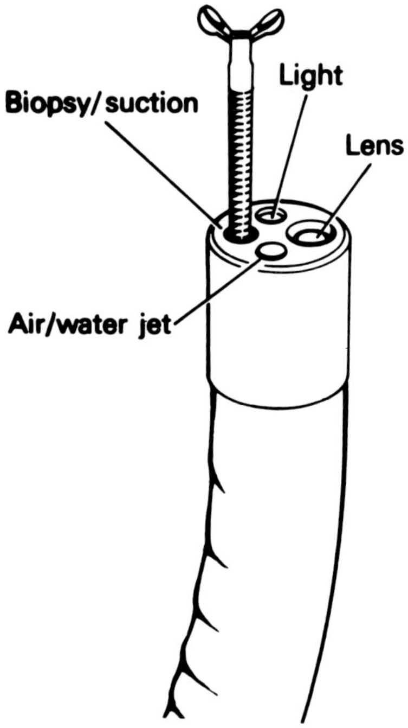

Figure 1–7. Distal end of flexible endoscope with facilities for illumination, lens and channels for air/water, and manipulation instruments.

and distorted views and could not be miniaturized.

The invention by Lamm in 1930, using bundles of fiber threads that could transmit both light and image through a flexible tube, became the starting point for flexible endoscopic instruments[11] (see Figure 1–5). In 1954, Hopkins and Kapany reported the first flexible fiberoptic gastroscope based on these principles.[32] In 1958 Hirschowitz and his co-workers published clinical experiences in the examination of the stomach.[33] In time, remote control of the tip, fixed focus, enlarged field of view, and channels for water, air, suction, biopsy, and cautery were added and improved (Figure 1–7).

In 1971 we started using an adult flexible *fiberoptic bronchoscope* for gastroduodenoscopy in infants and small children (Figure 1–8). The size and weight were more appropriate, but it did not have the capabilities of the larger sizes. We could look around corners and gain limited views. At the same time Freeman initiated trials of a similar instrument and reported his experience in 1973.[34] In June 1972, I was asked by the Olympus Company to meet their engineers in Tokyo to assist in the design of a flexible endoscope for pediatric use. A few months later they provided me with a prototype instrument. We used it for gastroduodenoscopy, colonoscopy, and a number of other situations in which it appeared to be appropriate. Our initial report was presented at the meeting of the Surgical Section of the American Academy of Pediatrics in 1974 and published in 1975.[35] This was the first published description of the use of pediatric flexible fiberscopes for gastroduodenoscopy and colonoscopy.

Here, as with the rigid endoscopes, the problem was that the instruments were still too large and too heavy for pediatric use and flexible endoscopy in children remained difficult. Miniaturization of the equipment presented serious problems. In the adult sizes, the image quality is obtained by the large number of threads in the image carrying fiber bundle. When the number of these threads is decreased to reduce the size of the instrument, the quality of the image suffers. Compromises were also necessary as compared with the other functions of the large scopes. Subsequent generations of these endoscopes have provided many technical changes and improvements and have brought us to the technology that exists today.

SUMMARY

We have come a long way since Bozinni peered into cavities by candle light, but each step was necessary to achieve our present technology. At first the open-tube and crude lighting systems prevailed and were reasonably satisfactory in adults but not for pediatric patients. The addition of the conventional telescope provided a wider viewing angle, but the considerable loss of transmitted light again made them less than satis-

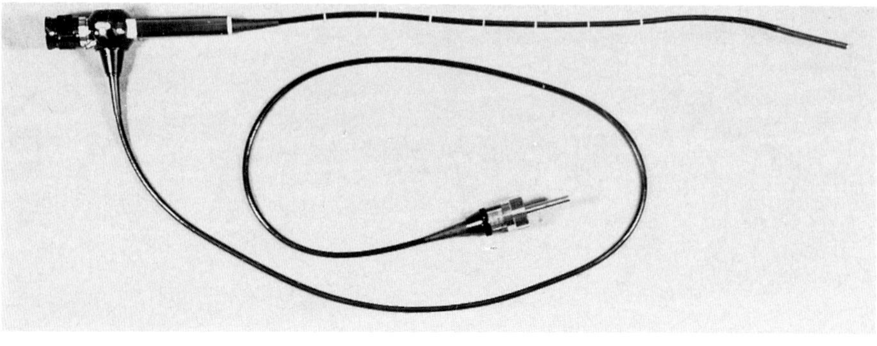

Figure 1–8. Adult flexible bronchoscope, early model.

factory for use in infants and children. Invention of fiberoptic illumination and the Hopkins rod-lens telescope made it possible to provide miniaturized endoscopes with exceptional performance. Continued technical improvements in fiberoptics have also allowed flexible endoscopic procedures to be performed in infants and children.

REFERENCES

1. Bozzinni PH. Lichtleiter, eine Erfindung Zur Anschauung innerer Teile und Krankheiten. *J Prak Heilk.* 1806;24:107.
2. Kussmaul J: Über Magenspiegelung. *Verh Naturforschenden Ges Freiburg.* 1870;5:112.
3. Huizinga E. On esophagoscopy and sword-swallowing. *Ann Otol Rhinol Laryngol.* 1969;78:32.
4. Von Mikulicz J. *Zur Technik der Gastroskopie und Oesophagoskopie.* Vienna: Wiener Med Press; 1881:1438.
5. Kelly HDB. Origins of oesophagology. *Proc R Soc Med.* 1969;62:781.
6. Berci G. History of endoscopy. In: Berci G, ed. *Endoscopy.* New York: Appleton-Century-Crofts; 1976.
7. Nitze M. Veraenderungen an meinem elektroendoskopischen Instrumentum zur Untersuchung der mannlichen Harnblase, III. *Monat Arztl Polytechn.* 1887;3:60.
8. Gans SL, Berci G. Inside tracheoesophageal fistula: New endoscopic approaches. *J Pediatr Surg.* 1973;8:205.
9. Gans SL. Principles of optics and illumination. In: Gans SL, ed. *Pediatric Endoscopy.* New York: Grune and Stratton; 1983.
10. Nitze M. Eine neue Beobachtungs Methode für Harnröhre und Harnblase. *Wien Med Wochenschr.* 1879;24:650.
11. Lamm H. Biegsame Optische Geräte. *Z Instrumentenkunde.* 1930;50:579.
12. Berci G, Kont LA. A new optical system in endoscopy with special reference to cystoscopy. *Br J Urol.* 1969; 41:564.
13. Gans SL, Berci G. Advances in endoscopy of infants and children. *J Pediatr Surg.* 1971;6:199.
14. Kelling G. Uber Oesophagaskopie, Gastroskopie und Celioskopie. *Munchen Med Wochenschr.* 1902;49:21.
15. Jacobaeus HC. Kurze Ubersicht uber meine Erfahrungen mit der Laparoskopie. *Munchen Med Wochenschr.* 1911;58:2017.
16. Kalk H, Bruhl W. *Leitfaden der Laparoskopie und Gastroskopie.* Stuttgart: Thieme; 1951.
17. Gans SL, Berci G. Peritoneoscopy in infants and children. *J Pediatr Surg.* 1973;8:399.
18. Gans SL, Johnson D, Berci G. Laparoscopy in infants and children. In: Berci G, ed. *Endoscopy.* New York: Appleton-Century-Crofts; 1976.
19. Gans SL. A new look at pediatric endoscopy. *Postgrad Med.* 1977;61:91.
20. Gans SL. The present status of pediatric endoscopy. *Z Kinderchir.* 1977;21:103.
21. Gans SL. Special problems in neonatal endoscopy. *Z Kinderchir.* 1979;27:81.
22. Gans SL, Austin E. Method and wide application of laparoscopy in infants and children. *J Jpn Soc Pediatr Surg.* 1981;17:1165.
23. Gans SL. Laparoscopy in pediatric surgery. *Chin J Pediatr Surg.* 1982;March:51.
24. Gans SL, Austin E. The technique of laparoscopy. In: Gans SL, ed. *Pediatric Endoscopy.* New York: Grune and Stratton; 1983.
25. Gans SL, Austin E. Laparoscopy in infants and children. In: Spitz L, Nixon HH, eds. *Operative Surgery: Paediatric Surgery.* 4th ed. Stoneham, MA: Butterworths; 1988.
26. Stauffer UG. Laparoscopy in hepatology and hepatobiliary diseases. In: Gans SL, ed. *Pediatric Endoscopy.* New York: Grune and Stratton; 1983.
27. Leape LL. Laparoscopy for gynecologic disorders. In: Gans SL, ed. *Pediatric Endoscopy.* New York: Grune and Stratton; 1983.
28. Leape LL. Laparoscopy for abdominal pain. In: Gans SL, ed. *Pediatric Endoscopy.* New York: Grune and Stratton; 1983.
29. Rodgers BM, Vries JK, Talbert JL. Laparoscopy in the diagnosis and treatment of malfunctioning ventriculoperitoneal shunts in children. *J Pediatr Surg.* 1978;13:247.
30. Rodgers BM. Thoracoscopy. In: Gans SL, ed. *Pediatric Endoscopy.* New York: Grune and Stratton; 1983.
31. Austin E, Gans SL. Laparoscopy in abdominal trauma. In: Gans SL, ed. *Pediatric Endoscopy.* New York: Grune and Stratton; 1983.
32. Hopkins HH, Kapany NS. A flexible fiberscope, using static scanning. *Nature (London).* 1954;173:39.
33. Hirschowitz BI, Curtis LE, Peters CW, et al. Demonstration of a new gastroscope. *Gastroenterology.* 1958;35:50.
34. Freeman NV. Clinical evaluation of the fiberoptic bronchoscope (Olympus BF5B) for pediatric endoscopy. *J Pediatr Surg.* 1973;8:213.
35. Gans SL, Ament M, Christie DL, Liebman WM. Pediatric endoscopy with flexible fiberscopes. *J Pediatr Surg.* 1975;10:375.

CHAPTER 2

Diagnostic Laparoscopy: Equipment, Technique, and Special Concerns in Children

GEORGE W. HOLCOMB III

Although the technique of laparoscopy has been available since the early part of this century, modern technology has improved the equipment, allowing the procedure to be performed safely and efficiently in children. With the proliferation of indications for minimally invasive procedures, technology should continue to advance and improved equipment should be produced.

Companies such as Wisap, Karl Storz, Olympus, and Richard Wolf, which produce flexible and rigid endoscopic instruments, also manufacture reusable laparoscopic equipment. Ethicon, Inc, and U.S. Surgical Corporation produce the majority of the disposable equipment. Disposable instruments have some advantages. For example, the point of a disposable trocar is very sharp and some have retractable sleeves. In addition, disposable scissors are usually sharper than reusable ones as they are used on one patient and discarded. Some instruments such as clip appliers and scissors can be rotated for easier use. Moreover, clip appliers are multiple-fire instruments and endostaplers are available to be used three or four times in the same patient. The disadvantage of disposable instruments is, however, cost. The disadvantages of the reusable equipment include a higher initial expenditure for purchase and progressive dullness with continued use; however, they can be used repeatedly.

The names of the equipment are peculiar to this innovative technology. The Veress needle is a long thin needle with a blunt retractable tip which can be employed to achieve a pneumoperitoneum (Figure 2–1). As the blunt tip touches tissue such as fascia or peritoneum, it retracts, exposing the sharp point. Once a space such as the abdominal cavity is entered, the retractable blunt tip extends, thereby protecting underlying structures from the sharp point of the needle. Insufflation tubing is connected to the Veress needle and pneumoperitoneum achieved.

Following insufflation, it is necessary to insert cannulas or ports, which are the cylinders through which instruments are passed into the abdominal or thoracic cavity (Figures 2–2 and 2–3). Often, a stopcock is connected to the cannula to allow flow of carbon dioxide for insufflation. In addition, there is a one-way valve within the cannula which permits introduction of instruments through the cannula but prevents gas escape. The trocar is the sharp stylette that accompanies the cannula. To insert the cannula, the trocar is placed through the cannula and both are inserted. Following insertion, the trocar is removed and instruments can then be passed through the cannula.

Cannulas are either disposable or reusable. The disposable ones frequently have accompanying trocars with safety shields, which protect intraabdominal structures from the sharp point of the trocar (Figure 2-2). Reusable trocars and cannulas do not usually have this safety shield advantage; however, they have been used safely and efficiently for a number of years by gynecologic surgeons.

Usually the initial cannula is placed in the umbilicus, which is the port through which the telescope is inserted. The most commonly used telescopes are 5 and 10 mm and require the appropriate-size cannula (Figure 2–4); however, a 2.8-French telescope, which has been used by pediatric surgeons for a number of years for rigid bronchoscopy, can be inserted through a 3-mm cannula for diagnostic peritoneoscopy in small

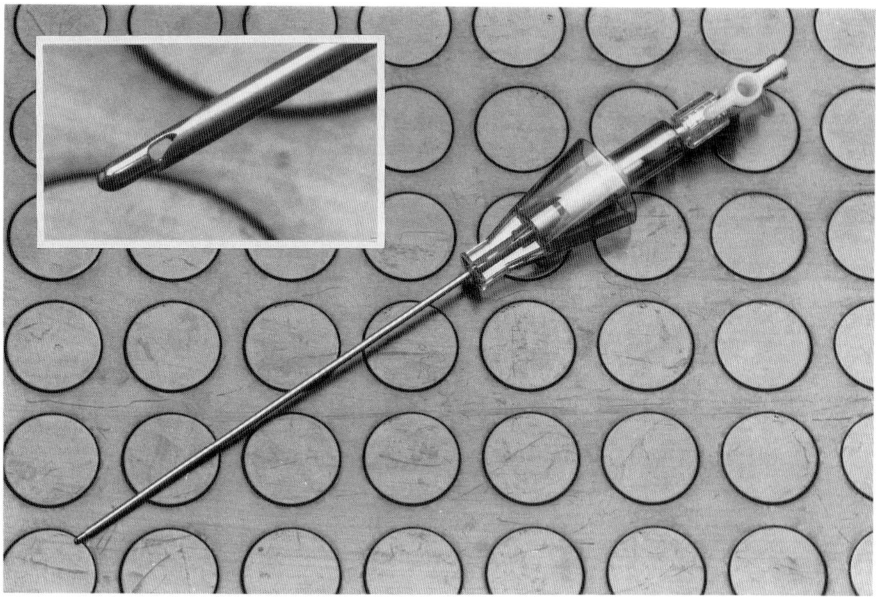

Figure 2–1. The Veress needle is often employed for creation of a pneumoperitoneum. Note the blunt, retractable tip which extends past the sharp needle (*inset*).

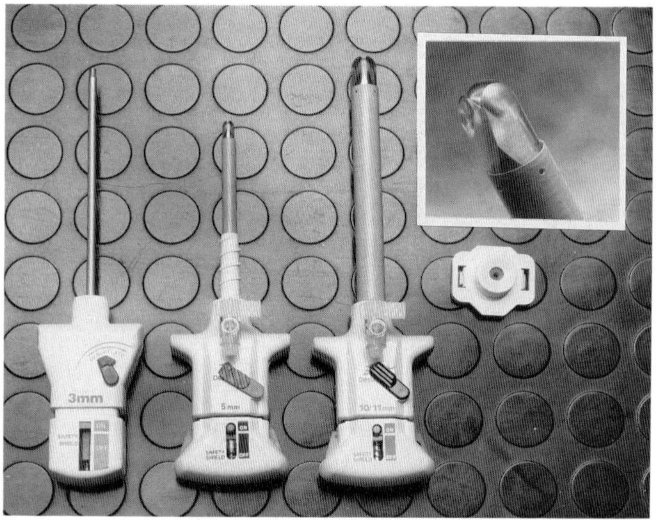

Figure 2–2. Three different-size disposable cannulas and trocars are shown. A 3-mm cannula (U.S. Surgical Corporation) is shown on the left and 5-mm and 10/11-mm cannulas (Ethicon, Inc) are shown on the right. Insufflation is possible on the two Ethicon cannulas through the stopcock. Also shown is a reducer cap, which is placed on the 10/11-mm cannula for insertion of smaller instruments to prevent loss of the pneumoperitoneum. *Inset* shows the safety shield surrounding the sharp stylette.

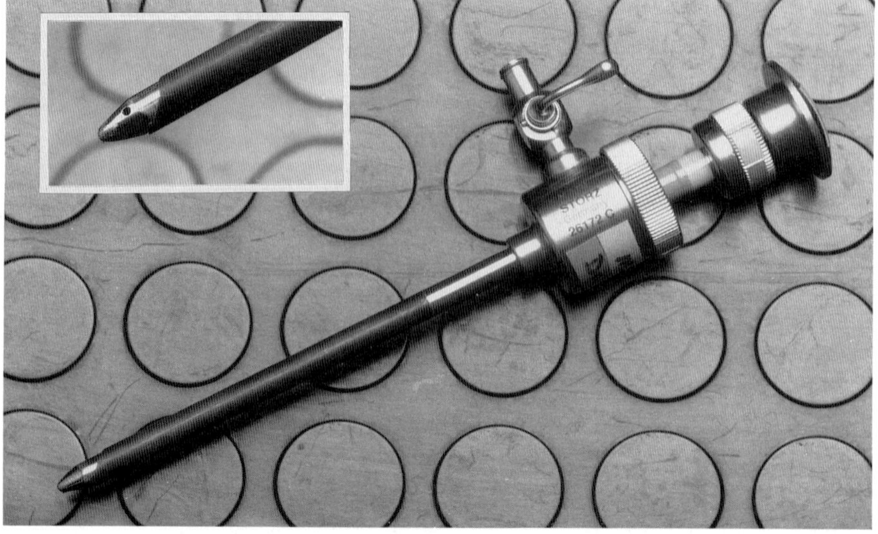

Figure 2–3. This reusable, metal 5-mm cannula and trocar have been specially designed by Karl Storz Company. The stylette has been modified to a blunt tip to prevent injuries with its insertion (*inset*). This equipment is used when the umbilical cutdown technique is performed for access to the abdominal cavity.

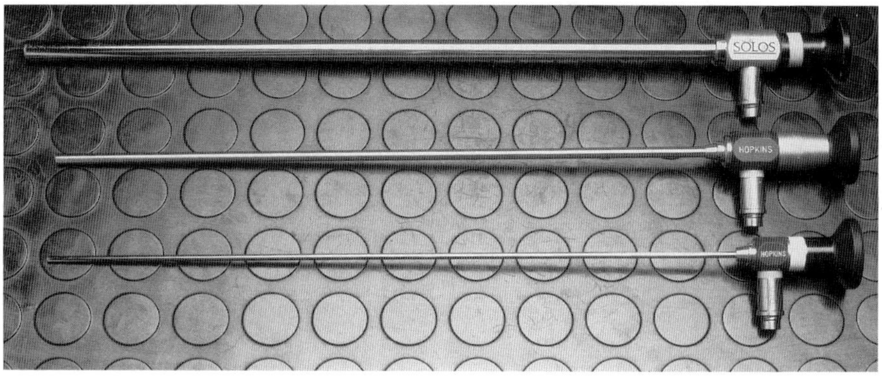

Figure 2–4. Three telescopes are identified: a 10-mm Solos telescope, a 5-mm Storz telescope, and a 2.8-mm Storz telescope. These can be introduced through a 10-, 5-, and 3-mm cannula, respectively.

infants if desired. Telescopes have several viewing angles ranging from 0 to 60 degrees (Figure 2–5). The camera connects to the eyepiece of the telescope and is connected to the video monitor to display the image.

The video monitors are employed at either the foot or head of the operating table and usually number one or two. Typically, for a procedure such as a splenectomy, fundoplication, or cholecystectomy, two video monitors are located at the head of the table (Figure 2–6), but for a diagnostic laparoscopy, laparoscopy for a nonpalpable testis, or laparoscopic appendectomy, a single monitor is positioned at the foot of the table (Figure 2–7). In addition, tubing is necessary for insufflation with connection to a carbon dioxide source. Pressure monitors are used to prevent overdistention of the abdominal cavity with resulting sequelae. Often, a case cart is assembled in which the video monitors, insufflators, light source, and pressure gauges are all arranged (Figure 2–8).

Grasping and dissecting forceps are used for tissue retraction, exposure, and dissection (Figure 2–9). Typically, a grasping forceps holds an organ for exposure. Grasping forceps can be either atraumatic or traumatic. Atraumatic forceps would be used when trauma to the organ is not desired, as for intestine or stomach. A traumatic forceps is used to grasp a specimen to be extracted and generally gives a stronger grip to the tissue than an atraumatic forceps.

Electrocautery instruments are also available. Hook and spatula tips are the most common tips available. In addition to forceps and cautery, scissors are needed and are either disposable or reusable (see Figure 2–9). Some scissors can be connected to electrocautery which allows the cautery to be employed during cutting or allows the closed scissors to be used as a blunt coagulation instrument. Suction equipment is generally effective. Again, reusable and disposable instruments are available. Endoloops (Ethicon, Inc) and Surgitie (U.S. Surgical Corporation, Norwalk, CT) are pretied ligatures. They can be applied to the appendix either for retraction during dissection or for ligation of the stump. In addition, they can also be used to close a perforation of the gallbladder if this occurs during dissection. Moreover, they can be used for vascular control. In Europe a pre-tied ligature is known as a Roeder sling.

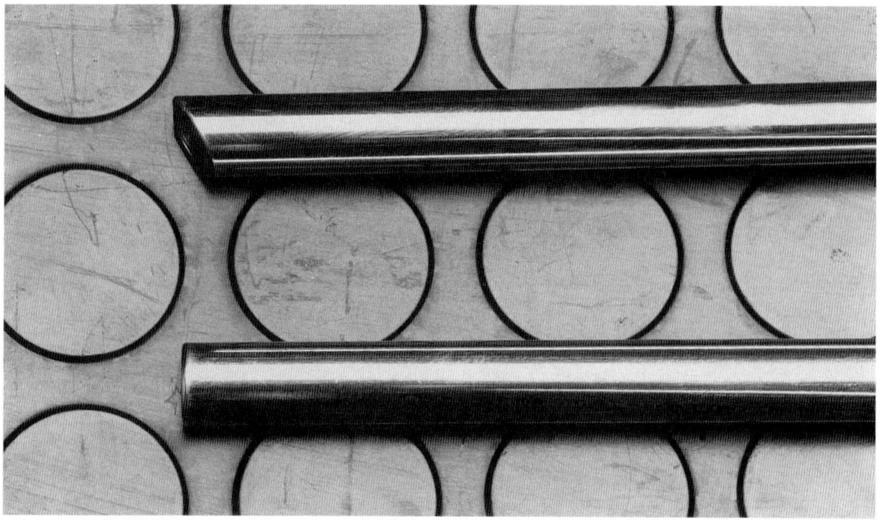

Figure 2–5. Telescopes have several viewing angles ranging from 0 to 60 degrees. A 0-degree lens is shown with a 30-degree lens above it.

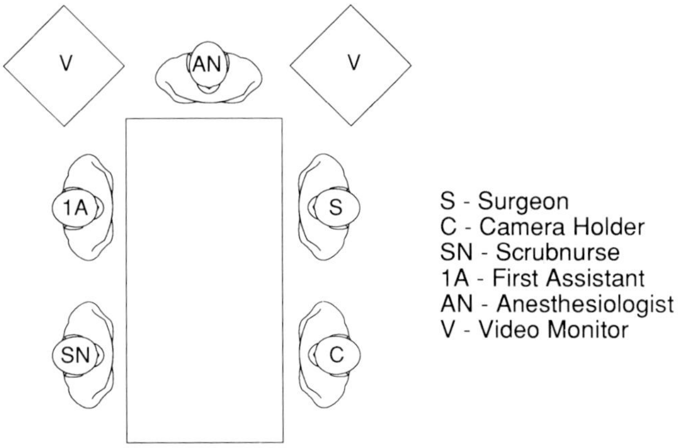

Figure 2–6. This diagram depicts placement of two video monitors for splenectomy, fundoplication, or cholecystectomy. With upper abdominal procedures, the monitors are usually placed at the head of the operating table.

Vascular control can be accomplished with endoclips or endostaples. Endoclips are typically used for ligation of small arteries and veins such as the cystic artery during laparoscopic cholecystectomy, but can also be applied to larger vessels such as the renal artery and vein or splenic artery and vein during nephrectomy or splenectomy. In addition, clips can be employed for division of the mesoappendix for appendectomy. Presently, endoclip appliers require a 10-mm cannula but 5-mm clip appliers may be available in the future (Figure 2–10).

The Endo-GIA (U.S. Surgical Corporation) is presently the only endostapler available (Figures 2–11A

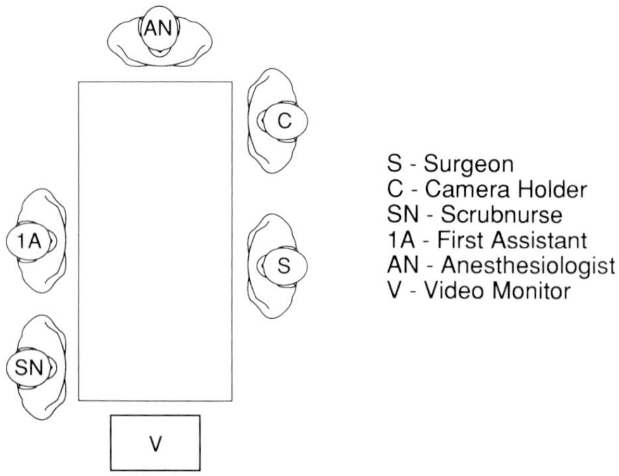

Figure 2–7. A single video monitor at the foot of the operating table is often employed for procedures such as diagnostic laparoscopy, laparoscopic appendectomy, and laparoscopy for a nonpalpable testis. In addition, the personnel are arranged differently for these procedures as compared with Figure 2–6.

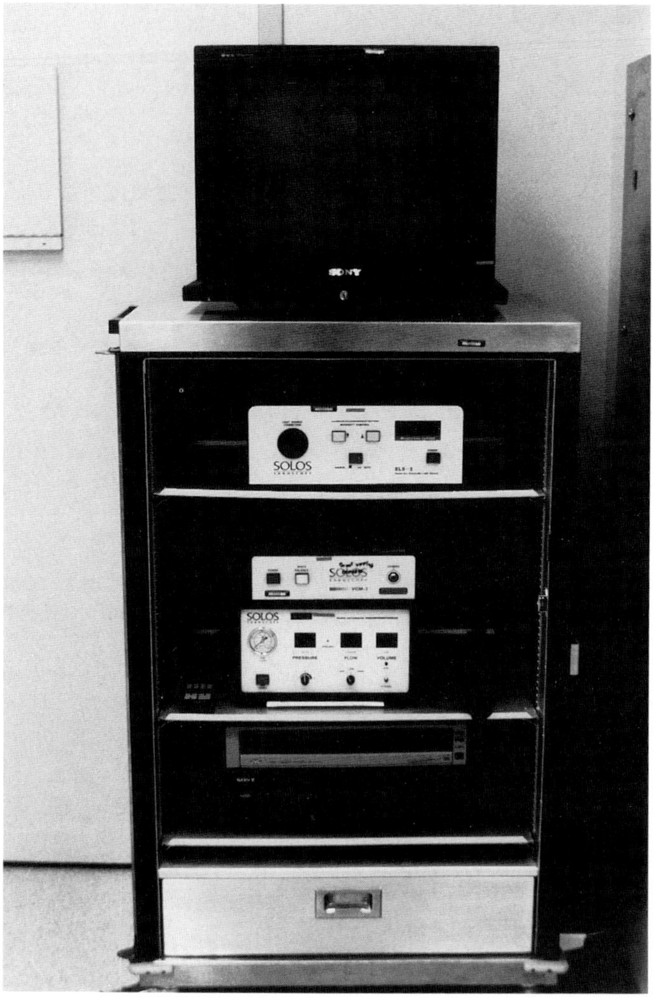

Figure 2–8. A case cart has been designed that contains the video monitor (*top*), telescope light source, camera light source and pressure monitor, and VCR/printer (*bottom*).

and 2–11B). Three rows of overlapping staples are placed along each edge of the cut. It can be used for ligation and division of the mesoappendix and appendix for appendectomy or for control of the splenic vasculature during splenectomy. Moreover, it is quite effective for thoracoscopic segmental lung resections and biopsies. Because of its size, the Endo-GIA requires a 12-mm cannula. In the near future, a roticulating instrument will be available.

Two other devices peculiar to endoscopic surgery include a specimen retrieval bag and a morcellator. Specimen retrieval bags are often used for removal of solid organs such as appendix, spleen, and kidney. Placement of an acutely inflamed appendix in the specimen bag is intended to decrease wound infection as the organ is delivered through one of the abdominal ports. To extract a larger solid organ, such as spleen or kidney, it is necessary to place it within a bag and disrupt it. This can be accomplished either with the

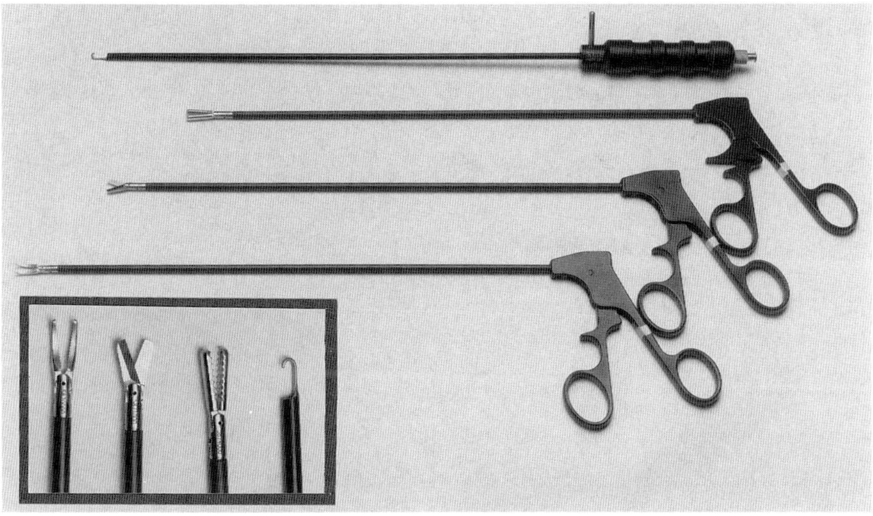

Figure 2–9. Several different reusable instruments including a curved dissector, scissors, atraumatic grasper, and hook cautery, are shown.

finger fracture technique or with a morcellator (Figure 2–12). The morcellator is a power-driven machine that disrupts the tissue and allows removal of the organ through a small incision.

DIAGNOSTIC LAPAROSCOPY

Prior to the laparoscopic procedure, a thorough preoperative conference should be held with the patient and/or parents detailing the advantages and disadvantages of the laparoscopic operation compared with the open procedure. Specific advantages are applicable to specific procedures but, in general, the laparoscopic procedure usually has reduced postoperative discomfort, decreased hospitalization, and a better cosmetic effect. Moreover, for more involved procedures, there is a faster return to regular activities such as sports and recreation and, often, reduced cost to the family.

During the preoperative conference, it should be emphasized that the laparoscopic procedure may need to be converted to an open procedure for a variety of reasons. Probably the most common reason for conversion is the inability to define the anatomy accurately for a safe laparoscopic procedure. This may be the result of an unusual anatomic variation or inflammation from an inflammatory process such as appendicitis or cholecystitis. Although excessive bleeding and bowel perforation are known complications, their occurrence is not frequent and should be minimal when proper technique is used.

The preoperative preparation for a laparoscopic procedure is the same as for an open one. If the child is to be admitted preoperatively for an open procedure, then he or she should be admitted in a similar fashion for the laparoscopic operation. This might include preoperative transfusions for sickle cell patients undergoing cholecystectomy or preoperative evaluation for lung biopsy or abdominal masses. Similarly, outpatient procedures performed with an open technique can be performed using the laparoscopic route as well.

The first step in performing any laparoscopic pro-

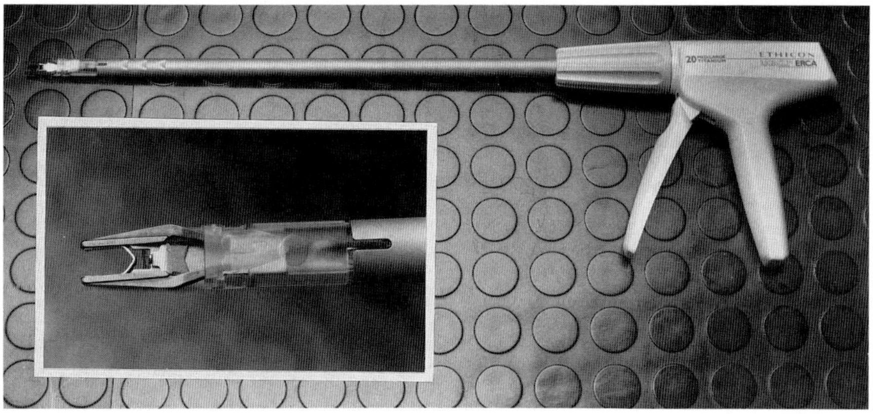

Figure 2–10. Endoclip appliers are available and are typically used for ligation of small arteries and veins.

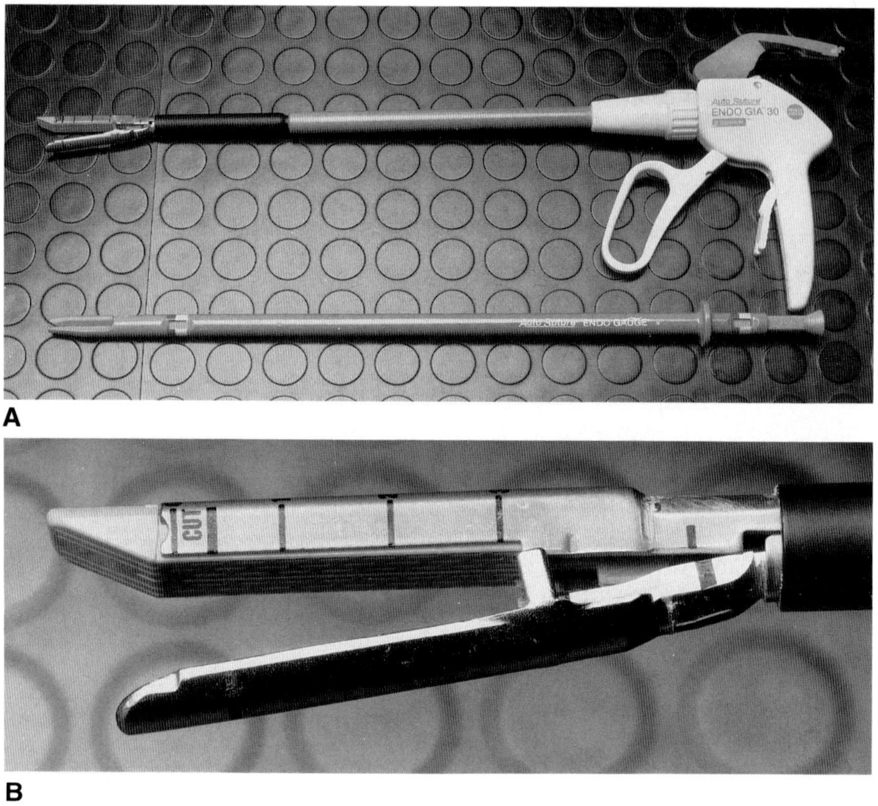

Figure 2–11. **A.** Presently, the Endo-GIA (U.S. Surgical Corporation) is the only endostapler available. Below the endostapler is an EndoGauge (U.S. Surgical Corporation), which measures the tissue thickness to determine the appropriate staple size. **B.** The staple line is 3 cm long. Three rows of overlapping staples are placed along each edge of the cut.

cedure is diagnostic laparoscopy. The patient is prepared for an open procedure and is positioned supine on the operating table. Video monitors are placed according to the needs of the particular procedure. Intravenous access is established and general anesthesia administered. Following anesthetic induction, an orogastric tube is inserted for decompression. In older patients, a Foley catheter is used for a prolonged procedure, but in smaller children, a Credé maneuver is adequate for bladder decompression. Gastric and bladder decompression are important to prevent inadvertent injury to these structures during passage of the umbilical trocar and cannula. The patient is then prepped and draped widely. Special attention is given to cleansing the umbilicus.

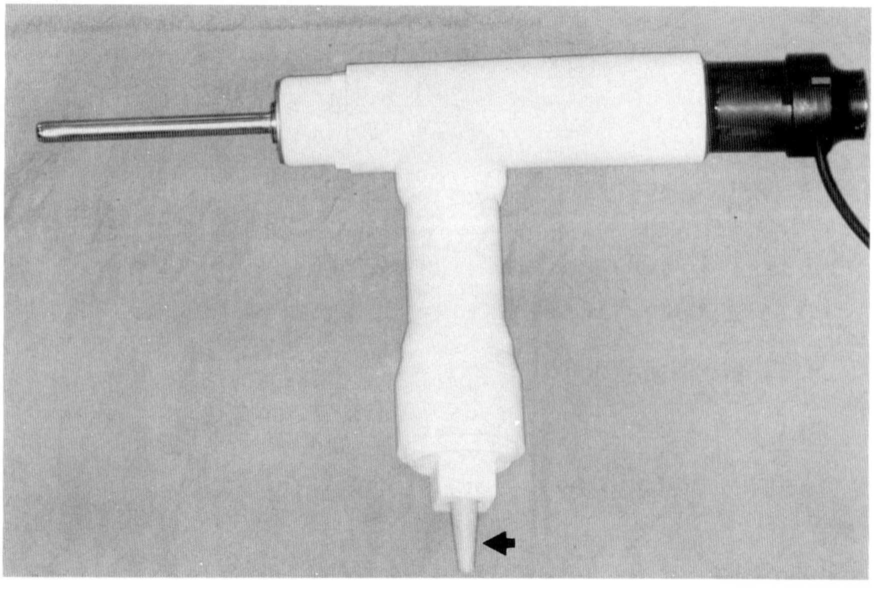

Figure 2–12. A power-driven morcellator is available for removal of solid organs such as spleen and kidney. A suction port (*arrow*) is also used during morcellation.

Umbilical Cutdown Technique

The umbilicus is the site of initial cannula insertion. Primarily two techniques are used for introduction of this cannula. In my early experience, I employed the Veress needle technique; however, an umbilical cutdown is now preferred on almost all children as this is the safest means for access into the peritoneal cavity. A vertical incision is made within the umbilicus and extended through the fascia and peritoneum. The opening into the abdominal cavity is visualized while the periumbilical skin is manually grasped and elevated. A 5-mm reusable metal cannula with a blunt trocar (Karl Storz, Culver City, CA) is gently rotated through the fascial and peritoneal incision into the abdominal cavity (Figure 2–3). The insufflation tubing is then connected to the metal stopcock and pneumoperitoneum quickly established.

Veress Needle Technique

An alternative technique employs the Veress needle following umbilical skin incision. Again, the abdominal wall is elevated by manually grasping the skin and the needle is inserted through the fascia and peritoneum, aiming toward the sacral promontory. Abdominal wall elevation may be facilitated in older or obese patients with the use of towel clips on each side of the umbilicus. If used, these clips are left in place for cannula placement. With insertion of the Veress needle, there should be a slight "pop" through the fascia and another one as the needle pierces the peritoneum. The angle of needle passage is roughly 45 degrees to the retroperitoneum, and one should conceptualize insertion of the needle just through the peritoneum (Figure 2–13). A lesser angle of insertion risks preperitoneal placement; a greater angle risks injury to bowel or large vessels. Care must be taken not to insert the needle too deeply toward the retroperitoneum, because if it contacts the vena cava or aorta, the blunt tip will automatically retract and the sharp point will puncture the vessel.

Following needle insertion, a few milliliters of saline is instilled with a small syringe. There should be no resistance to injection and only air should return with aspiration. If saline returns with aspiration, the needle tip is probably preperitoneal. If colored fluid (red or brown) returns, the needle is in an unacceptable location and should be removed. With each subsequent pass of the Veress needle, the risk of complication increases substantially. If the needle is not satisfactorily positioned after one or two attempts, it would be wise to switch to the cutdown technique previously described.

Another equally satisfactory test to determine if the needle is intraperitoneal is the "saline drop test." A drop of saline is placed in the hub of the Veress needle and the abdominal wall is lifted. The saline should quickly flow into the abdominal cavity with abdominal wall elevation, indicating proper intraperitoneal placement.

Another procedure used by some surgeons for

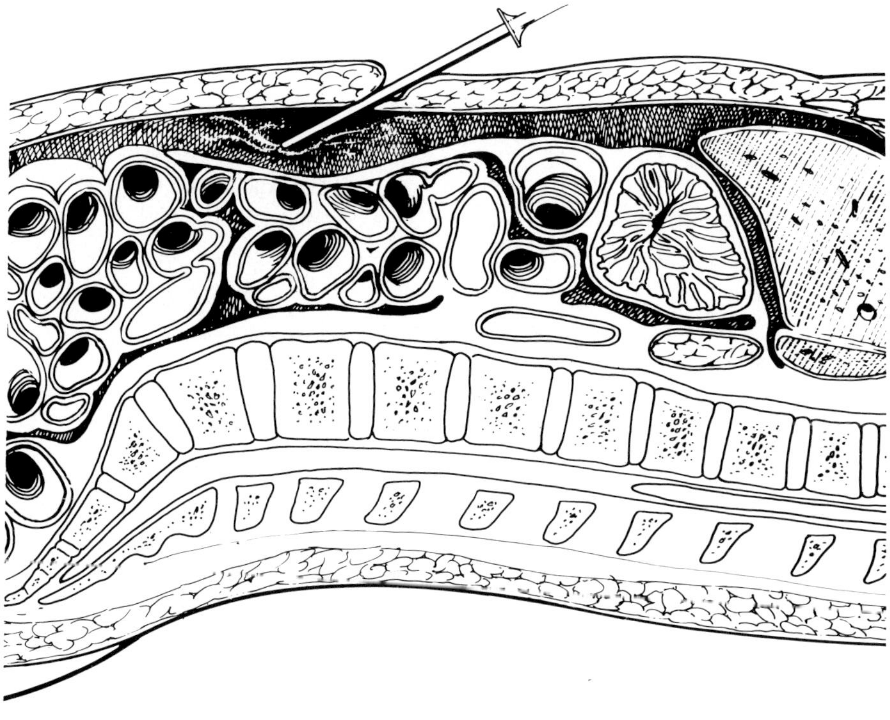

Figure 2–13. The Veress needle is inserted through the umbilical fascia and just through the peritoneum at a 45-degree angle. (*Reproduced, with permission, from Holcomb et al.*[1])

entry into the peritoneal cavity is the Lazarus–Nelson technique. With this approach, a short, hollow needle is placed just inside the fascia and a soft-tip guidewire is inserted through the needle into the abdomen. A multihole catheter is then passed into the abdomen over the guidewire (Figure 2–14).

Following entry of the Veress needle or multihole catheter into the abdominal cavity, carbon dioxide insufflation is initiated. Infants and small children require only modest flow rates (0.5 to 1.0 L/min). Initial and subsequent filling pressures should be less than 15 mm Hg, and early filling is normally attended by virtually no increase in pressure. In other words, the filling curve should be flat. An elevated initial pressure would indicate improper placement of the needle or catheter.

During insufflation, all four abdominal quadrants are assessed for tympany to ensure proper filling of the general abdominal cavity. A three-sense monitoring technique should be employed: an eye should be focused on the insufflator pressure gauge, an ear should be attuned to the pulse rate monitor, and a hand should be placed on the abdominal cavity. Distention of the peritoneal cavity should be symmetric. Percussion over the liver reveals a tympanitic sound because the pneumoperitoneum has lifted the abdominal wall away from the right hepatic lobe. Adequate pneumoperitoneum is assessed by loss of hepatic dullness, generous distention of the abdominal cavity, and modest palpable tension on the abdominal wall. Should the lower abdominal cavity be tympanitic but the upper portion dull and not distended, extraperitoneal placement of the Veress needle or catheter is likely and they should be removed and reinserted.

Once the needle tip or catheter is documented to lie within the peritoneal cavity with low-pressure measurements and symmetric tympany, higher flow rates (3–4 L/min) may be instituted in older children. Intraabdominal pressures exceeding 15 mm Hg during insufflation should raise suspicion about the position of the needle or catheter. The amount of carbon dioxide needed to insufflate the abdominal cavity adequately for laparoscopy will vary depending on the size of the child. From 1 to 4 L may be needed for initial insufflation.

Following satisfactory pneumoperitoneum, an umbilical incision is made adjacent to the Veress needle or catheter large enough to accommodate the umbilical trocar and cannula. The Veress needle or catheter is removed and the cannula and trocar are inserted safely into the pneumoperitoneum. With this technique, it is preferable to use a trocar with a sharp conical tip, but with a safety shield to protect the tip against the underlying structures once it has penetrated the peritoneum (see Figure 2–2). The trocar and cannula should be passed into the abdominal cavity at the same angle as the Veress needle. A "pop" and "gush" of gas should be heard with proper entry into the abdominal cavity. The camera and light cord are connected to the telescope and the telescope is inserted through the cannula. It is important not to move the cannula following insertion so that the underlying intestine can be inspected for possible injury at the site of the trocar insertion. Insufflation tubing is connected to the umbilical cannula and gas flow resumed.

Following insertion of the telescope, laparoscopy is performed. Laparoscopy can be employed for a number of reasons including evaluation of a child with

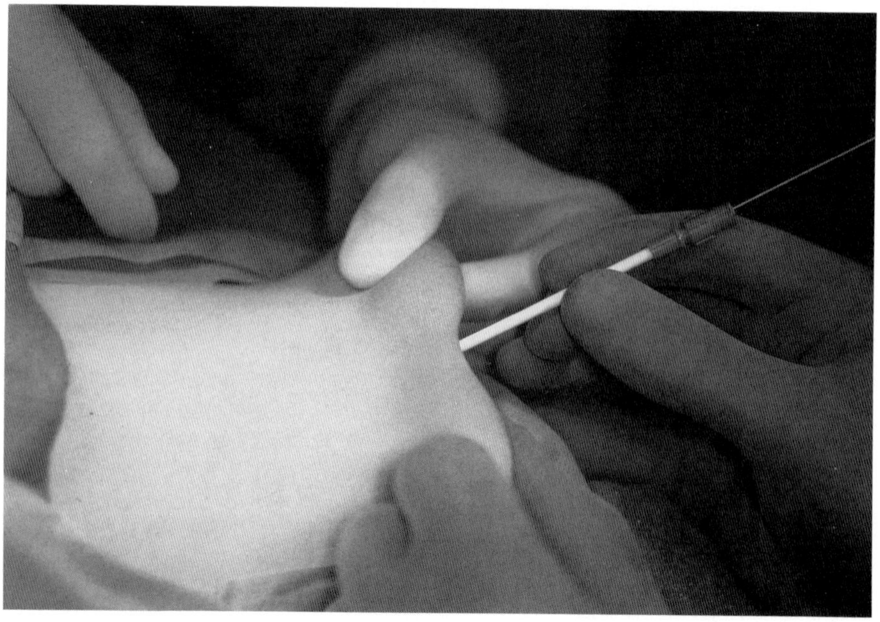

Figure 2–14. With the Lazarus–Nelson technique, a soft-tip guidewire is inserted through the umbilical needle into the abdomen. A multihole catheter is then passed into the abdomen over the guidewire.

a nonpalpable testis, for chronic abdominal pain, for possible contralateral inguinal hernia, for abdominal masses, and for evaluation of ovarian cysts. After complete endoscopic evaluation of the abdominal cavity, other cannulas can be inserted for procedural laparoscopy. Placement of these ports will depend on the nature of the procedure. Following insertion of the other cannulas, it is often helpful to change the insufflation tubing from the umbilical cannula to the largest accessory port, as the cool carbon dioxide used to insufflate the abdominal cavity may fog the telescopic lens.

SAFETY AND CONCERNS IN CHILDREN

With any procedure, it is important to use a safe and efficient technique. Because of the small size of the pediatric patient, there are several concerns peculiar to this age group. In most children under anesthesia, a Credé maneuver will adequately empty a distended bladder. As the bladder is an intraabdominal organ in infants and young children, it is important to decompress it prior to insertion of the Veress needle and cannula; however, insertion of a urinary catheter in a small infant may lead to iatrogenic urethral injury. For this reason, it is preferable to avoid catheterizing boys younger than age 10 and to catheterize older children only if a prolonged procedure is contemplated. It is also important to decompress the stomach with an orogastric tube.

A child's abdominal cavity has a much smaller surface area than an adult patient's cavity. Therefore, it is important to space the ports as widely as possible to allow adequate working space between them. If the cannulas are positioned too close, an efficient procedure will not be possible. Proper location of the ports can be difficult in small children for certain operations such as cholecystectomy and nephrectomy. For these procedures, at least four ports are usually necessary and it is important to separate them as widely as possible.

Emphasis on proper technique for insertion of trocars and cannulas cannot be overemphasized. Use of the umbilical cutdown has been mentioned with the advantage of direct visualization during insertion of the umbilical cannula. By using this technique, injuries to the underlying intestine should be minimized. Following creation of the pneumoperitoneum, if other ports are required, it is important to pay careful attention when the sharp conical tip of the trocar is penetrating the abdominal cavity. In small children with a very pliable abdominal wall, it is easy to push the peritoneum too deeply and injure the viscera during insertion of the trocar. One useful maneuver to prevent intestinal injury is to direct the trocar away from the viscera when the sharp tip is about to penetrate the peritoneum. Another technique to prevent trocar injuries is to use the Seldinger principle. This cannula is manufactured by Cook (Bloomington, IN) (Figure 2–15). With this technique, first a needle is inserted at the cannula site and then a guidewire is inserted through the needle. The needle is removed and the blunt trocar and cannula are inserted into the peritoneal cavity over the guidewire, dilating the tract as the insertion progresses. With this approach, sharp trocars are not used and this may be advantageous in infants and children.

Another potential concern is rapid intestinal insufflation during anesthetic induction. Anesthetic gas and air can be forced into the small intestine at a rapid rate with vigorous mask induction, which may make the laparoscopic procedure more difficult. This is especially important if the anesthesiologist does not appreciate the importance of minimal intestinal distention during the endoscopic procedure.

A final concern regards closure of the fascial incisions. In general, the 5- and 10-mm umbilical incisions should be closed to prevent an umbilical hernia. The 5-mm fascial incisions outside the umbilicus do not need to be sutured; however, it is important to close the anterior rectus sheath and, if possible, the

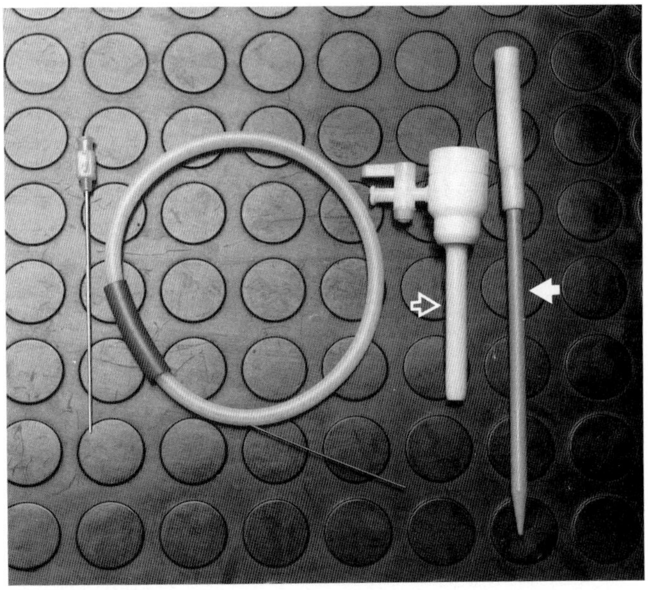

Figure 2–15. The Seldinger principle is used with insertion of the needle followed by the guidewire. The needle is removed and the dilator (*solid arrow*) and cannula (*open arrow*) are then introduced into the abdominal cavity over the guidewire. This laparoscopic sheath set is made by Cook (Bloomington, IN).

posterior sheath for 10- and 12-mm incisions, to prevent an incisional hernia.

With proper technique and experience, diagnostic and procedural laparoscopy will be a safe operation in children. It may be that one individual in a group practice will become interested in this new technology and will perform the majority of the operations for the group. With this approach, one surgeon gains a greater experience as the number of procedures increases, which ultimately should result in improved patient safety and operative efficiency.

COMPLICATIONS

As with any surgical technique, laparoscopy is a potentially lethal procedure and requires careful technique and safety precautions. The greatest risk for complications probably comes from placement of the Veress needle. It is for this reason that an umbilical cutdown is recommended for entry into the peritoneal cavity of children. Complications of improper Veress needle insertion include preperitoneal insufflation, which allows carbon dioxide to diffuse into the retroperitoneum and anterior abdominal wall, quickly obscuring the anatomic landmarks. Moreover, injury to underlying structures such as omentum, bowel, mesentery, or vessels is also possible. With insertion of the needle, if blood is noted in the needle or returns with aspiration, a vascular injury should be suspected. The safest approach is to remove the needle and assess the injury. Depending on the skill of the laparoscopist, this could be performed either endoscopically or through an open abdominal exploration. Fatal consequences may occur if the surgeon inadvertently insufflates while the needle is in a large vessel. At this point, immediate deterioration of the vital signs may result from an air embolus (see Chapter 18).

Intestinal injury may also occur as the needle enters the abdomen, but this may not be recognized until the laparoscope is placed and bowel contents are observed. Intestinal injury usually requires an open laparotomy for repair because maintenance of an adequate pneumoperitoneum in these circumstances may not be possible. If the insufflating needle is placed in the omentum, "omental emphysema" may be produced. Again, it is often impossible to proceed because the omentum cannot always be aspirated and deflated safely.

Injury may also occur as the trocars and cannulas are inserted. The intestine may be injured with placement of the umbilical cannula if this is a "blind puncture." As such, the trocar is not being viewed as it enters the abdomen. In addition, injury may occur to the underlying bowel from accessory trocars and cannulas because of the pliability of the abdominal wall.

Epigastric vessels can be injured as they are pierced by the sharp trocar. This is sometimes visualized endoscopically as the point is seen to pierce the vessels. With a thin patient, this injury may be repaired by extending the puncture incision and placing a suture ligature cephalad and caudad to the trocar site. This injury sometimes occurs in more obese patients because of the difficulty in visualization of the epigastric vessels. Nowzaraden et al have described the technique of placing a large deflated Foley catheter through the cannula[2] (Figure 2–16). The cannula is withdrawn over the balloon and the Foley balloon inflated. The balloon is then lifted against the abdominal wall and the tubing clamped at the skin level (Figure 2–17). It can remain for up to 24 hours if necessary. If the surgeon is experienced with laser coagulation, the epigastric vessels can be coagulated intraperitoneally

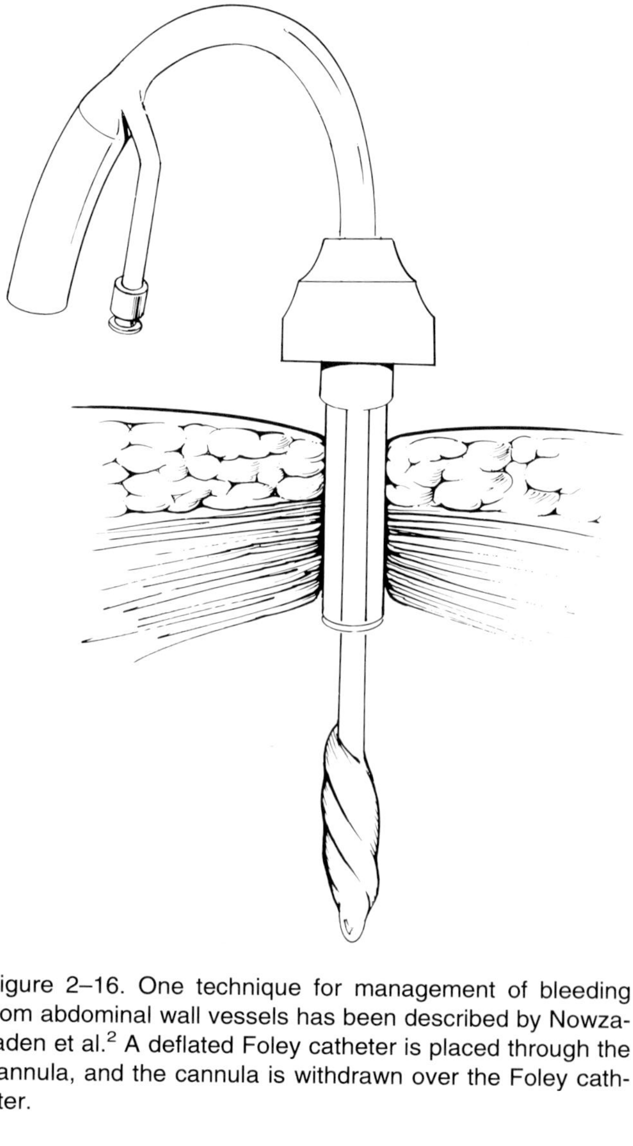

Figure 2–16. One technique for management of bleeding from abdominal wall vessels has been described by Nowzaraden et al.[2] A deflated Foley catheter is placed through the cannula, and the cannula is withdrawn over the Foley catheter.

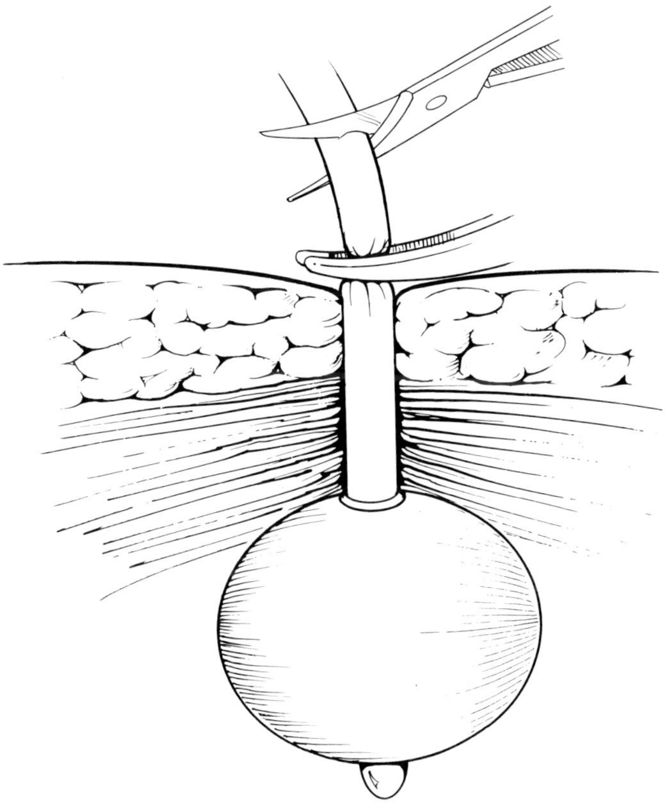

Figure 2–17. The Foley balloon is inflated and lifted against the abdominal wall. The tubing is then clamped at the skin level and the bleeding is tamponed.

using the Nd:YAG laser set at 40 watts. Alternatively, endoscopic suture techniques may be used for ligation of the vessels on each side of the bleeding point.

Postoperatively, complications may also be noted. Most commonly, these would include incisional hernia and omental evisceration if the skin was not completely closed. Delayed abdominal wall hematomas may also occur as small muscular arterial branches injured by trocar insertion may bleed in the postoperative period. Finally, postoperative peritonitis with abdominal distention, nausea, and vomiting may herald a "missed" bowel injury. It is noteworthy that a bowel perforation resulting from a monopolar electrocautery arc injury may not develop postoperatively for several days.[3]

TABLE 2–1. INITIAL LAPAROSCOPIC EXPERIENCE AT CHILDREN'S HOSPITAL, VANDERBILT UNIVERSITY MEDICAL CENTER, 1990–1992

Indication	Number of Patients
Contralateral inguinal hernia evaluation	170
Nonpalpable testis	35
Cholecystectomy	22
Appendectomy	20
Ventriculoperitoneal shunt problems	5
Gastrostomy	3
Peritoneal dialysis catheter	2
Partial ovarian cystectomy	1
Splenectomy	1
Diagnosis	3
Total	262

THE VANDERBILT EXPERIENCE

Over 250 laparoscopic procedures in infants and children have been performed at Children's Hospital, Vanderbilt University Medical Center, by several surgeons (Table 2–1). No intraoperative complications occurred and no short- or long-term complications have developed.

REFERENCES

1. Holcomb GW III, Olsen DO, Sharp KW. Laparoscopic cholecystectomy in the pediatric patient. *J Pediatr Surg.* 1991;26:1186.
2. Nowzaradan Y, Westmoreland J, McCarver C, et al. Laparoscopic appendectomy for acute appendicitis: Indications and current use. *J Laparoendosc Surg.* 1991;1:247.
3. Naffis D. Laparoscopic appendectomy. In: Holcomb GW III, ed. *Seminars in Pediatric Surgery.* Philadelphia: WB Saunders; 1993.

CHAPTER 3

Laparoscopic Appendectomy

KURT P. SCHROPP • THOM E LOBE

General surgery has undergone a revolution in the last decade. The explosion of laparoscopic technology has allowed minimally invasive surgery to become not only a feasible alternative modality for performing an operation, but the standard of care for many procedures.

Laparoscopy has existed in various forms over the last century, but within the last few decades this diagnostic method gained widespread popularity as a therapeutic technique. For years, gynecologists have performed many simple laparoscopic procedures including tubal ligations and myomectomies. Over the last few years, as instrumentation improved with ultralight video cameras and innovations such as the endoscopic linear stapler, the general surgeon has embraced this method as a primary technique for many complex surgical procedures.

Laparoscopic appendectomy was first reported as an incidental adjuvant to diagnostic laparoscopy by the German gynecologist, Semm, in 1983.[1] Various reports of laparoscopic-assisted appendectomy for acute appendicitis were published over the next few years.[2,3] Finally, in 1987, Schreiber reported a laparoscopic appendectomy for acute appendicitis.[4] In the following years a number of series, in the United States and abroad, were published and attest to the widespread popularity of this procedure.[5–10]

CLINICAL PRESENTATION/DIAGNOSES

Any patient with suspected diagnosis of acute appendicitis is a candidate for laparoscopic appendectomy. Very little can be added to the volume of material written about the presentation of patients with acute appendicitis. Signs and symptoms include crampy abdominal pain that migrates to the right lower quadrant (RLQ), symptoms less than 48 hours, anorexia, localized RLQ tenderness, tenderness on rectal exam, and low-grade fever. A number of pathologic entities are included in the differential diagnosis of appendicitis that may or may not be amenable to the laparoscopic approach depending on the circumstances. These include complicated appendicitis (ruptured or gangrenous), ovarian pathology such as cysts and torsion, mesenteric adenitis, Meckel's diverticulitis, and Crohn's disease. If any of these entities are discovered during diagnostic laparoscopy, the appendix may be removed incidentally if there are no contraindications to removing it had the procedure been an open laparotomy. We do not intentionally laparoscope patients if we believe perforated appendicitis to be present for several reasons. Patients with perforated appendicitis usually require a longer operative procedure because of the difficulty of finding and dissecting the perforated appendix. The theoretic disadvantage of placing a patient with a pneumoperitoneum in Trendelenburg position, allowing purulent fluid to settle over the liver and spleen, has been unsettling to many surgeons. Similarly, in a patient with a localized perforation that would be amenable to a small drainage procedure, pus would spread throughout the abdomen during a laparoscopic procedure. Also, as patients with perforation and diffuse peritonitis already require a prolonged hospital stay, little is gained by performing the procedure laparoscopically. Our preference at this time, therefore, is to avoid laparoscopic exploration if a patient has signs and symptoms of ruptured appendicitis, including free air, symptoms greater than 48 hours, and diffuse abdominal tenderness. If a perforated appendix is unexpectedly encountered while laparoscoping a patient for acute appendicitis, an attempt is made to remove the appendix laparoscopically, as there is little additional morbidity with the actual procedure of removing the appendix.

TREATMENT OPTIONS

Because there is no medical treatment for acute appendicitis, only surgical options exist for these patients. The surgical options include open appendectomy, laparoscopic appendectomy, or a combination of the two (laparoscopic-assisted open appendectomy). Elective laparoscopy may be useful, though, in selected patients with ruptured appendicitis. It may be employed in patients that initially have been managed medically with antibiotics and return at 6 to 8 weeks for an interval appendectomy. Also, laparoscopic drainage of multiple abscesses in some complicated patients as a sequela of ruptured appendicitis may be indicated and less dangerous than radiologic drainage.

RISKS AND BENEFITS

Most surgeons who perform laparoscopic procedures believe that laparoscopic appendectomy has a number of advantages over the open technique. It is an easy extension of diagnostic laparoscopy for abdominal pain. Once a surgeon is over the "learning curve" of laparoscopic procedures, it may be faster to accomplish these cases laparoscopically, as layered closure of an abdominal incision is not necessary. In addition, there is an improved ability to visualize the remainder of the pelvis and abdomen to search for incidental pathology. Usually, there is a decreased recovery period for the patient, including a decreased hospital stay and a faster return to normal activity.[9] As the incisions are hidden in the umbilicus and below the bikini line, there is a better cosmetic result. At this time, there appears to be a similar complication rate, but some surgeons feel that as a greater number of laparoscopic procedures are performed, there will be fewer complications in the laparoscopic group.

In a prospective randomized trial of laparoscopic versus open appendectomy, Attwood and colleagues concluded that patients undergoing laparoscopic appendectomy had (1) significantly decreased hospital stay (2.5 days versus 3.8 days), (2) decreased postoperative complications, (3) decreased pain, and (4) quicker return to preoperative activity. They concluded that laparoscopic appendectomy is the procedure of choice in patients with acute appendicitis.[10]

TECHNIQUE

As in most other laparoscopic procedures, the immediate preoperative preparation for the case and of the patient is crucial. The surgeon should assist the scrub nurse in choosing the correct laparoscope, cannulas, and instruments, appropriate for the patient's size and weight. The operating room is usually arranged so the primary surgeon can stand on the patient's left side, with the assisting surgeon standing opposite. Most surgeons feel comfortable with two video monitors, but unlike laparoscopic cholecystectomy, the procedure can be done with a single monitor at the foot of the bed (Figure 3–1). The child should have an orogastric tube and a urinary catheter appropriate for his or her size. After the patient is placed supine, a full antimicrobial preparation of the abdomen should be done from nipples to genitalia and from table to table on the sides. Special attention should be given to cleaning the umbilicus. Drapes should be placed to expose the umbilicus, right and left anterior superior iliac spines, and the area just above the pubis.

Abdominal insufflation and insertion of umbilical trocar are next accomplished. One of several techniques can be employed depending on the surgeon's preference as discussed in Chapter 2. We use a 5-mm laparoscope for children less than 10 years and a 10-mm scope and cannula for older children. A quick inspection of the pelvis and abdomen is accomplished starting in the RLQ. We usually take a quick glance at the other quadrants to rule out other obvious pathology. If there is inflammation in the RLQ we make the decision to proceed with the operation and must then determine which technique we will use to remove the appendix because it will influence the placement and size of the remaining two cannulas.

An appendectomy may be performed by using the linear stapler, endoscopic loops, surgical clips, laser, or suture, all requiring slight variation in the can-

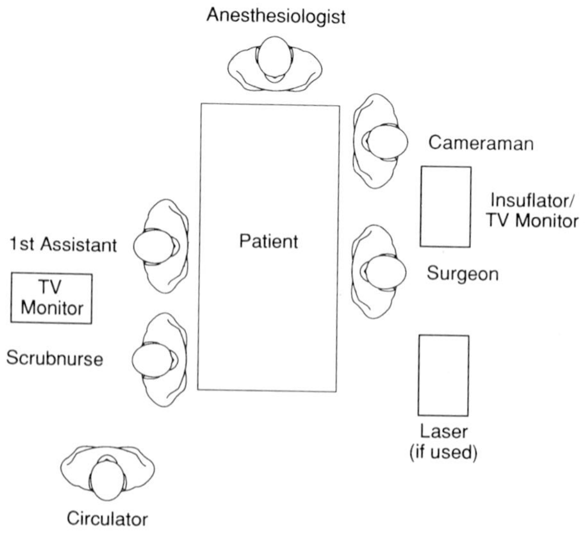

Figure 3–1. This diagram depicts proper room arrangement for a typical laparoscopic appendectomy. If a single TV monitor is used, it can be placed at the foot of the bed where all participants can view the procedure.

nula size and fine technique. Probably the quickest and easiest method is to use the endoscopic linear stapler. Additional cannulas, placed symmetrically in each lower quadrant below the beltline and lateral to the epigastric vessels, will be necessary (Figure 3–2). The linear stapler now available requires a 12-mm cannula in the left lower quadrant (LLQ). A 5-mm cannula can then be inserted into the RLQ. Before proceeding, the insufflation tubing should be switched from the umbilical port to the largest RLQ or LLQ port, because the cool carbon dioxide may fog the laparoscope lens as it cools the scope with high-volume insufflation as when suction is being used. By use of a 5-mm reducer on the 12-mm cannula, two 5-mm instruments are used to mobilize the appendix. Two atraumatic graspers, one ratcheted, are always useful. After the patient is rotated into the Trendelenburg position, grasping forceps are used to run the bowel until the cecum is identified. An irrigator–aspirator inserted through the LLQ port is useful in taking down thin adhesions while the appendix is grasped from the right side. Alternatively, more dense adhesions may be cut with Metzenbaum-type endoscopic scissors, electric cautery (monopolar or bipolar), or a bare laser fiber. Great caution must be used when employing monopolar cautery, though, as increasing numbers of injuries are being seen with this mode of hemostasis. Also, the laser should be employed only by surgeons experienced in its use. We have found the KTP/YAG (Laserscope, San Jose, CA) laser to be quite helpful set in the KTP mode at about 5 W, continuous mode. Dissection is continued until the full length of the appendix is visualized. If possible, the ratcheted forceps from the RLQ is used to grasp the tip of the appendix (Figure 3–2). Traction is placed on this until the mesentery is well visualized. Depending on the surgeon's preference, the mesentery can be ligated in a number of ways. If a stapler is to be used to ligate the appendix, two options exist. If the appendix and mesentery are not extremely inflamed, one firing of the linear stapler, usually using 30-V staples which give better hemostasis, can be accomplished across the mesentery and the base of the appendix. There is, however, increasing concern that leaks will occur at the junction of the mesentery and appendix if only a single firing of the stapler is used. If there is a large amount of inflammation at the base, it is safer to dissect the mesentery free from the base and fire the stapler once across the mesentery and once across the appendix (Figure 3–3). Caution should be exerted when using

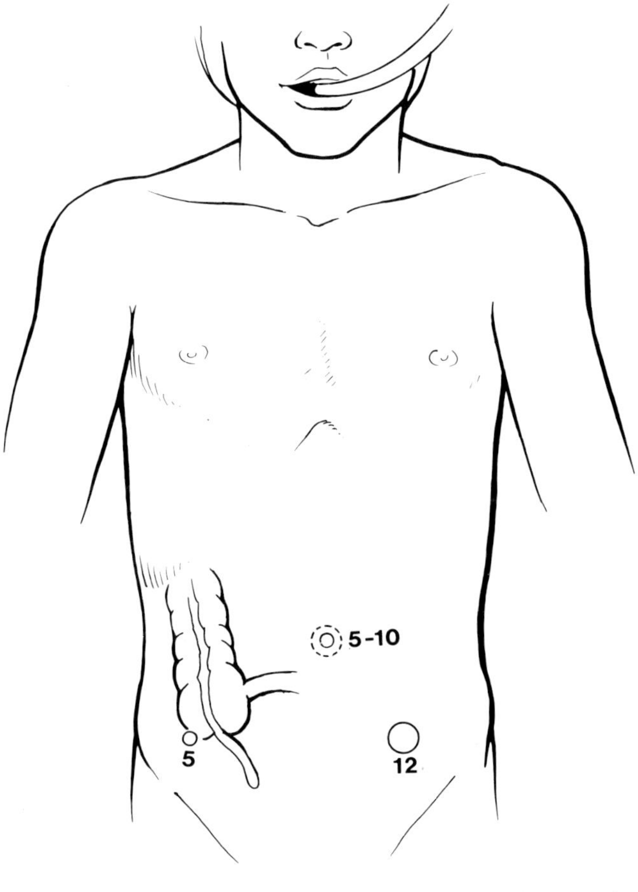

Figure 3–2. Usually, a three-port technique is adequate for laparoscopic appendectomy. Either a 5- or 10-mm umbilical port is employed for placement of the telescope. This depends on whether a 5- or 10-mm telescope is used. A 12-mm incision is made in the left lower quadrant if an endostapler is used. If endoclips are to be used, only a 10-mm incision is needed at that site. The appendix is retracted through a grasper placed in the 5-mm right lower quadrant port.

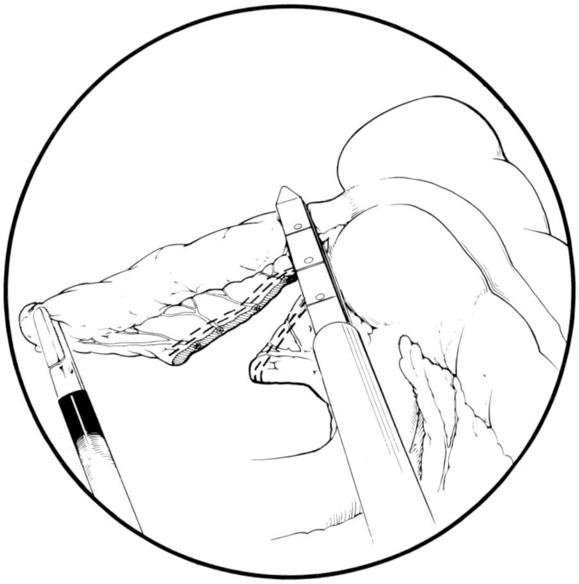

Figure 3–3. An endostapler has been used to ligate and divide the mesoappendix and is now placed across the base of the appendix.

the stapler by always taking a close look at both sides of the jaws after they are closed around the tissue to make sure no other structures are involved. Also, all tissue must be proximal to the "cut" mark to ensure a single firing (Figure 3–4).

An alternate method of ligating the mesoappendix is to use an endoscopic clip applier multiple times through the LLQ cannula, which requires placement of a 10-mm cannula (Figure 3–5). Electrocautery may also be used through this trocar. Again, the KTP/YAG laser may be used by starting with the KTP set at 5 W, continuous duration. The appendix is elevated with the RLQ grasping forceps while a suction/irrigation instrument with a laser fiber channel is placed through the LLQ cannula. The laser fiber is then passed through the instrument with its tip 1 to 2 mm from the tissue. After KTP is used to score the peritoneum, Nd:YAG is set to 40 W with a duration of 1 second and 0.2-second intervals. The fiber is directed up and down to thoroughly coagulate any vessels in the mesoappendix (Figure 3–6). As the fat "melts," vessels become apparent and easy to coagulate. Care must be taken to ensure the fiber is directed at the intended tissue at all times and the aiming beam can always be seen. Also, intermittent aspiration of the laser plume must be done to ensure adequate visualization.

Using any of these alternate methods of ligating the mesentery will necessitate another manner to ligate the appendix. A simple method is to use an endoscopic ligature such as the Surgitie (U.S. Surgical Corporation, Norwalk, CT) (Figure 3–5). To do this, the tip of the appendix is released from the RLQ grasping forceps and the loop applier is passed through the LLQ cannula. Under laparoscopic vision, the loop is advanced into the abdomen, the RLQ grasping forceps is passed through the loop, and the tip of the appendix is again secured. The appendix is then retracted through the loop and the loop directed to the base. The knot is tightened by breaking off the external end of the push rod and pulling as the tip of the push rod is placed at the base of the appendix, where the ligature will be placed. Great care must be taken to ensure that no bowel or other tissue is included in the loop. The passer is then removed, scissors are passed down the same cannula, and the tail of the loop is cut. Two loops can be placed on the appendiceal stump and one on the specimen side. The appendix is divided between the second and third ties. When the laser has been used to take down adhesions or the mesoappendix, we have found it convenient to use the KTP laser at 10 W, continuous duration, to divide the appendix (Figure 3–7).

Next, the appendix is removed. If a stapler has been used, the stapled end of the appendix can be grasped with the LLQ grasper and pulled through the 12-mm cannula. If one of the other methods is used, the appendix can be removed from the largest cannula. If the surgeon does not feel comfortable pulling the "hot" appendix through a cannula or if it is too large, a sterile condom or Endobag (Dexide, Fort Worth, TX) can be passed through the cannula. The appendix is placed into the bag with one grasping forceps while the bag is held with the other (Figure 3–8). Next the bag is retracted into the cannula. Both the cannula and sac are exteriorized as far as possible.

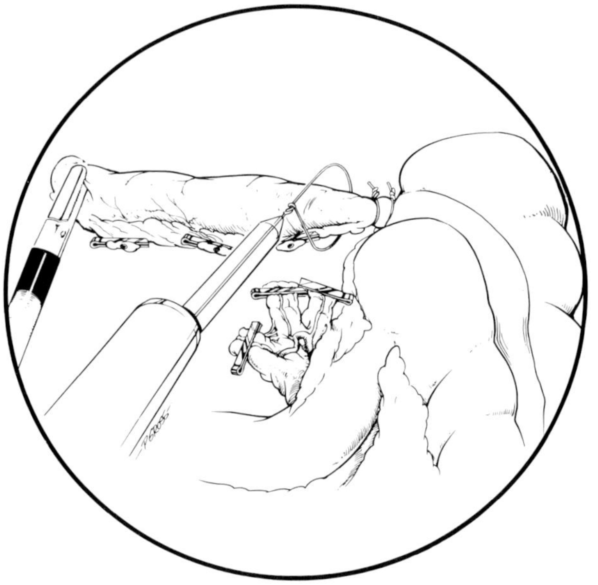

Figure 3–5. Another technique for vascular control of the mesoappendix involves endoclips. Following division of the mesoappendix, pretied chromic endoloops are placed across the base of the appendix and the appendix is divided between the second and third endoloops.

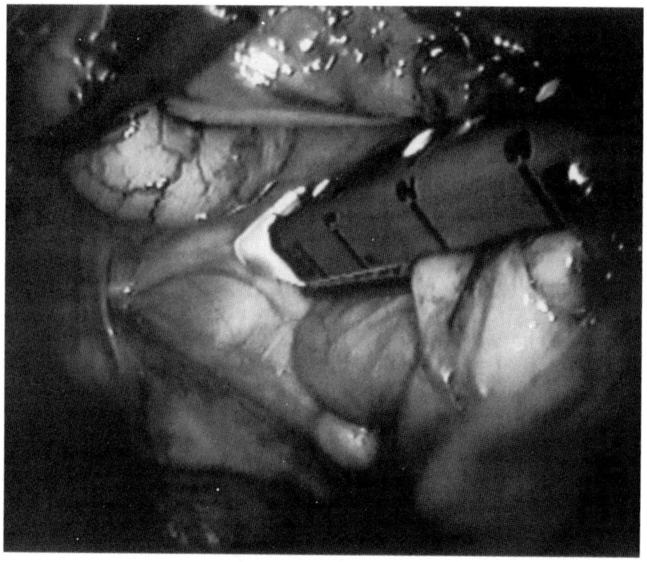

Figure 3–4. This intraoperative photograph shows the endostapler situated across the mesoappendix.

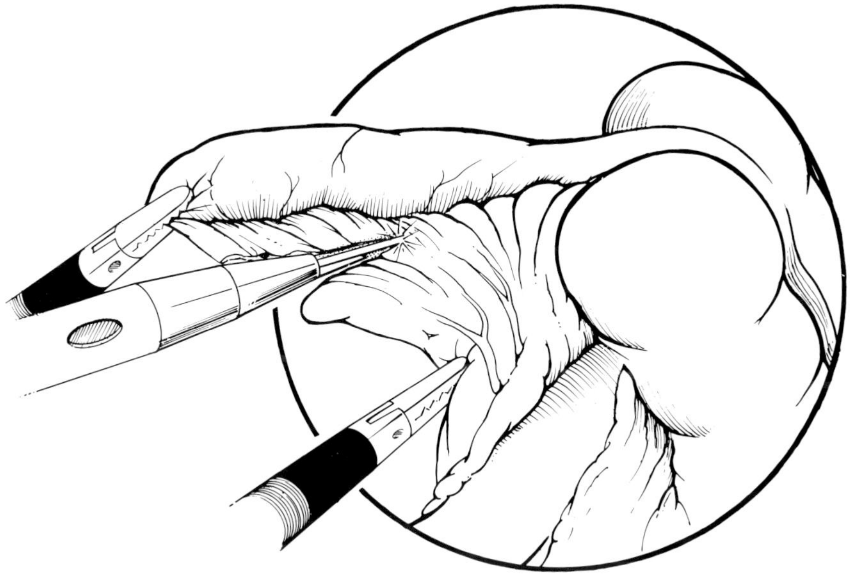

Figure 3–6. The laser can also be used to divide the mesoappendix if the endoscopist is experienced with this modality.

When it is evident that the neck of the sac is outside the abdominal wall, it can be released and grasped externally, minimizing contamination of the cannula tract. A similar device is the EndoCatch (U.S. Surgical Corporation, Norwalk, CT). It can be placed through a 10-mm cannula and deployed by activating the pusher. It then looks like a butterfly net. It is easier to insert the specimen into the device because the opening to the bag stays open without manipulation. Occasionally, it is necessary to enlarge the cannula site slightly to allow removal of a large appendix.

Following specimen removal, a copious amount of irrigant saline is instilled into the pelvis using the irrigator–aspirator. A careful check for hemostasis is made. The patient is placed in reverse Trendelenburg position so the irrigation fluid can be completely removed, which avoids the loculated abscesses that may form if the fluid is not completely evacuated.

Some surgeons prefer avoiding an exposed appendiceal stump but many have done this for years without complications. Common laparoscopic suture techniques can be used to perform a "Z" stitch or to pursestring the cecum. It is usually easier to apply either of these sutures after the appendix is removed and irrigation is finished.

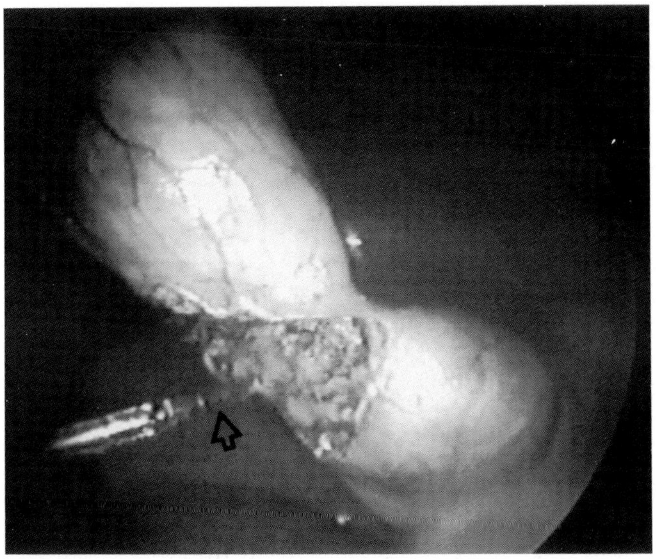

Figure 3–7. Intraoperative photograph of the KTP laser fiber (*open arrow*) being used to divide the appendix.

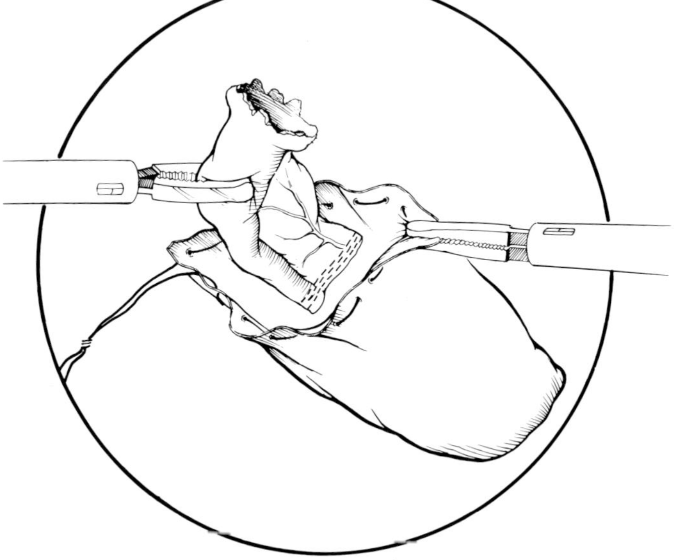

Figure 3–8. After the appendix is freed, it may be placed into an endoscopic retrieval bag.

Occasionally, especially with a retrocecal appendix, it is difficult to mobilize the tip of the appendix. In these cases we have found it easier to divide the appendix and mesoappendix and to remove the appendix in a retrograde fashion (Figure 3–9). This can be accomplished by dissecting between the mesoappendix and the appendix and either using the stapler, firing across each separately, or using the laser to cut the appendix 1 cm from its base, after clips have been applied to each side. The other alternative is to use a Surgitie around each of the two open ends.

In some cases, laparoscopic-assisted appendectomy may be beneficial. This involves an identical procedure up to the point of transecting the appendix. It usually can be accomplished with an umbilical cannula and two 5-mm cannulas, one in the RLQ and one in the LLQ. The appendix is dissected until the tip can be seized with the RLQ grasping instrument. The appendix is then delivered through the RLQ port. Often, this port may need to be enlarged, and if a large appendix is seen during exploration of the abdomen, a 10-mm cannula should be used in the RLQ. Once the appendix is exteriorized, the mesentery can be clamped and ligated, as in an open procedure. The appendix also can be ligated as in an open procedure and a pursestring placed, if desired.

Although suspected perforated appendicitis is a relative contraindication to laparoscopic removal, a perforated or gangrenous appendix may be seen in a child initially thought to have only acute appendicitis.

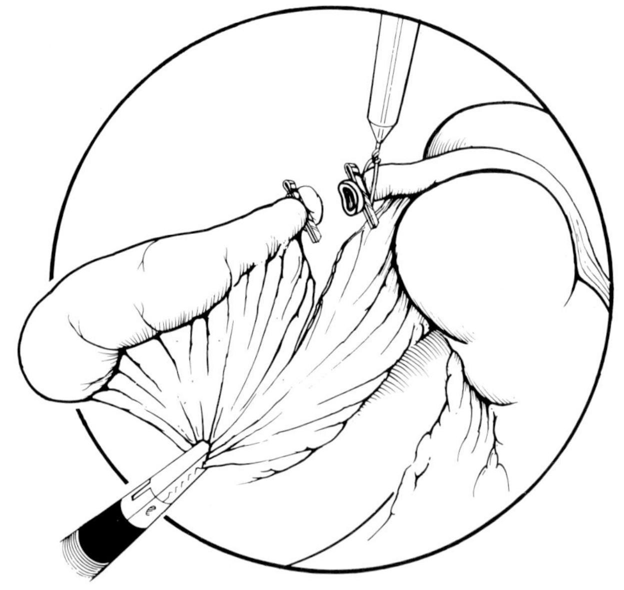

Figure 3–9. It may be necessary to divide the appendix and mesoappendix in a retrograde fashion. This diagram shows initial division of the base of the appendix with endoclips and a chromic endoloop. The next steps are ligation and division of the mesoappendix.

When encountering such a situation the surgeon must be very cautious. If a fecalith has extruded into an abscess or is loose in the peritoneal cavity, it must be found by using copious irrigation and careful inspection of the pelvis and peritoneum. It also should be remembered that while the patient is in a Trendelenburg position with a pneumoperitoneum, it is easy for pus to gravitate over the dome of the liver and produce localized inflammation. This is probably the greatest theoretical disadvantage of operating on perforated appendicitis laparoscopically and is the reason to initiate intravenous antibiotic therapy intraoperatively and continue it postoperatively.

Finally, after the appendix is removed, the terminal ileum is examined for a Meckel's diverticulum. Also, both inguinal regions should be inspected for an inguinal hernia. When the surgeon is confident that hemostasis is secure and the peritoneal cavity has been adequately aspirated, the cannulas are removed under laparoscopic visualization to make sure there is no intraabdominal bleeding from the cannula sites. The laparoscope and umbilical cannula are removed last. At least one fascial suture is used in each cannula site and the skin is closed with one interrupted stitch per cannula site. Steristrips and dressing are then applied.

POSTOPERATIVE CARE

Immediate postoperative care of patients who have had a laparoscopic appendectomy is very similar to the care given patients who have undergone open procedures. We usually allow patients to have clear liquids as they request them. Diet can be advanced quickly as tolerated. Metoclopramide 1 to 2 mg/kg twice daily and a Scopolamine patch seem to decrease postoperative nausea.

Patients are allowed to return to their preoperative activity very rapidly. They may return to school almost immediately and sports within the week. If a transparent occlusive dressing is used, the child may shower or bathe and is instructed to remove it in 1 week. Patients may require a prescription for narcotics for a few days (acetaminophen with codeine)[7]. They are also instructed to take their temperature for 1 week and call for rising temperature evaluations. Routine postoperative visits are scheduled at 2 and 6 weeks.

COMPLICATIONS

The complications of laparoscopic appendectomy fall into two categories: those resulting from the technique of laparoscopy itself and those resulting from appendectomy. Complications associated with the technique of diagnostic laparoscopy are discussed in Chapter 2.

Wound infections are not common and do not necessarily occur at the cannula site used to withdraw the appendix. To avoid this complication, the site of cannula insertion should be copiously irrigated before skin closure (in addition to irrigation of the puncture site). Placing the appendix in a bag before withdrawing it through the abdominal wall minimizes infection.

Abdominal infection may be observed, just as in an open procedure, if an appendicolith is retained in the abdomen. Some surgeons believe it is easier to search for the fecalith with the laparoscope as the entire abdomen may be viewed easily. Also, some surgeons worry about the possible danger of having the cat gut suture at the base of the appendix dissolve too early or come loose and cause a fecal fistula. This has prompted the use of a linear stapler, multiple loops, or a "Z" stitch with stump inversion.

Lastly, postoperative bowel obstruction is possible. Subjectively, many surgeons feel that this may be more common when laparoscopic appendectomy is performed. Only after thousands of cases are performed using similar techniques will this hypothesis be confirmed or refuted. This obstruction is theoretically possible because the stump is not inverted as it often is during open appendectomy.

REVIEW

Even though laparoscopic appendectomy is a relatively new technique, a few large series have been published confirming the safety and appropriateness of the procedure in both adults and children. In 1991, Nowzaradan et al described their experience in 43 adults and children with suspected acute appendicitis. The only complication was a bleeding epigastric vessel in an obese patient. There were no wound infections or other major complications.[6]

In a multi-institutional retrospective review from France in 1991, Valla and colleagues reported 465 laparoscopic appendectomies in children.[7] There was a 3.6% incidence of minor intraoperative complications and a 3.0% incidence of postoperative complications. Five procedures (1%) had to be converted to open procedures, and 1.3% required a repeat laparoscopy or open laparotomy, which is less than half the incidence of reoperation in other reports.[11,12] They concluded that the laparoscopic approach provided numerous advantages to the open technique.

We recently reported our experience with this technique and reviewed complications and cost of all laparoscopic appendectomies (acute and complicated) compared with open appendectomies.[8] In comparing 14 laparoscopic appendectomies with 50 open procedures, we found a lower overall complication rate (16% versus 20%) in the laparoscopic group, but most of the complications with either technique occurred in the complicated patients. The laparoscopic technique costs an average of $1000.00 more, but the total cost was less because of the shorter hospital stay in the laparoscopic group (1.2 days in patients with acute appendicitis versus 3.9 days for the open procedure). Therefore, we believe that laparoscopic appendectomy is a safe and cost-effective procedure and may someday be considered the "standard of care."

REFERENCES

1. Semm K. Endoscopic appendectomy. *Endoscopy.* 1983;15:59.
2. Fleming J. Laparoscopically directed appendectomy. *Aust NZ Obstet Gynaecol.* 1985;25:238.
3. Wilson T: Laparoscopically-assisted appendectomies. *Med J Aust.* 1986;145:551.
4. Schreiber J. Early experience with laparoscopic appendectomy in women. *Surg Endosc.* 1987;1:211.
5. Pier A, Gotz F, Bacher C. Laparoscopic appendectomy in 625 cases: From innovation to routine. *Surg Laparosc Endosc.* 1991;1:8.
6. Nowzaradan Y, Westmoreland J, McCarver C, et al. Laparoscopic appendectomy for acute appendicitis: Indications and current use. *J Laparoendosc Surg.* 1991;1:247.
7. Valla J, Limonne B, Valla V, et al. Laparoscopic appendectomy in children: Report of 465 cases. *Surg Laparosc Endosc.* 1991;1:166.
8. Gilchrist B, Lobe T, Schropp K, et al. Is there a role for laparoscopic appendectomy in pediatric surgery? *J Pediatr Surg.* 1992;27:209.
9. O'Regan P. Laparoscopic appendectomy. *Can J Surg.* 1991;34:256.
10. Attwood S, Hill A, Murphy P, et al. A prospective randomized trial of laparoscopic versus open appendectomy. *Surgery.* 1992;112:497.
11. Putnam T, Gagliano N, Emmens R. Appendicitis in children. *Surg Gynecol Obstet.* 1990;170:527.
12. Chevalier J, Durand A. Reflexions sur une serie homogene de 3200 appendicectomies. *Lyon Chir.* 1980;76:251.

CHAPTER 4

Laparoscopic Cholecystectomy

GEORGE W. HOLCOMB III

Laparoscopy was initially reported by Von Ott in 1901, but this report failed to stimulate much interest and the technique did not become refined until about 1960.[1] One of the early pioneers with the pediatric age group was Stephen Gans, who described a large experience in the use of peritoneoscopy in infants and children in 1973[2]; however, until a recent report by Reddick and Olsen on laparoscopic cholecystectomy, laparoscopy remained the domain of gynecologic surgeons.[3] Since that report, laparoscopic procedures in adults and recently in children have proliferated. In a few short years, laparoscopic cholecystectomy has become the preferred procedure by many surgeons for removal of the gallbladder in adults and is rapidly gaining acceptance in children.

CHOLELITHIASIS

The reported incidence of cholelithiasis in the pediatric patient has increased during the past two decades.[4–6] Clinicians should consider gallstones in the differential diagnosis for any child with vague upper abdominal symptoms and especially those patients with associated risk factors (Table 4–1). Historically, biliary disease has been assumed to occur primarily in children with hemolytic disease. In a 1980 review, however, 85% (74/85) of children had nonhemolytic cholelithiasis.[4] Since that time, an increasing number of children and adolescents have been found to have nonhemolytic gallstones.

Cholelithiasis and Nonhemolytic Disease

Nonhemolytic gallstones can be seen in infants, children, and adolescents regardless of age. Infants with gallstones are being detected in greater numbers largely because of the frequent use of ultrasonography. Infants with gallstones often have associated diseases such as necrotizing enterocolitis, extensive small bowel resection, prolonged total parenteral nutrition (TPN), and anomalies of the biliary system. A common finding in infants with gallstones is the loss of active alimentation with subsequent development of biliary stasis and disappearance of the normal enterohepatic circulation of bile salts. At ultrasonography, gallstones or "sludge" is frequently found. Sludge consists of calcium bilirubinate and layers in the dependent portion of the gallbladder, resulting in low-amplitude echoes. Sludge balls often can be distinguished from multiple small gallstones by the acoustic shadowing effect of the latter, but this differential finding is not always distinguishable. Moreover, children initially thought to have sludge have been noted later to have gallstones. Whether the stones were present initially or developed is not always certain.

Interestingly, several reports have documented spontaneous resolution of gallstones in infants without treatment.[7–10] Some investigators have wondered if these suspected stones may actually have been sludge balls instead of true stones. Several authors have advocated expectant treatment and observation of nonradiopaque gallstones but there is not uniform agreement on this approach. A 6- to 12-month period of observation in the asymptomatic infant is not unreasonable, but cholecystectomy is recommended after that period should gallstones with true shadowing persist on ultrasound studies. In addition, cholecystectomy is recommended in infancy for radiopaque stones and symptomatic patients.

Gallstones also are being noted increasingly in children between 2 and 10 years of age. Many of these patients have associated anatomic abnormalities such

TABLE 4–1. MAJOR RISK FACTORS FOR DEVELOPMENT OF CHOLELITHIASIS IN CHILDREN

Hemolytic	Nonhemolytic
Hereditary spherocytosis	Total parenteral nutrition
Sickle cell disease	Cholestasis
Thalassemia major	Ileal resection
	Teenage pregnancy
	Oral contraceptives
	Obesity
	Biliary tract anomalies

as extensive small bowel resection with total parenteral nutrition (TPN)-associated disease, but others have developed gallstones for unknown reasons. Many of the younger children complain of epigastric or vague abdominal pain and seem unable to specifically localize the discomfort to the right subcostal region as do older children. Gallstones in this age group are composed primarily of mixtures of calcium bilirubinate with varying amounts of calcium carbonate and cholesterol. Again, diagnosis is best accomplished with ultrasound although radiopaque gallstones may be seen on plain roentgenograms.

In children older than 10 years, the symptoms and physical findings are more similar to those found in adults. Pain is frequently described as being in the right upper quadrant or epigastric area with accompanying nausea and vomiting. Intolerance to fatty foods is also an occasional component of the symptom complex. The cholesterol content of gallstones is often elevated in teenagers, as diets that are high in cholesterol and low in fiber predominate in the Western world and this diet contributes to the increased occurrence of mixed cholesterol stones. The female-to-male ratio of adults with gallstones is generally accepted at 4:1. In several pediatric studies, an even higher ratio has been noted.[4,11–13] Other associated risk factors for the development of gallstones in adolescents include teenage pregnancy, obesity, choledochal cysts, and abnormalities of the cystic duct.

Cholelithiasis and Hemolytic Disease

Hereditary spherocytosis, sickle cell anemia, and thalassemia major are the most frequently associated hemolytic disorders associated with biliary calculi. The incidence of cholelithiasis in children with spherocytosis is approximately 50%.[14] As intermittent jaundice is part of the hemolytic process in these children, cholelithiasis may be a silent condition and may be detected only by diagnostic studies. As many children with spherocytosis eventually undergo a splenectomy, evaluation of the gallbladder should be performed prior to splenectomy, allowing cholecystectomy to be performed simultaneously if stones are noted.

A 20 to 30% prevalence of cholelithiasis in patients with sickle cell disease likewise indicates the need to screen for gallstones in these children who complain of upper abdominal pain. Commonly, the abdominal cramping is diagnosed as being caused by abdominal vaso-occlusive crises when, in fact, the children are experiencing symptoms of cholecystitis. By late adolescence, cholelithiasis may occur in as many as 40% of these patients, with 75% becoming symptomatic.[15]

Gallstones are relatively infrequent in children with thalassemia primarily because of the use of a hypertransfusion regimen.[16] Abdominal symptoms may, however, be related to calculi in these patients and symptoms should be evaluated by ultrasonography.

Acalculous Biliary Disease

Mention should be made of the occasional child with acalculous disease. In an earlier review, seven children were reported with documented gallbladder inflammation without stones.[4] At operation, the gallbladder was markedly inflamed and distended in each patient, with gangrenous changes noted in three children. Obstruction of the cystic duct from enlarged lymph nodes and congenital narrowing or tortuosity of the cystic duct and other idiopathic causes have been mentioned as contributing to gallbladder distention and acalculous cholecystitis.

Radiographic Evaluation

Evaluation of the child with upper abdominal discomfort should begin with supine and erect abdominal films (Table 4–2). Radiopaque gallstones (seen in up to 20% of children) can be detected, abdominal masses are suspected, and intestinal abnormalities are considered from the abdominal film (Figure 4–1). Should the plain films fail to reveal a specific etiology, then ultrasound is the next step. Ultrasonography will docu-

TABLE 4–2. RADIOGRAPHIC EVALUATION FOR GALLBLADDER DISEASE

Abdominal films—supine/erect
Abdominal ultrasound
Oral cholecystogram
Cholescintigraphy
Cholecystokinin-assisted ultrasound

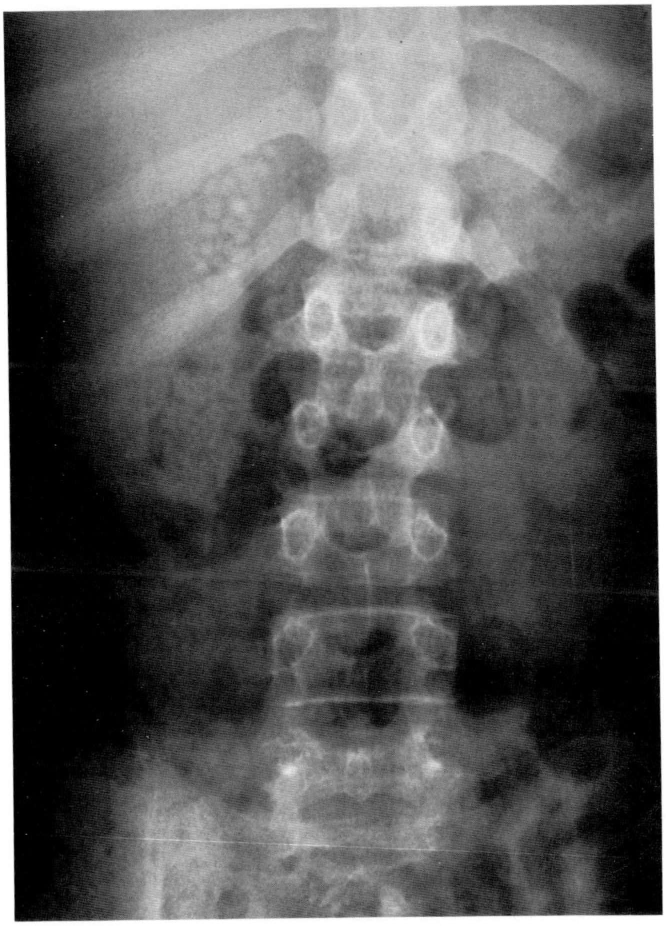

Figure 4–1. Radiopaque gallstones can be seen in about 20% of children and are noted on this abdominal film.

ment stones with layering and shadowing on the sonogram, whereas pericholecystic fluid will suggest cholecystitis (Figure 4–2). Moreover, ultrasonic evaluation for choledochal dilation is important in the preoperative planning for a laparoscopic procedure. Cholescintigraphy with radiolabeled iminodiacetic acid (IDA) compounds is the most useful means for diagnosing acute cholecystitis. With occlusion of the cystic duct, the gallbladder will not visualize.

For the child with acalculous biliary disease, the abdominal film and ultrasound will be negative for stones. Although this is not a common preoperative diagnosis, it may occur occasionally. This condition can be evaluated by oral cholecystogram and cholecystokinin-stimulated ultrasound. The oral cholecystogram evaluates functional disorders of the gallbladder as well as cystic duct obstruction. The cholecystokinin-stimulated ultrasound attempts to reproduce the patient's pain when gallbladder contraction is visualized by ultrasound. These two studies can be performed in the same morning. For oral cholecystography, the patient ingests the iopanoic acid tablets the night before the procedure and abdominal films are taken the following morning. Opacification of the gallbladder should be noted if the cystic duct is patent and the gallbladder is functional. Nonvisualization of the gallbladder on two occasions is an indication for cholecystectomy.

The patient is then moved to the ultrasonography suite where intravenous cholecystokinin at 0.02 μg/kg is injected over a 30- to 60-second period. The gallbladder is scanned at 2- to 4-minute intervals for contraction and is scanned if the patient's pain is reproduced. If the pain has not been reproduced at 15 minutes or if the gallbladder has not contracted, then the test is repeated with 0.04 μg/kg and the patient scanned intermittently for the next 15 minutes. Gallbladder contraction without pain is a negative test, whereas reproducibility of symptoms with gallbladder contractions is considered a positive test and an indication for cholecystectomy.

Treatment

A nonoperative approach to treatment of gallstones has been used in a number of adults with mixed results and some later complications. Dissolution of gallstones with high oral doses of chenodeoxycholic and/or ursodeoxycholic acid has been attempted with less than satisfactory success.[17,18] Its use in children has been very limited. Biliary lithotripsy has also been used in selected adults[19]; however, complications such as pancreatitis and gross hematuria have been reported. Lithotripsy has been used primarily in elderly patients and not in children. Moreover, neither dissolution therapy nor lithotripsy has been successful in resolving calcified stones.

For children with a long life expectancy, cholecystectomy is the treatment of choice for gallbladder disease. Biliary pancreatitis is a definite complication of cholelithiasis, with the possible development of hemorrhagic or necrotizing pancreatitis. Moreover, common duct obstruction without pancreatitis is also a potential complication leading to more complex management. Therefore, elective cholecystectomy is recommended once gallstones are confirmed. Cholecystectomy is also indicated for patients with biliary symptoms and failure of gallbladder visualization on two oral cholecystograms or with a positive cholecystokinin-assisted ultrasound study.

Until recently, open cholecystectomy in children has been the procedure of choice; however, reports of laparoscopic cholecystectomy are increasing and its safe utilization in children has been documented in several small studies.[20–22]

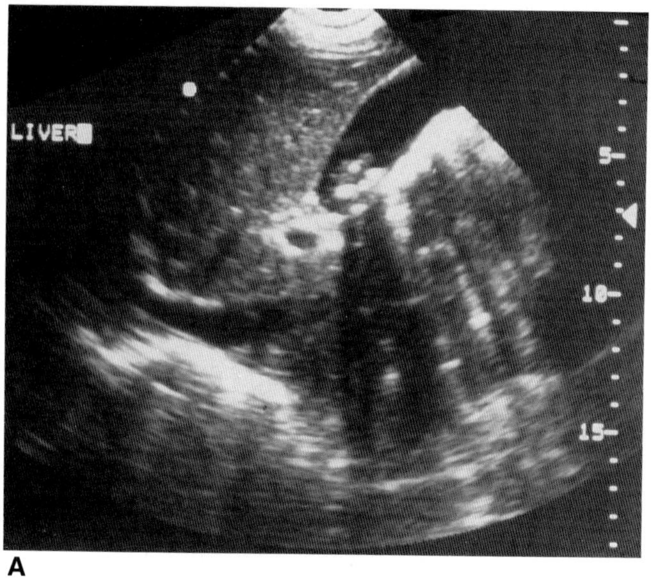

A

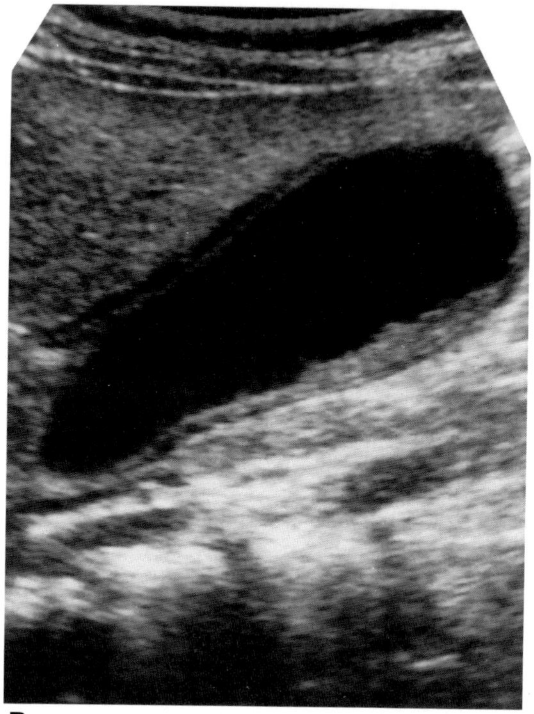

B

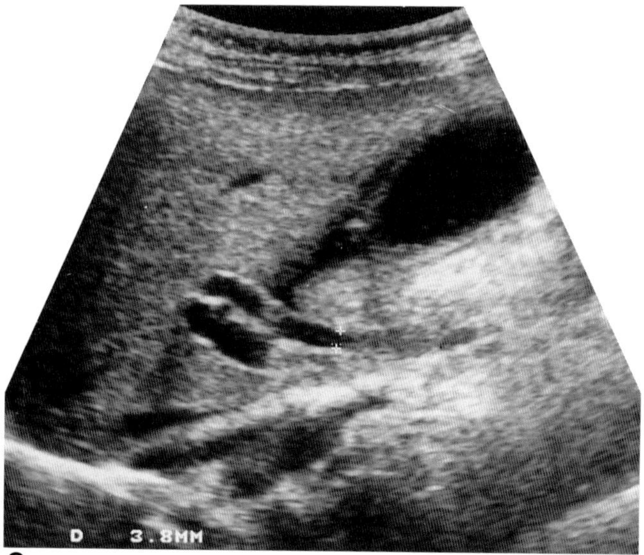

C

Figure 4–2. **A.** Gallbladder ultrasound revealing multiple gallstones with echogenic shadowing. **B.** Ultrasound revealing a distended gallbladder with pericholecystic fluid, indicating acute cholecystitis. Although sludge rather than gallstones is seen on this view, gallstones were observed on a sonogram 1 month earlier. **C.** Ultrasound study of the distal common bile duct reveals ductal dilation as the duct passes through the head of the pancreas. This patient (in B) presented with acute cholecystitis and jaundice. Although a stone was not visualized, it was presumed to have passed into her duodenum.

Contraindications

Absolute contraindications to laparoscopic cholecystectomy include an uncorrectable coagulopathy, generalized peritonitis, and abdominal wall sepsis at the site for cannula insertion. Acute cholecystitis is not a contraindication. Common bile duct stones constitute a relative contraindication in children. Additional experience with endoscopic sphincterotomy (ES) or laparoscopic choledochoscopy is needed for management of choledocholithiasis in children; however, ES has been reported in infants with removal of common duct stones and can be employed preoperatively if this expertise is available.[23,24]

Risks and Benefits

The risks of laparoscopic cholecystectomy should be the same or less than those of an open procedure. Moreover, it may be necessary to convert the laparoscopic procedure to an open operation, and this possibility should always be discussed with the patient and family. One major advantage of laparoscopic cholecystectomy results from the small incisions needed for the procedure and the avoidance of intestinal manipulation with resultant ileus (Table 4–3). The children are ready for liquids or solid food the night of the procedure and usually a regular diet on the first postoperative morning. A 24-hour hospitalization for elective procedures substantially decreases the total cost for management of gallbladder disease. In addition, there is decreased postoperative discomfort and a reduced need for analgesics. Moreover, there is a much shorter interval between the surgical procedure and return to normal activities such as school or play. Adolescents engaging in athletic activities can be released to full contact sports within a week or possibly sooner. A final distinct advantage is the minimization of scarring, especially in children with a tendency toward keloid formation.

LAPAROSCOPIC CHOLECYSTECTOMY

Preoperative Preparation

For children undergoing elective cholecystectomy, without associated hemolytic disease, preoperative admission is not necessary. The patient arrives the morning of the procedure with an empty stomach for at least 6 hours. For children with sickle cell disease, it is important to decrease the hemoglobin S concentration to at least 30%. Therefore, these children can be admitted to the outpatient clinic 7 to 10 days prior to the cholecystectomy and transfused with 1 to 2 units of packed red cells to ensure a hemoglobin level of 8 to 10 g/dL. Hospital admission the day before surgery is necessary for infusion of intravenous fluids at 1 to 1.5 maintenance volume to ensure adequate hydration. An additional transfusion can be performed at this time if desired.

For those patients who present with acute cholecystitis without evidence of common duct obstruction or complicating pancreatitis, medical management is initially recommended. A period of bowel rest, intravenous hydration, analgesics, and antibiotics usually result in resolution of the acute inflammation. Cholecystectomy can be performed within 5 to 7 days of the onset of acute cholecystitis provided the patient responds to medical management. Alternatively, the patient may be discharged for 2 to 3 weeks and return for elective cholecystectomy. The concern regarding discharge and readmission is the opportunity for development of complications in the intervening time. Although this does not usually occur, it is a possibility.

TABLE 4–3. ADVANTAGES OF LAPAROSCOPIC CHOLECYSTECTOMY

24-hour hospitalization for elective cases
Less postoperative discomfort and analgesic requirement
Faster return to regular activities
Early return to athletic participation
Minimal scarring, smaller incisions

Operative Technique

Cefazolin is administered preoperatively for antibiotic prophylaxis in uncomplicated cases. General endotracheal anesthesia is used and an orogastric tube and Foley catheter are inserted to decompress the stomach and bladder, thus minimizing the risk of injury with trocar insertion. Metoclopramide (0.2 mg/kg) and droperidol (0.06 mg/kg) are given intravenously after induction of anesthesia to minimize postoperative nausea and vomiting. The abdomen is then prepped and draped widely similar to the regimen used for open cholecystectomy. The operation is observed with two video cameras displayed at the head of the operating table. One video monitor is placed on the side of the surgeon and the other on the side of the first assistant. The operating surgeon stands to the patient's left with the first assistant opposite.

Abdominal insufflation and diagnostic laparoscopy are performed through a 5-mm umbilical incision as discussed in Chapter 2. Attention is next directed toward the gallbladder, and 5-mm incisions are made in the midclavicular line (MCL) just over the dome of the gallbladder and in the anterior axillary line slightly above and medial to the right anterior superior iliac crest (ASIC). Under video inspection, a 5-mm trocar and cannula are inserted through each of these two incisions. As each trocar is seen to penetrate the posterior abdominal fascia and peritoneum, it should be directed anteriorly and away from the underlying intestine. The trocars are inserted with a slow twisting motion and gentle pressure until entry into the peritoneal cavity is noted.

The site of insertion of the fourth trocar and cannula is individualized depending on the patient's size (Figure 4–3). This 10-mm cannula will be the port through which the operating surgeon performs the procedure. In smaller children, the port needs to be toward the left MCL line and on a plane even with the third port over the dome of the gallbladder. In older and larger children, however, this epigastric cannula should be placed more in the midline epigastrium, similar to adults. The only difficulty with placing it in the left upper abdominal quadrant is having to work under the falciform ligament; however, placing this port in the midline epigastrium in a small child means that the working forceps will be too close together to perform the procedure easily.

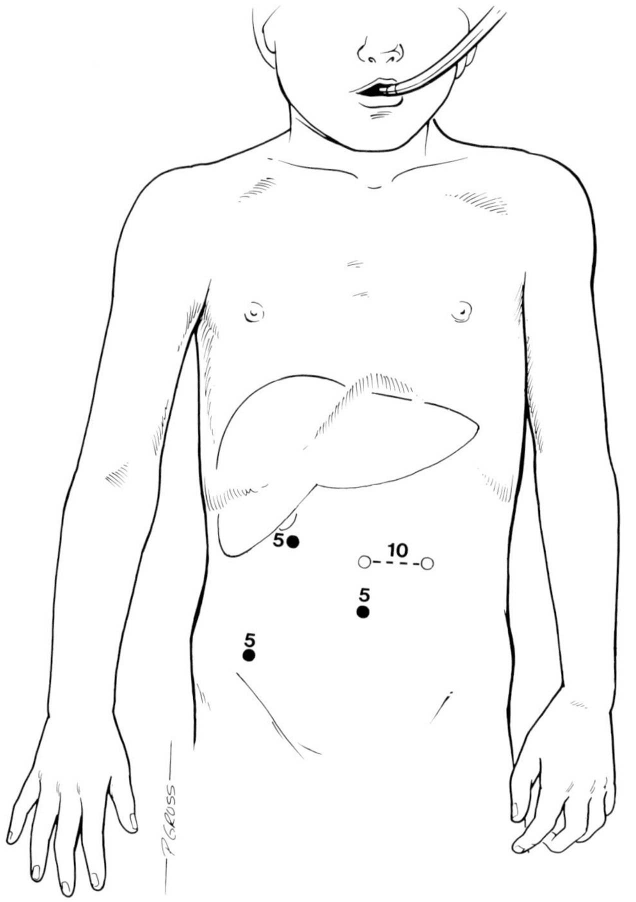

Figure 4–3. This diagram depicts the sites of the various ports for laparoscopic cholecystectomy in a child. A 5-mm cannula is used in the umbilicus through which the video laparoscope is inserted. Similar 5-mm cannulas are inserted over the dome of the gallbladder in the midclavicular line and just medial and superior to the anterior superior iliac crest. Placement of the fourth port in the epigastric area varies according to the patient's size. In infants and small children, this cannula should be placed in the left upper abdominal quadrant, whereas in the older child it can be placed in the midline epigastrium, as in adults.

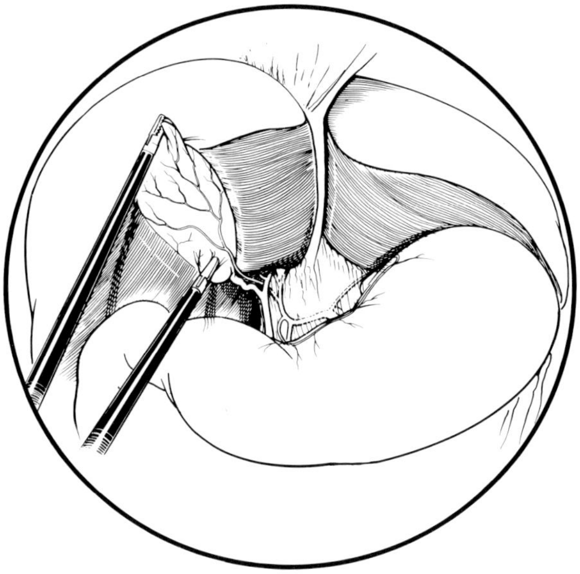

Figure 4–4. Through the right inferior port, a forceps is inserted and the gallbladder rotated ventrally and superiorly over the liver. Another forceps is inserted through the port over the dome of the gallbladder and Hartmann's pouch is retracted to the patient's right. This exposes the cystic duct, cystic artery, and common bile duct.

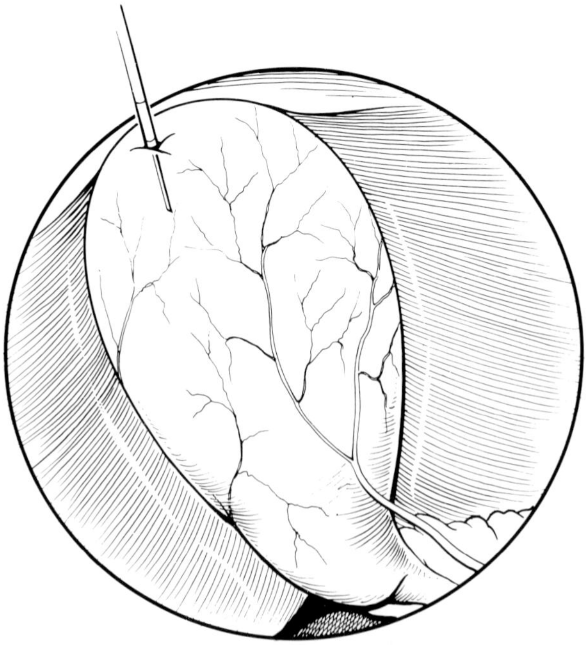

Figure 4–5. In cases of acute cholecystitis with extensive edema and inflammation surrounding the gallbladder, it may not be possible to easily grasp the gallbladder for retraction. Therefore, the gallbladder can be aspirated, resulting in decompression. The gallbladder may then be grasped for retraction.

The patient is now placed in 40-degree reverse Trendelenburg position and turned slightly to the patient's left to allow the transverse colon and small bowel to drop away from the gallbladder. An atraumatic ratcheted forceps is inserted through the right inferior port (ASIC). The gallbladder is grasped and rotated ventrally and superiorly over the liver. Another forceps is inserted through the right MCL port, and Hartmann's pouch is retracted to the patient's right (Figure 4–4). In some cases of acute cholecystitis, there is extensive edema and inflammation, making it difficult to grasp the gallbladder for retraction. Therefore, the gallbladder should be aspirated and the bilious contents removed (Figure 4–5). This will enable the gallbladder to be more easily grasped and retracted to expose the cystic and common ducts.

The anatomy of the cystic duct and common duct triangle is carefully assessed. Specifically, the course of the common duct is usually easily visualized, and the cystic duct coursing to the gallbladder is also seen. The peritoneal attachments to the cystic duct and gallbladder are stripped using the dissecting forceps. Hemostasis is controlled with the electrocautery, avoiding any contact between the cautery tip and the common bile duct or cystic duct. Often a lymph node lies in the triangle of Calot and requires excision during this dissection. After this triangle is skeletonized and the cystic duct, cystic artery, and common bile duct are carefully identified, attention is directed to cholangiography. Cholangiography should be used in all patients prior to division of the cystic duct for two reasons. It will document unsuspected choledocholithiasis and will define the anatomy and course of the cystic and common bile ducts. Correct identification of these structures will prevent most injuries to the common bile duct.

Several techniques can be employed for cholangiography. One method involves placement of a surgical clip on the gallbladder at the cystic duct. A cholangiocatheter or 4-French ureteral catheter is directed through an Olsen clamp (Karl Storz, Culver City, CA). Following a small lateral incision in the cystic duct, the catheter is directed into the duct (Figure 4–6). The catheter is secured with the Olsen clamp and two cholangiograms are performed in a standard fashion.

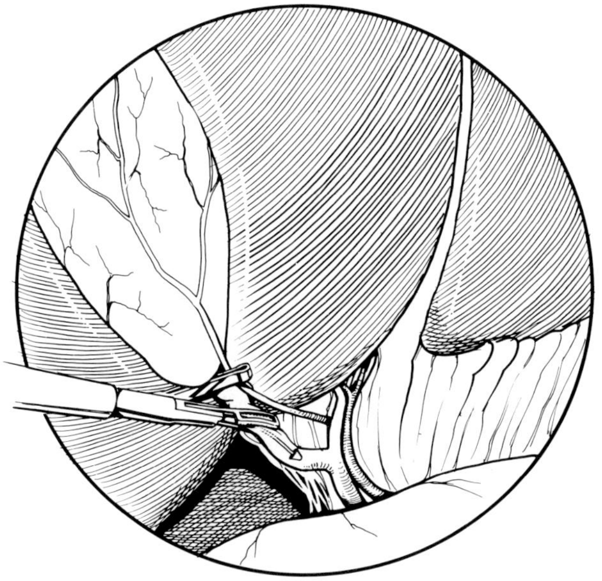

Figure 4–6. Several techniques can be used for cholangiography. This diagram depicts a technique using clip occlusion of the proximal cystic duct with insertion of a cholangiocatheter through a lateral incision in the cystic duct. The catheter is secured to the cystic duct with an Olsen clamp.

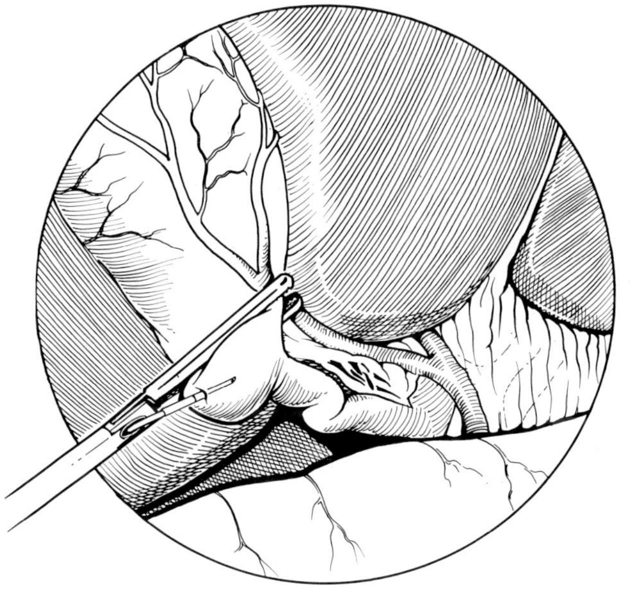

Figure 4–7. An alternative method uses a Kumar clamp with occlusion of the gallbladder infundibulum. Through a side port in the clamp, a small sclerotherapy needle is inserted directly into the gallbladder and a contrast study is obtained. This method has the advantage that the catheter does not have to be threaded through the small cystic duct which can be very difficult in small children.

Alternative methods may be more easily performed in smaller children because of the difficulty in threading the catheter into a narrow cystic duct. In one such technique, a cholangioclamp with a side port is used for placement of a cholangiocatheter (Kumar clamp). A 23-gauge sclerotherapy needle works well with this technique. The clamp is inserted through the right inferior cannula (ASIC) and the neck of the gallbladder gently palpated and clamped to prevent migration of stones. The sclerotherapy needle is then threaded through the side-arm and the gallbladder is punctured just above the cystic duct junction (Figure 4–7). Cholangiography is then performed fluoroscopically (Figure 4–8).

Two other techniques involve percutaneous puncture of the gallbladder for cholangiography. The gallbladder fundus can be punctured with a small needle and cholangiography performed through the gallbladder, similar to the technique used for four decades by pediatric surgeons to visualize the biliary tract in biliary atresia patients. This method has been advocated in adults recently by Graves et al.[25] Alternatively, a clip can be placed across the gallbladder at the cystic-duct junction and the needle directed into the more dilated portion of the cystic duct (Figure 4–9).

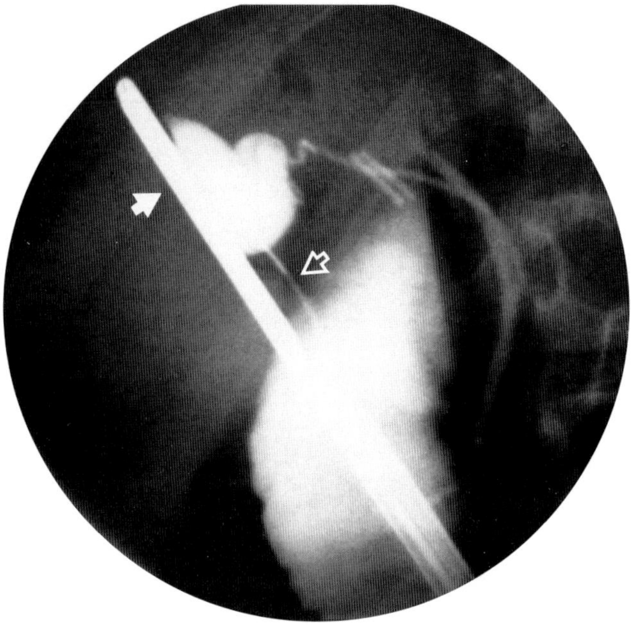

Figure 4–8. This cholangiogram performed using the Kumar technique depicts the clamp placed across the infundibulum of the gallbladder (*solid arrow*), with the sclerotherapy needle inserted into the gallbladder infundibulum(*open arrow*). The cholangiogram shows a very small cystic duct and common duct with free flow into the duodenum. Clips have been placed on the cystic artery as it coursed on top of the cystic duct and needed to be divided prior to dissection of the cystic duct.

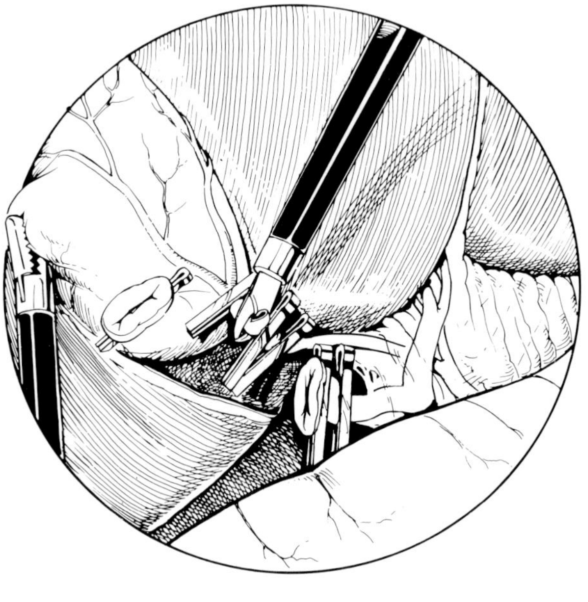

Figure 4–10. The cystic duct has been divided with two clips placed on the duct near its entrance to the common bile duct. In a similar fashion, the cystic artery is clipped and is being divided. (*Reprinted, with permission, from Holcomb et al.*[20])

The cholangiogram is then reviewed. If no indication of injury to the cystic or common ducts and no evidence of obstruction to the common duct are seen, the cholangiocatheter is removed. Two surgical clips are then placed on the cystic duct away from the com

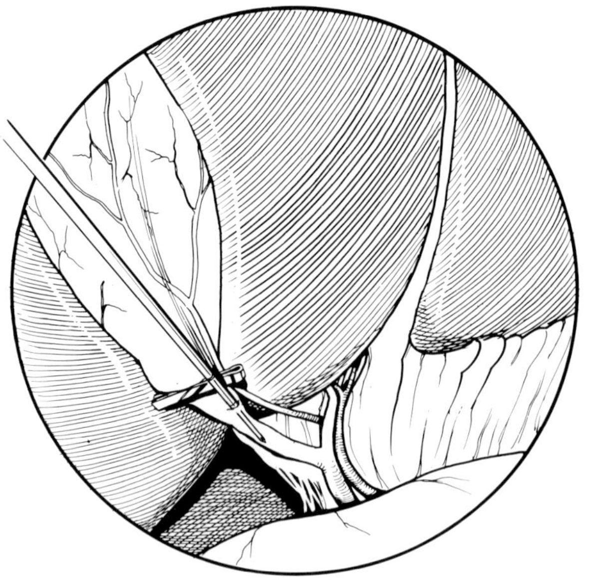

Figure 4–9. Another technique uses clip occlusion of the proximal cystic duct with direct puncture of the more dilated cystic duct with a fine needle.

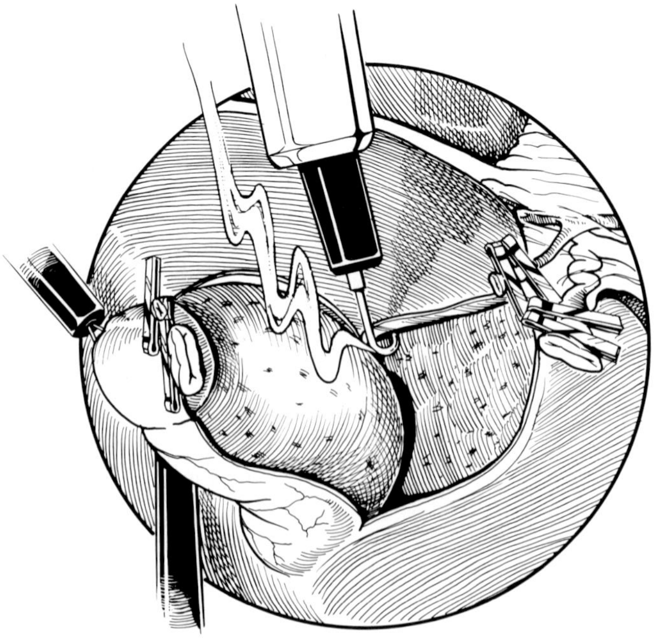

Figure 4–11. The gallbladder is dissected in a retrograde fashion from the liver bed using the electrocautery. (*Reprinted, with permission, from Holcomb et al.*[20])

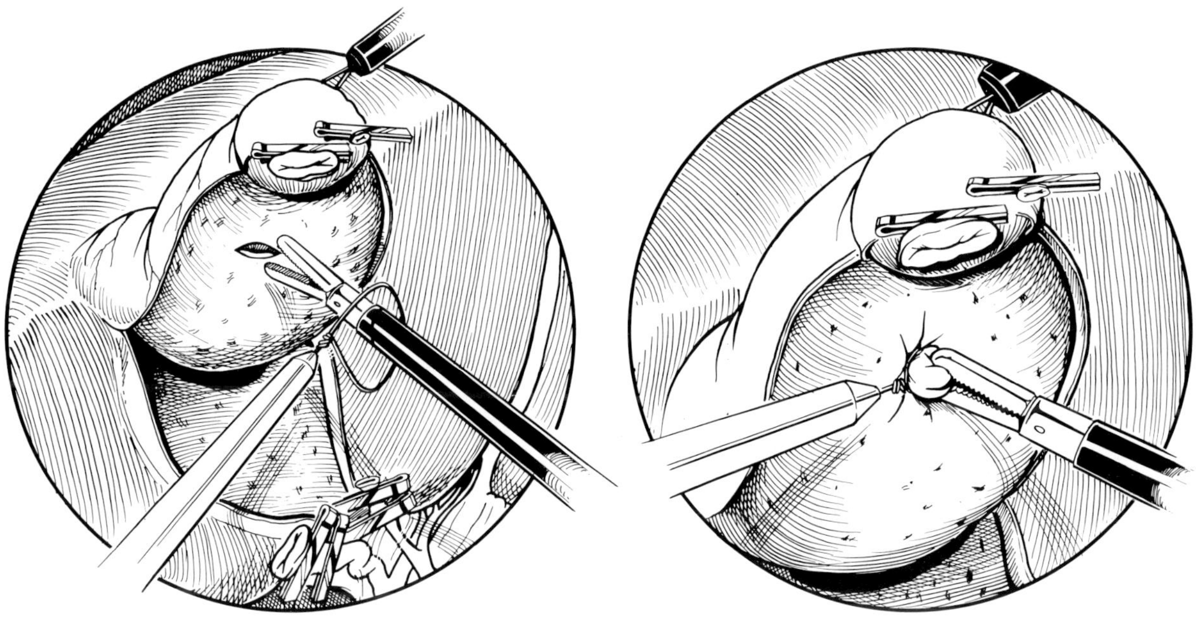

Figure 4–12. During retrograde dissection, entry into the gallbladder may occur. This is managed by placing a grasping forceps through an endoloop and securing the perforation. The endoloop is then secured around the perforation and leakage is controlled.

mon duct so as not to injure the latter. The cystic duct is divided proximal to these two clips by scissors. The cystic artery is similarly divided after two clips are placed distally and one clip is placed proximally toward the gallbladder (Figure 4–10).

The gallbladder is removed in a retrograde fashion using the electrocautery (Figure 4–11). During this part of the procedure, it is extremely important to maintain hemostasis in the liver bed as dissection proceeds superiorly. Should entry into the gallbladder lumen occur, it can easily be controlled with a chromic endoloop. This is accomplished by grasping the perforation with a forceps and securing the endoloop around the hole (Figure 4–12). The excess chromic suture is then cut. When the gallbladder is almost detached from the liver bed, the porta hepatis is inspected for hemostasis and for proper placement of the surgical clips. This inspection should be performed prior to complete removal of the gallbladder as it is much easier to retract the liver superiorly and inspect the operative bed with the gallbladder partially attached. The suprahepatic and subhepatic spaces are copiously irrigated with heparinized saline and the irrigant is inspected for blood or biliary contents. With a clear effluent, the gallbladder is extracted through the 10-mm epigastric trocar (Figure 4–13).

In children, the gallbladder can often be removed through the cannula. If, however, the gallbladder is too distended with bile or stones to permit removal in this manner, the cannula is removed and the gallbladder exteriorized through the fascial opening. Should it still not be possible to remove the gallbladder, its neck is grasped on two sides with clamps and opened. The bile is aspirated, the stones are removed, and the shrunken gallbladder is advanced through the fascial

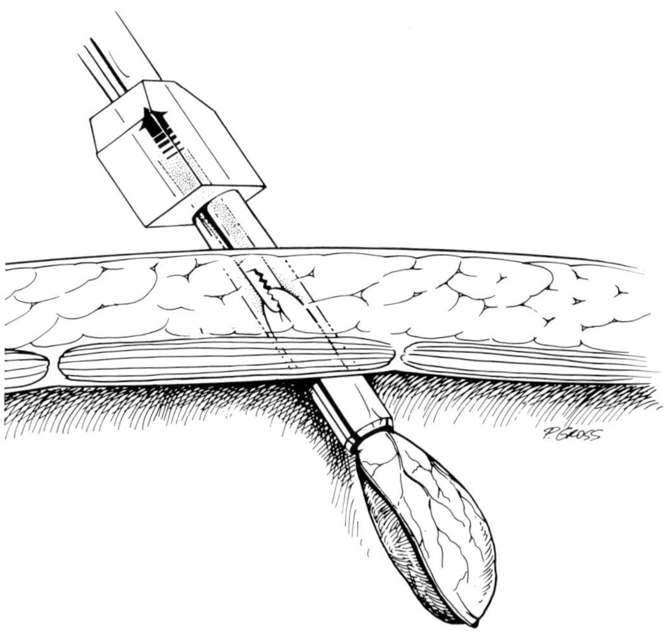

Figure 4–13. Following cholecystectomy, the gallbladder is extracted through the 10-mm epigastric cannula. Often, the gallbladder can be removed without the need for aspiration in children.

opening. If problems persist, the fascial opening can be enlarged.

Great care is taken to inspect the peritoneal surface at the sites of cannula insertion for hemostasis and evidence of spillage. With hemostasis secured, the abdomen is desufflated and all ports removed. The umbilical fascial opening is closed with an absorbable suture and all four skin incisions are approximated in a subcuticular fashion. The patient is transported to the recovery room where the orogastric tube and Foley catheter are removed. Cefazolin is administered postoperatively 6 hours after the initial dose. The children are usually discharged the following morning. They are allowed to resume regular activities within 3 days and to participate in contact sports within 1 week.

Each patient is seen in the pediatric surgical clinic 2 weeks following discharge. Postoperative laboratory studies, ultrasound, or other evaluations are not routinely performed in the absence of symptoms. To date, no patient has developed a complication following the procedure.

Previous Operations

In children with previous upper abdominal incisions, insufflation can be initiated through the subcostal MCL port over the gallbladder because the right upper quadrant is usually free of adhesions. Video laparoscopy can then be initiated through this port and the umbilicus visualized. If the umbilicus is free of adhesions, then a 5-mm trocar and cannula may be inserted under direct visualization and the laparoscope placed through this cannula. Any adhesions noted at the umbilical area may be removed by a dissecting forceps inserted through the right lateral port just above the ASIC. Cholecystectomy is then performed in a standard fashion.

Choledocholithiasis

The preoperative documentation of common bile duct stones has been a relative contraindication to laparoscopic cholecystectomy in children. With advanced technology and smaller endoscopes, however, this may no longer be a contraindication. Preoperative endoscopic sphincterotomy is being increasingly used in adults and has been applied successfully in a few children.[23,24] Following relief of the common bile duct obstruction, laparoscopic cholecystectomy can be performed.

If common duct stones are detected on intraoperative cholangiography, choledochal exploration is indicated. Laparoscopic choledochoscopy through the dilated cystic duct and common bile duct with basket retrieval of choledochal stones is now possible and has been performed in a 15-year-old (personal experience). Another option is completion of the laparoscopic cholecystectomy followed by postoperative endoscopic sphincterotomy. At this time, attempted basket retrieval using a nephroureteroscope in patients with a dilated cystic duct is recommended (Figure 4–14). If not successful, postoperative endoscopic retrograde cholangiopancreatography and sphincterotomy would be indicated if available. If expertise with endoscopic sphincterotomy is not available, then open cholecystectomy and common duct exploration should be employed.

Complications

As this is a new approach for cholecystectomy, complications may occur. In several adult studies, the complications are thought to be more common in the initial experience of the surgeon but this has not been uniform.[26–28] Nevertheless, for laparoscopic cholecystectomy to become the standard of care, it must be performed with the same complication rate as the open operation. Complications may occur at any point during the procedure. With introduction of the Veress needle and trocar insertion, injury to the intestine or mesentery is a potential danger. Therefore, it is important to insert the Veress needle into the peritoneal cavity carefully to avoid this occurrence. Similarly, it is necessary that the surgeon maintain a secure grasp of

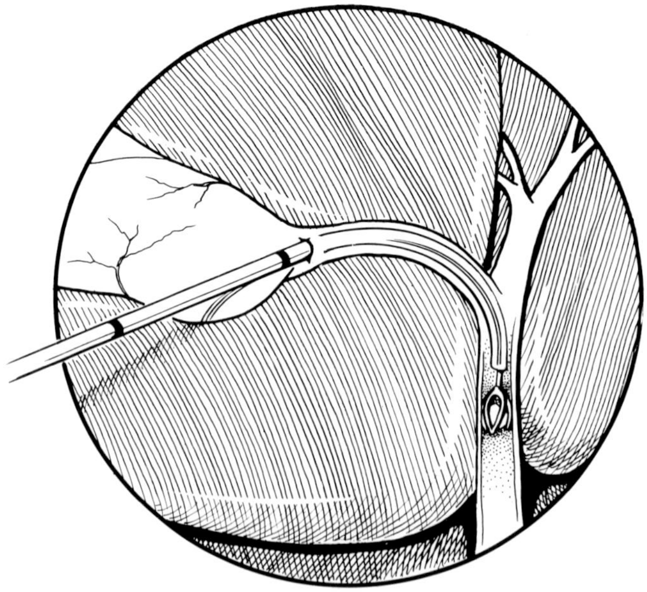

Figure 4–14. Laparoscopic choledochoscopy through the dilated cystic duct and common bile duct may be possible by an experienced laparoscopist. With this technique, basket retrieval of common bile duct stones may be possible in the older child and teenager.

the cannula during penetration so that his or her hand does not slip and insert the trocar/cannula too deeply. Many trocars have retractable plastic sleeves which offer protection from their sharp points once the abdominal cavity is entered. If an injury occurs, it can be assessed laparoscopically and the operation converted to an open procedure when necessary; however, contusion to the bowel or mesentery is usually not an indication for conversion to an open procedure. Although laparoscopic intestinal suturing techniques are now available, this should not be attempted by the inexperienced surgeon.

As dissection proceeds along the triangle of Calot, potential complications include injury to the common bile duct with either sharp dissection or contact with the cautery tip. The incidence of this complication should be small if dissection and cautery tip are kept sufficiently distant from the common bile duct. Injury to the common bile duct is an indication for conversion to an open procedure. Bleeding is a potential hazard during this part of the procedure but usually can be controlled with clips or cauterization and rarely should be a reason for open cholecystectomy.

Probably the most frequent reason for conversion to open cholecystectomy is the inability to discern the anatomy with certainty during the dissection. Confusion regarding the course of the cystic and common ducts can be clarified in most instances with the cholangiogram; however, anomalous variations in the course of the cystic artery or right hepatic artery or edema and inflammation from acute cholecystitis may be reasons for uncertainty and the need for open cholecystectomy. Once the anatomy is carefully defined, removal of the gallbladder is relatively straightforward. Entry into the gallbladder and leakage of its contents can be controlled with endoloop ligatures laparoscopically. Spillage can quickly be evacuated with irrigation and suction. Following detachment of the gallbladder, complications should be few and easily managed.

In summary, care to every detail of the procedure and meticulous attention to safety should lead to minimal, if any, complications with this procedure.

THE VANDERBILT EXPERIENCE

Between June 1990 and June 1993, 27 children aged 2 to 19 years have been evaluated for biliary colic. Nine children weighed less than 45 kg, with the smallest weighing 15 kg. Gallstones were documented by ultrasonography in all patients except one. In this patient, biliary dyskinesia was diagnosed after an upper gastrointestinal series, computed tomography (CT) scan, and ultrasound failed to document an etiology for her recurring right upper abdominal pain related to meals. A cholecystokinin-stimulated ultrasound study was found to reproduce the pain with gallbladder contraction. This was considered a positive study and cholecystectomy was recommended. Moreover, this patient had a prominent family history of gallbladder disease requiring cholecystectomy.

Risk factors for the development of cholelithiasis were noted in nine patients. Three males and one female presented with sickle cell disease and symptomatic cholelithiasis. Two females had documented spherocytosis and one presented with acute cholecystitis and common bile duct obstruction. Three teenagers developed symptomatic cholelithiasis during pregnancy and underwent cholecystectomy following delivery. In addition, three patients had undergone previous operative gastrostomy and one had a ventriculoperitoneal shunt.

Five patients presented with acute cholecystitis based on clinical and ultrasound evaluation. Each was admitted for intravenous hydration, antibiotics, and analgesics with resolution of the acute cholecystitis. Common duct dilation without a definite calculus was noted in one patient at ultrasound but this dilation resolved prior to cholecystectomy. Laparoscopic cholecystectomy was performed in these five patients within 5 days of admission. The remaining 22 children underwent elective laparoscopic cholecystectomy. Four patients with sickle cell disease were admitted the day prior to the procedure for intravenous fluids and transfusions. The other 18 patients were admitted the day of the operation, and all patients undergoing elective procedures were discharged the first postoperative day.

Intraoperative cholangiography was possible in 17 patients using various clamp and catheter techniques. A stone was noted in the distal common bile duct in one teenager and was extracted laparoscopically. In the remaining 10, cholangiography was attempted but it was not possible to insert the cholangiocatheter into the cystic duct. It appeared that the cystic duct was too small to accept either a Taut cholangiocatheter or a 4-French ureteral catheter. Cholangiography has been much more easily accomplished in the last 11 patients using the Kumar clamp technique.

In the first two patients, the KTP-532 (Laserscope, San Jose, CA) laser was used for dissection of the gallbladder from the liver bed. In the remaining patients, the electrocautery was found to be as effective as the laser for hemostasis and dissection and had the added advantage of being less expensive.

The total operative time ranged from 70 to 200 minutes (mean, 116 minutes). One of the patients with acute cholecystitis required 3 hours for the procedure mainly because of edema from the acute inflammatory process.

All gallbladders were removed intact and entry into the gallbladder did not occur during dissection from the liver bed in any patient. Neither operative common duct injury nor postoperative cystic duct leaks occurred and conversion to an open procedure was not necessary in any patient. No operative or postoperative complications of any type have been noted.

Twenty-six gallbladders exhibited cholelithiasis and chronic cholecystitis on pathologic examination. Five also showed acute cholecystitis. In the patient with biliary dyskinesia, chronic cholecystitis was noted without cholelithiasis.

REFERENCES

1. Gordon AG, Magos AL. The development of laparoscopic surgery. *Clin Obstet Gynecol.* 1989;3:429.
2. Gans SL, Berci G. Peritoneoscopy in infants and children. *J Pediatr Surg.* 1973;8:399.
3. Reddick EJ, Olsen DO. Laparoscopic laser cholecystectomy. *Surg Endosc.* 1989;3:131.
4. Holcomb GW Jr, O'Neill JA Jr, Holcomb GW III. Cholecystitis, cholelithiasis and common duct stenosis in children and adolescents. *Ann Surg.* 1980;191:626.
5. Holcomb GW Jr, Holcomb GW III. Cholelithiasis in infants, children and adolescents. *Pediatr Rev.* 1990;11:268.
6. Rescorla FJ, Grosfeld JL. Cholecystitis and cholelithiasis in children. *Semin Pediatr Surg.* 1992;1:98.
7. Keller MS, Markle BM, Laffey PA, et al. Spontaneous resolution of cholelithiasis in infants. *Radiology.* 1985;157:345.
8. Pope CV, Bidula MM, Kirks DR, et al. Rapid spontaneous resolution of cholelithiasis in a newborn. *South Med J.* 1988;81:672.
9. Akierman A, Elliott PD, Gall DG. Association of cholelithiasis with total parenteral nutrition and fasting in a preterm infant. *Can Med Assoc J.* 1984;131:122.
10. Jacir NN, Anderson KD, Eichelberger M, et al. Cholelithiasis in infancy: Resolution of gallstones in three of four infants. *J Pediatr Surg.* 1986;21:567.
11. Odom FC, Oliver BB, Kline M, et al. Gallbladder disease in patients 20 years of age and under. *South Med J.* 1976;69:1299.
12. Soderlund S, Zetterstrom B. Cholecystitis and cholelithiasis in children. *Arch Dis Child.* 1962;37:174.
13. Strauss RG. Cholelithiasis in childhood. *Am J Dis Child.* 1969;117:689.
14. Bates GC, Brown CH. Incidence of gallbladder disease in chronic hemolytic anemia (spherocytosis). *Gastroenterology.* 1952;21:104.
15. Sarnaik S, Slovis TL, Corbett DP, et al. Incidence of cholelithiasis in sickle cell anemia using the ultrasonic grayscale technique. *J Pediatr.* 1980;96:1005.
16. Borgna-Pignatti C, DeStefano P, Pajno D, et al. Cholelithiasis in children with thalassemia major: An ultrasonographic study. *J Pediatr.* 1981;99:243.
17. Danzinger RG, Hofmann AF, Schoenfield LJ, et al. Dissolution of cholesterol gallstones by chenodeoxycholic acid. *N Engl J Med.* 1972;286:1.
18. Schoenfield LJ, Lachin JM, Steering Committee, National Cooperative Gallstone Study Group. Chenodiol (chenodeoxycholic acid) for dissolution of gallstones: The National Cooperative Gallstone Study: A controlled trial of efficacy and safety. *Ann Intern Med.* 1981;95:257.
19. Sackmann M, Delius M, Sauerbruch T, et al. Shock-wave lithotripsy of gallbladder stones: The first 175 patients. *N Engl J Med.* 1988;318:393.
20. Holcomb GW III, Olsen DO, Sharp KW. Laparoscopic cholecystectomy in the pediatric patient. *J Pediatr Surg.* 1991;26:1186.
21. Newman KD, Marmon LM, Attorri R, et al. Laparoscopic cholecystectomy in pediatric patients. *J Pediatr Surg.* 1991;26:1184.
22. Sigman HH, Laberge JM, Croitoru D, et al. Laparoscopic cholecystectomy: A treatment option for gallbladder disease in children. *J Pediatr Surg.* 1991;26:1181.
23. Man DWK, Spitz L. Choledocholithiasis in infancy. *J Pediatr Surg.* 1985;20:65.
24. Jonas A, Yahav J, Fradkin A, et al. Choledocholithiasis in infants: Diagnostic and therapeutic problems. *J Pediatr Gastroenterol Nutr.* 1990;11:513.
25. Graves HA Jr, Ballinger JF, Anderson WJ. Appraisal of laparoscopic cholecystectomy. *Ann Surg.* 1991;213:655.
26. The Southern Surgeons Club. A prospective analysis of 1518 laparoscopic cholecystectomies. *N Engl J Med.* 1991;324:1073.
27. Peters JH, Ellison EC, Innes JT, et al. Safety and efficacy of laparoscopic cholecystectomy: A prospective analysis of 100 initial patients. *Ann Surg.* 1991;213:3.
28. Wolfe BM, Gardiner BN, Leary BF, et al. Endoscopic cholecystectomy: An analysis of complications. *Arch Surg.* 1991;126:1192.

CHAPTER 5

Laparoscopy for the Nonpalpable Testis

DAVID A. BLOOM • MICHAEL L. RITCHEY
GIANTONIO MANZONI

Clinical recognition of the undescended testicle no doubt dates to the first medicine man who could count to two. Operative management had to await a time when elective surgery became reasonably safe as cryptorchidism is hardly an urgent necessity. Ambroise Paré recognized undescended testes and explained how they could mimic an inguinal hernia: "But let not the Chirurgion thrust himselfe upon his worke rashly without the advice of the Physition, for it diverse times comes to passe, that the testicles are not as yet fallen downe into the codde by the too great sluggishnese of natures in some of a pretty growth, but remaines long in the groines."[1] Three centuries later, orchidopexy remained risky. Adams reported death from a wound infection at the London Hospital 2 weeks after operation for an undescended testis in an 11-week-old and concluded that it might be wise to defer or avoid such surgery.[2] Only 7 years later the literature recorded a successful orchidopexy: "Professor Annandale then showed a photograph of a rare congenital malposition of the testicle in the perineum. . . . He believed his own success to be due to the use of antiseptics, meaning by this the Listerian method."[3] Within a few decades, most of the principles of modern orchidopexy had been established. The nonpalpable testis, however, continued to defy simple diagnosis and clear-cut therapy.

Throughout history physicians no doubt have dreamed of a magical way to inspect the interior of the living body. Optical and illumination technology in the nineteenth century permitted endoscopic inspection of natural body orifices such as ears, nose, throat, anus, vagina, and urethra. Francis Richard Cruise, medical officer at the Mater Misericordiae Hospital in Dublin, was among the very first in Ireland to use a cystoscope, and in 1865 he predicted that similar optical tubes would someday permit inspection of any body cavity.[4]

In 1910 Hans Christian Jacobaeus, Professor of Medicine at the Karolinska Institute in Stockholm, reported techniques for thoracoscopy and peritoneoscopy in cadavers and patients using air insufflation.[5] For the next 70 years, most innovations in laparoscopy were predominantly gynecologic, and peritoneoscopy picked up the inexact appellation *laparoscopy*.[6,7] In Kiel, Germany, Semm spent his career perfecting laparoscopic procedures and instruments that permitted a wide array of intracorporeal operative procedures.

The first major genitourinary application concerned nonpalpable testes. Cortesi in Modena and Paramo in Madrid were the first to use peritoneoscopy to locate intraabdominal testes. Nicola Cortesi (personal communication; 1992) had a long interest and extensive experience in peritoneoscopy, as he eventually preferred to call the procedure, for diagnosis of abdominal trauma, inflammatory disease and malignancies as early as 1962 (Figure 5–1). He and his colleagues made a peritoneoscopic diagnosis of Mayer–Rokitansky–Kuster syndrome in 1972.[8] Their diagnosis of intraabdominal testes in an 18-year-old man was the first report of laparoscopy for nonpalpable testes. "We think laparoscopy, a simple and harmless examination, is useful in any case, when one or both testes are not palpable; then surgery must follow, to verify real gonadal agenesis, or to perform orchidopexy in case of ectopia."[9] Cortesi was accurate in describing laparoscopy as harmless in his practice; only 3 years later he presented his total experience of laparoscopy in 1720 cases.[10] Paramo endoscoped six patients with cryptorchid testes, including a 10-year-old boy, between 1975 and 1977 and found intraperitoneal testes in two. His experience was reported by his colleague Uson as a letter in the *Journal of Urology*.[11] Since then, a number of large clinical experi-

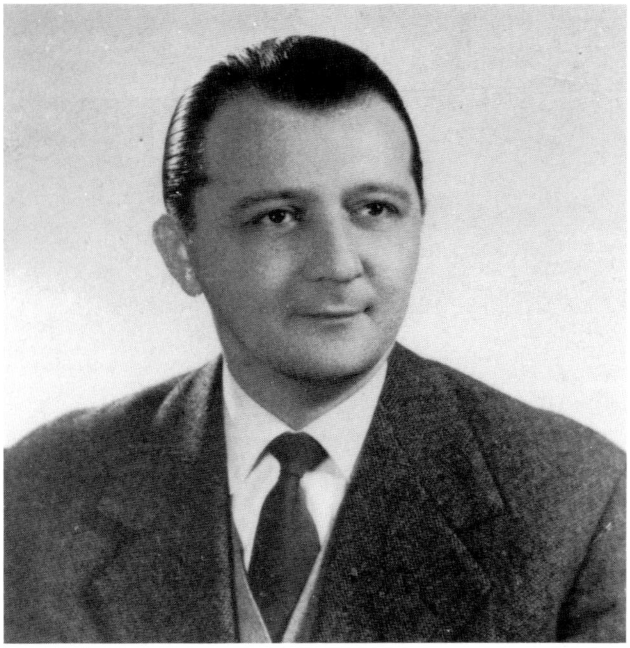

Figure 5–1. Professor Nicola Cortesi of the Emergency Surgery Department, University of Modena, Italy, has been a pioneer of surgical and genitourinary laparoscopy.

ences have validated the role of laparoscopy for nonpalpable testes.[12–16]

PATIENT EVALUATION

A testis cannot be declared nonpalpable until deliberate diagnostic maneuvers have been performed to rule out retractile or canalicular undescended testes. The patient should be cooperative; infants should be reexamined when calm, whereas for toddlers and older children, a few minutes invested in rapport may obviate an inconclusive examination. We begin by trying to milk a testis down from the internal ring. Lubricating jelly or liquid soap may elicit an obscure gonad by reducing tactile friction. Reexamination with the youngster in a cross-leg posture may reveal some testes. Only if these efforts fail to reveal a cryptorchid testis do we label the situation nonpalpable. Furthermore, these same steps are repeated under general anesthesia at the time of operation.

The role of the surgeon in patients with a nonpalpable testis is to locate the testis and deal with it appropriately or else to declare absence with a high degree of confidence. Inaccurate declaration of absence leaves a youngster with the potential time bomb of testicular cancer.[17] Although many imaging modalities have been used, none is completely dependable for locating an occult testis or proving absence. As the first operative step, peritoneoscopy is quite reliable in both objectives.[18] In some patients concomitant inguinal exploration will be necessary; in others, peritoneoscopy alone will prove absence.

The role of endocrinologic tests is still debated. In infants and children with bilateral nonpalpable testes, measurement of serum testosterone before and after stimulation with human chorionic gonadotropin (HCG) may give evidence that responsive testicular tissue is present somewhere. The issues of localization and management, however, remain to be answered. In addition, there have been occasions in which a HCG stimulation test was falsely negative or inconclusive. Levels of gonadotropin-releasing hormone in children with bilateral nonpalpable gonads may be elevated if there is no functioning gonadal tissue. High serum levels may therefore be regarded as proof of absence of testes; however, no single medical center has a very large experience with anorchid infants and, at present, we still favor laparoscopic investigation to absolutely exclude cryptorchid gonads because the penalty for an erroneous assumption of absence is great.

TREATMENT OPTIONS

Therapy is tailored to each patient and laparoscopic findings with reference to the normal male pelvic anatomic landmarks (Figure 5–2).

Blind-Ending Spermatic Vessels

Kogan et al believe that blind-ending spermatic vessels are the sine qua non of testicular absence.[19] The left side has the greater risk for this finding. When spermatic vessels have been seen ending blindly *above* (proximal to) the internal inguinal ring, peritoneoscopy has conclusively proven testicular absence: there is no distal or proximal testis on that side (Figure 5–3). In other instances laparoscopy reveals attenuated or hypoplastic vessels still present at the internal inguinal ring. Although suspicious that there was no viable distal gonad in this group of youngsters, we explored the inguinal canal in the first 100 laparoscopies for nonpalpable testes at the University of Michigan. In 48 patients tissue remnants at the end of blind-ending spermatic vessels in or below the inguinal canal were excised. Testicular parenchyma was identified in one child (a few immature seminiferous tubules with calcification and old hemorrhage) and suggested in a second child (vascular dense connective tissue with dystrophic calcification and hemosiderin-laden macrophages; no testis, but regions or architecture suggestive of severely distorted tubular structures). Other reports indicate a higher incidence of persistent tubular remnants in such nubbins, and

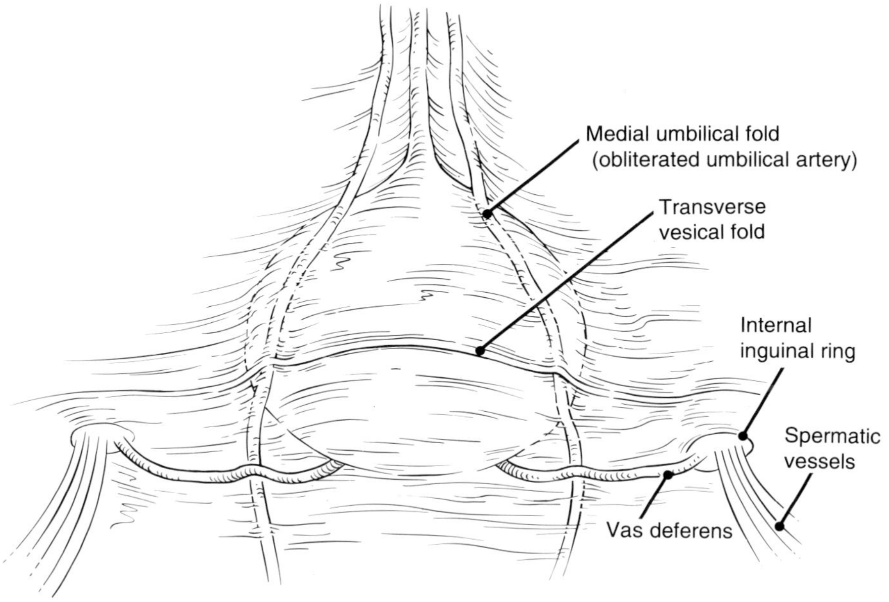

Figure 5–2. Normal male pelviscopic landmarks.

the authors recommend routine inguinal exploration for all nonpalpable testes with vessels that pass into the internal inguinal ring.[20] It is a reasonable hypothesis that an antenatal or perinatal vascular accident was responsible for the loss of these testes. None of our patients with blind-ending spermatic vessels have had visible müllerian remnants.

Unilateral Cryptorchism

When a diagnosis of unilateral testicular absence is made by peritoneoscopy, with or without concomitant inguinal exploration, we follow the advice of Kogan, Harris, and their co-workers to pex the contralateral solitary testis.[19,21] Although the remaining solitary go-

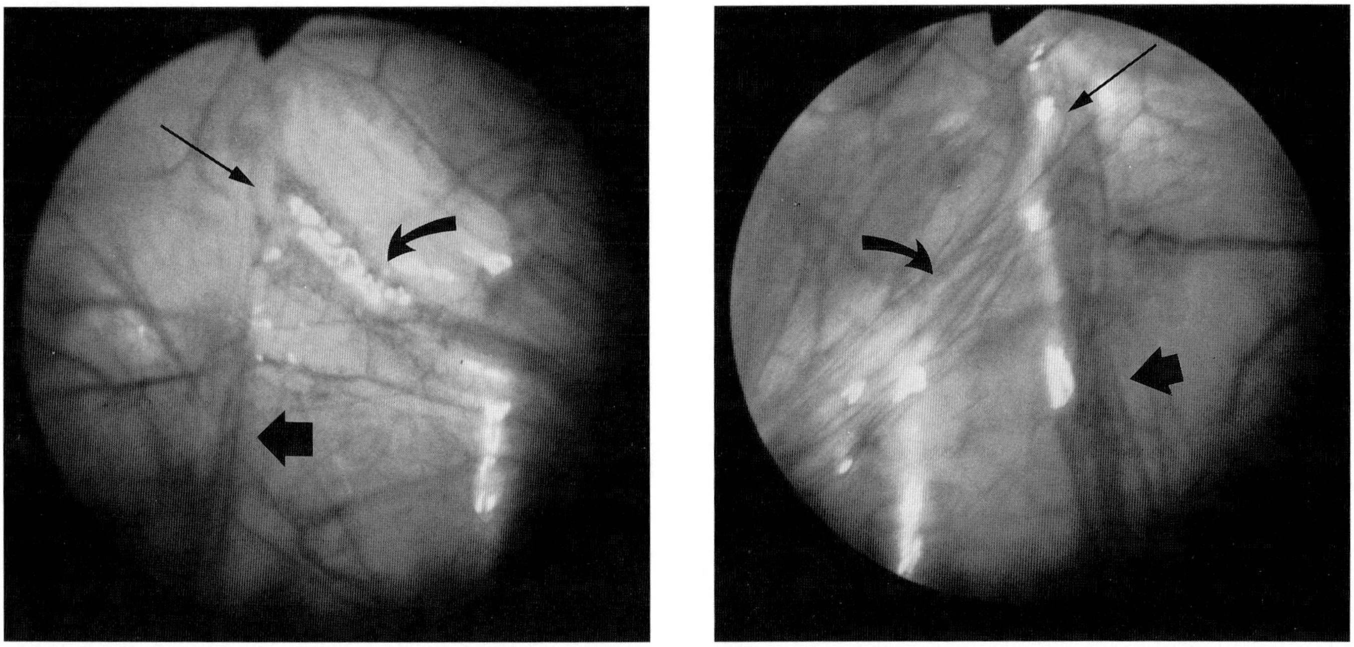

A B

Figure 5–3. Blind-ending spermatic vessels on the left side in a boy with a nonpalpable left testis and normal right testis. **A.** Left side: Spermatic vessels (*short thick arrow*) end above a closed internal inguinal ring (*thin arrow*). Normal vas deferens (*curved arrow*). **B.** Right side: Normal spermatic vessels (*short thick arrow*) cross into internal ring (*thin arrow*) adjacent to vas (*curved arrow*).

nad may not have an increased risk of torsion, its loss, however unlikely, would indeed be catastrophic. When a youngster is already asleep at the time of laparoscopy we carefully place a few extraparenchymal sutures for fixation within a dartos pouch to minimize the risk of subsequent intravaginal spermatic cord torsion. It is important to secure the testis without injury to the gonad.[22] We caution the families that nothing can guarantee against subsequent torsion, but dartos pouch fixation will decrease the incidence.

Controversy surrounds the role of testicular prostheses. Cosmetically, a prepubertal scrotum with a single testis does not look much different to the uneducated eye in a locker room than a scrotum with two testes. Furthermore, we have found only the rare teenager with a solitary testis interested in an operative procedure for a contralateral prosthesis. Therefore, only in unusual family or personal circumstances would we place a prosthesis in a youngster who already has one normal testis in the scrotum.

Bilateral Cryptorchism

Bilateral blind-ending spermatic vessels are uncommon. When this unfortunate diagnosis is made, careful and compassionate counseling is mandatory. Given normal penile morphology, these boys will be completely normal until puberty, but will then need hormonal initiation for puberty and maintenance of secondary sexual characteristics. Early pediatric endocrinologic consultation is necessary. Growth parameters are monitored closely near the time of anticipated puberty to gauge the best time to begin exogenous testosterone. Anorchid adults will, of course, be infertile but should have normal sexual interests and function if maintained on appropriate exogenous hormonal support. Because the completely empty scrotum is very obviously flat and small, we favor early placement of one or two small testicular prostheses and replacement with adult sizes after puberty. The present anxiety over risks from silicon gel prostheses has raised concerns among urologic patients and families as well.[23] An informal survey among pediatric urologists revealed not one patient among thousands with a documented long-term complication beyond an occasional traumatic rupture.[24] For patients with silicon gel prostheses, the risk of removal may be greater than the risk from leaving the device in place.

Missed Low Testes

In some boys, despite a careful preoperative and intraoperative examination, a testis that is at or below the internal inguinal ring may be missed to palpation. We found this situation in about 25% of our patients. In some instances peritoneoscopy revealed what we have called a *peeping testis*, that is, a testis just at the internal inguinal ring within a patent processus vagi-

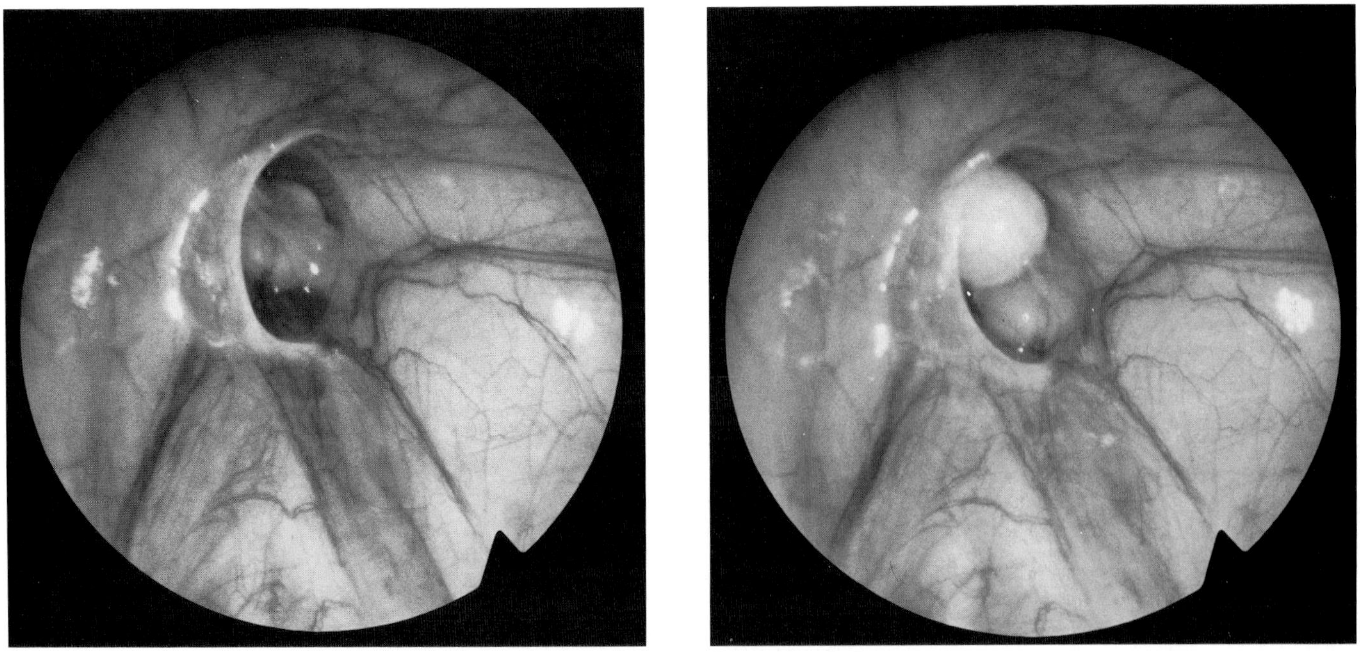

A B

Figure 5–4. Another explanation for a nonpalpable testis: a peeping testis at the internal inguinal ring. **A.** Initial pelviscopic view of internal ring showing inguinal hernia. **B.** View with slight external manual pressure in inguinal canal showing the peeping testis.

nalis (Figure 5–4). On physical examination such testes tend to be pushed proximally into the peritoneal cavity. When these patients underwent traditional inguinal exploration (without endoscopy) the gonads were typically defined as *intraabdominal*. Simple orchidopexy was possible in some cases, and when Fowler–Stephens orchidopexy was necessary, the success rate was likely to be high. In our paradigm of nonpalpable testes, however, we consider these not as abdominal testes, but as missed low testes. In a substantial number of children (5/24), the missed low testes were bilateral and hypoplastic, suggestive of an underlying endocrinopathy. Reitleman has commented that palpable membranes in the scrotum or inguinal canal predict an atrophic descended testic accurately enough to obviate laparoscopy.[25] Palpation of a hernia sac in the inguinal area, however, does not preclude the possibility of a high abdominal testis, which we prefer to manage with a two-step clip orchidopexy. Most missed low testes can be brought into the scrotum by conventional orchidopexy. Jordan has developed a laparoscopic method of orchidopexy that may be suitable for many of these testes.[26]

Abdominal Testes

In about one third of patients with a nonpalpable testis, the gonad will be situated above the internal inguinal ring. When these are completely above the internal ring and consistently within the peritoneal cavity, we describe them as abdominal testes (Figure 5–5). Peritoneoscopy is quite reliable in locating these gonads. Hinman advised that, given a normal contralateral gonad, most abdominal testes are best placed in a specimen jar.[27] Because of the doubtful fertility value and substantial malignancy risk of these testes, this advice is generally sound. Laparoscopy provides the advantage of precise localization. Transabdominal illumination of the site of the testis permits a small precise incision for quick and simple orchiectomy. Alternatively, with two additional trocar punctures, laparoscopic orchiectomy can be performed.

In some instances salvage of an abdominal testis is warranted. This is true in small children with a fairly normal-looking intraabdominal testis or in patients with bilateral abdominal testes. A variety of techniques are applicable including conventional orchiopexy, staged orchidopexy, microsurgical autotransplantation, and Fowler–Stephens orchidopexy.[28–31] The Fowler–Stephens procedure is presently the most popular. It requires division of the spermatic vessel leash and mobilization of the testis on a long vasal loop. Success rates vary with this procedure, in part because of the various types of undescended testes and vasal configurations. Pascual et al showed that ligation of the spermatic vessels removed 80% of the blood supply to the testis in an animal model; however, if the vasal collaterals were not compromised, full blood flow was restored within 2 months.[32] There was no diminution in gonadal weight or interstitial cell ratios, although varying degrees of tubular disturbances occurred. Salman and Fonkalsrud, however, reported more severe damage in their study.[33] We have found that endoscopic clip occlusion of the spermatic vessel leash with a Fowler–Stephens type of orchidopexy 6 months later is reliable and successful

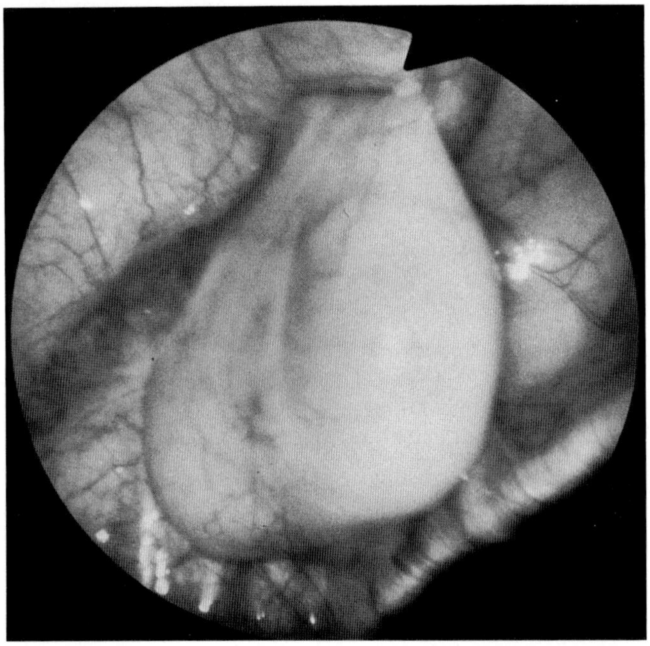

Figure 5–5. True abdominal testis lying above the internal inguinal ring. The vas did not have a long loop extending into the inguinal canal.

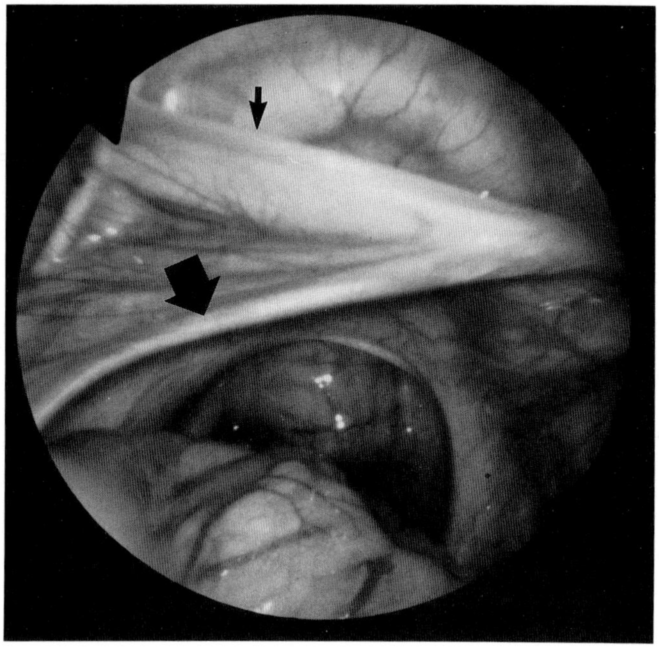

Figure 5–6. Rare explanation for a nonpalpable testis: transverse testicular ectopia (*small arrow* points to transverse vesical fold; *large arrow* indicates left spermatic vessel leash crossing to right internal inguinal ring).

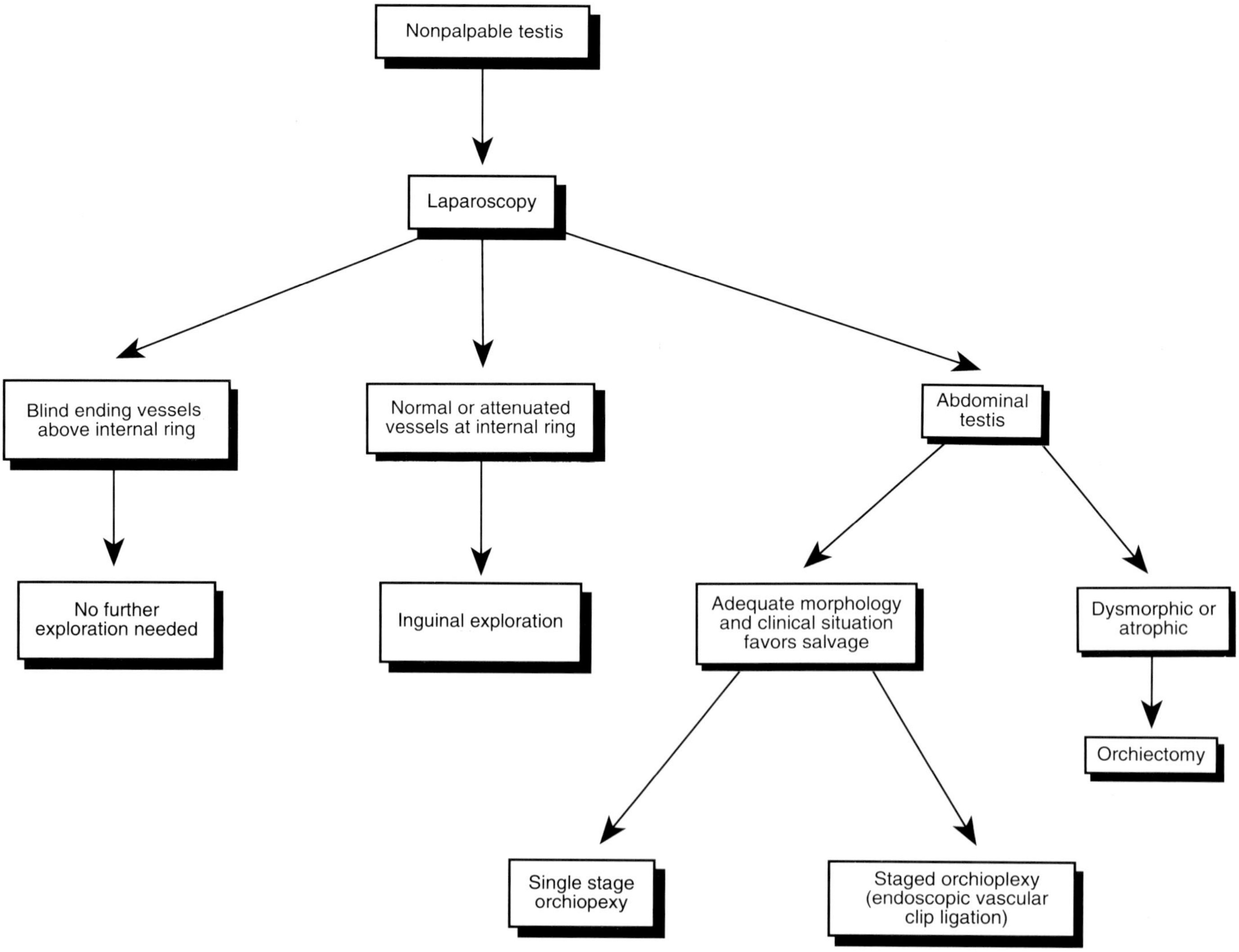

Figure 5–7. This algorithm depicts operative management for children with nonpalpable testes based on their initial laparoscopic findings.

even in children without long vasal loops.[34] In fact, the majority of true abdominal testes do not have long vasal loops. Jordan believes that even intraabdominal testes will be amenable to laparoscopic orchidopexy.[26]

Unusual Situations

Four patients among our first 115 had no visible spermatic vessels or remnants at laparoscopy. One of these children had an ipsilateral absent kidney and hemitrigone. Two children had concomitant surgical exploration of the retroperitoneal area, where atretic blind-ending spermatic vessels were observed. This was early in our clinical series and we probably were not experienced enough to identify the atretic vessels endoscopically. One patient without laparoscopically visible spermatic vessels had postoperative venography, which also failed to either identify a testis or prove absence. None of these patients had müllerian structures at peritoneoscopy. Two patients had transverse testicular ectopia, which has also been described elsewhere[35] (Figure 5–6).

LAPAROSCOPIC TECHNIQUE

The indication for laparoscopy, in our opinion, is the presence of one or two nonpalpable testes. The declaration of a nonpalpable testis is made only after the deliberate sequence of diagnostic maneuvers described earlier.

Under general anesthesia, abdominal insufflation is accomplished using the Veress needle technique as discussed in Chapter 2. A 5-mm umbilical trocar and cannula are inserted and diagnostic peritoneoscopy is performed. The focus of the endoscopic exam is the pelvis and the internal rings bilaterally.

On visualization of the internal ring, several points are observed. Is the internal ring closed or is there an associated hernia? Are the spermatic vessels of normal caliber and do they pass through the internal ring into the inguinal region? Is the vas deferens normal in size and appearance? Is a testis visualized either within an associated hernia sac or within the abdominal cavity?

The various treatment options based on the endoscopic findings are summarized in Figure 5–7. If the vessels end blindly without entering a closed internal ring, then no further exploration is needed because the absence of a testis has been documented. If, however, the spermatic vessels are attenuated but pass through the internal ring, then inguinal exploration is needed to excise any remnants of testicular tissue. It may be possible to excise this tissue laparoscopically as well.

Should a testis be located within the upper inguinal canal, then conventional single-stage orchiopexy will usually be successful. For a viable intraabdominal testis with an inadequate vascular leash for conventional orchiopexy, however, initial clip ligation of the testicular vessels followed by Fowler–Stephens orchidopexy 6 to 9 months later is recommended.

For clip ligation of the vascular leash, a second port is needed (Figure 5–8). A 1.1-cm incision is made in the suprapubic midline and a 1.0-cm trocar and cannula are inserted into the abdominal cavity under telescopic visualization. Through this suprapubic cannula, an endoscopic clip applier is inserted and the spermatic vessels are ligated as far from the testis as possible (Figure 5–9). A second clip can be placed for complete ligation if needed. The second step in this staged orchidopexy is delayed 6 months or longer and has been described previously.[19] We prefer to use the Hulka device for clip ligation of the vessels at the first stage and find the larger clips quite convenient at the second stage.

If a dystrophic abdominal testis or a testis in a teenager is noted on diagnostic pelviscopy, then laparoscopic orchiectomy can be performed. In addition to the 1.0-cm suprapubic incision, a 5-mm incision is needed in the ipsilateral lower abdomen (Figure 5–10).

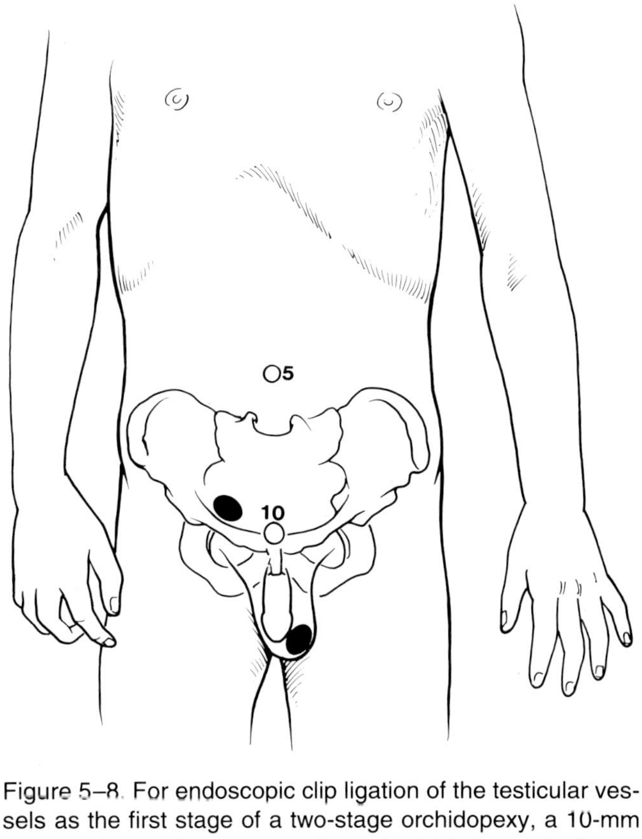

Figure 5–8. For endoscopic clip ligation of the testicular vessels as the first stage of a two-stage orchidopexy, a 10-mm suprapubic port is necessary through which the endoclip applier is inserted.

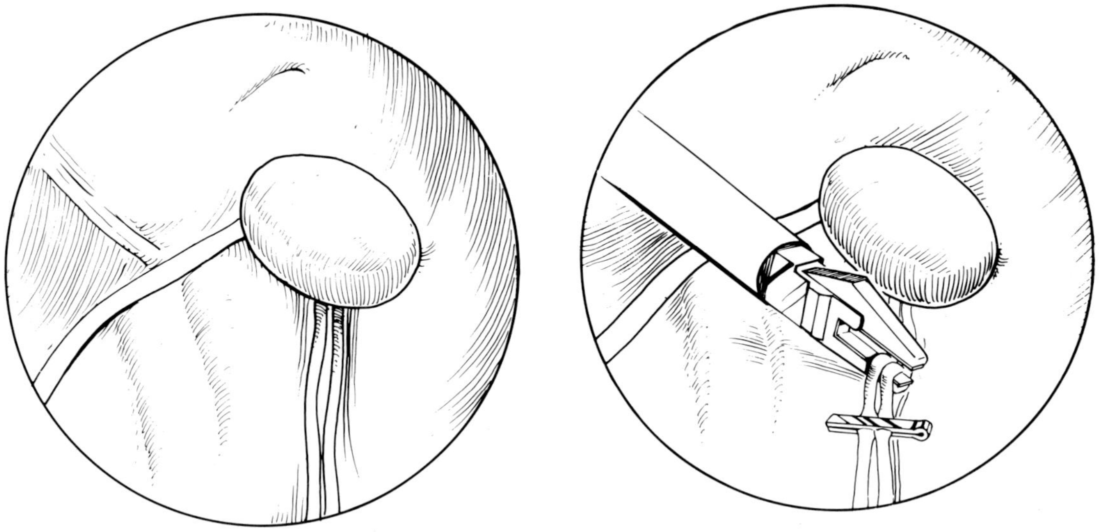

Figure 5–9. This drawing depicts an intraabdominal right testis with laparoscopic clip ligation of the spermatic vessels.

A grasping forceps is inserted through this cannula to handle the testis while clips are placed endoscopically using the suprapubic port (Figure 5–11). The electrocautery can also be used for hemostasis if necessary.

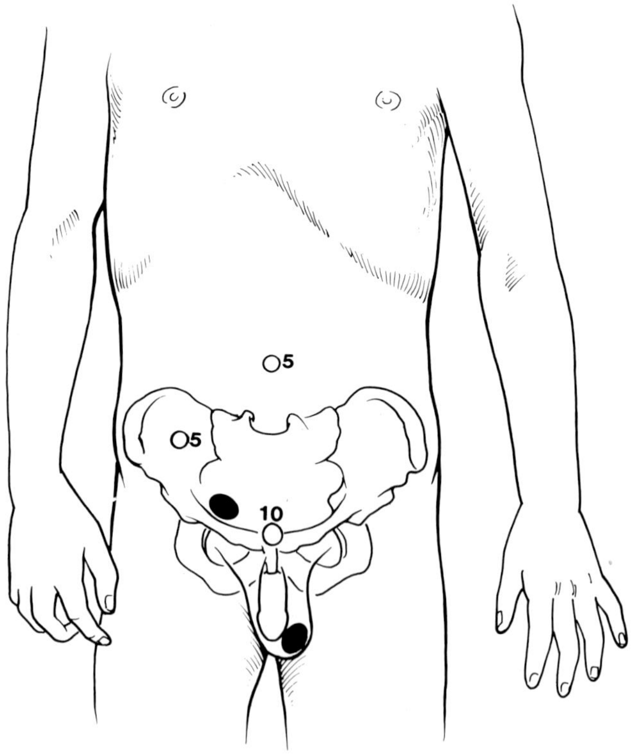

Figure 5–10. Laparoscopic orchiectomy can also be performed when indicated. A third port is needed for assistance with manipulation of the testis and associated structures. This 5-mm port is placed in the ipsilateral lower quadrant.

Orchiectomy can also be performed through a small incision located over the intraabdominal testis.

COMPLICATIONS

Laparoscopy in children is a potentially lethal procedure. Careful technique using the safety steps of Semm lowers the risk to nearly zero and permits experts like Semm and Cortesi to report that laparoscopy, in their hands, is harmless.[36]

The major risks of laparoscopy for nonpalpable testes lie in the creation of the pneumoperitoneum and the insertion of the umbilical trocar as discussed in Chapter 2. Omental evisceration following this procedure has been reported.[37] Complications from the vascular clip ligation or orchiectomy should be rare.

THE UNIVERSITY OF MICHIGAN EXPERIENCE

Our experience with laparoscopy for evaluation of children with nonpalpable testes from 1985 to 1992 is summarized in Table 5–1. One hundred fifteen children have been evaluated endoscopically. Fifty-two patients had attenuated vessels and underwent inguinal exploration to excise any testicular remnants. In 25 cases, the testis was visualized within the inguinal canal and either conventional or single-stage Fowler–Stephens orchiopexy was performed.

In 31 exams, an abdominal testis was found. Four patients underwent conventional orchiopexy. Eighteen patients with 23 intraabdominal testes have undergone endoscopic vascular clip ligation, and 16 chil-

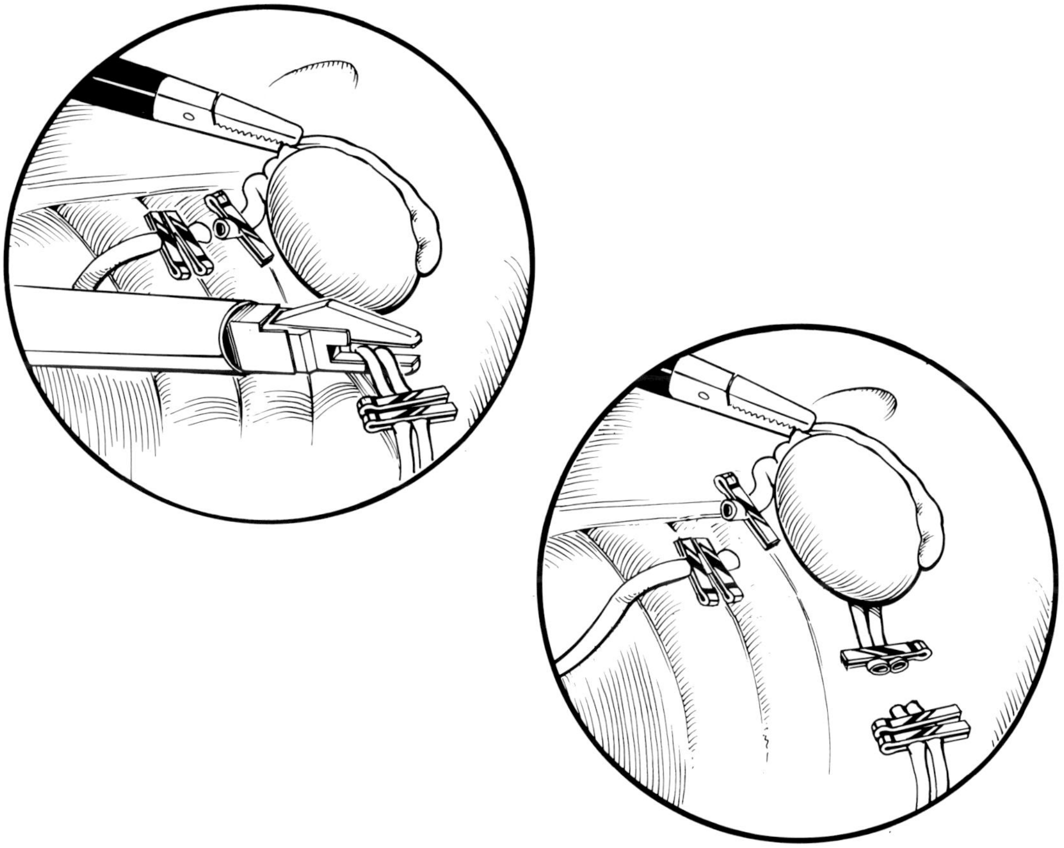

Figure 5–11. This diagram depicts laparoscopic orchiectomy with ligation of the vas deferens and testicular vessels with endoclips. The electrocautery can also be used for hemostasis of the collateral vessels when needed.

dren have subsequently had a second-stage Fowler–Stephens orchiopexy. In 4 patients, orchiectomy was performed.

Five patients did not have visible spermatic vessels on the left side. Two patients underwent retroperitoneal exploration early in our experience, but we would not perform this additional procedure today. In two patients, transverse testicular ectopia was found at endoscopy and single-stage orchiopexy was performed.

TABLE 5–1. REVIEW OF THE MICHIGAN EXPERIENCE WITH LAPAROSCOPY FOR NONPALPABLE TESTES, 1985–1992: LAPAROSCOPIC FINDINGS IN 115 PATIENTS

	Number of Patients	Right	Left	Bilateral
Attenuated vessels	52	16	30	6
Missed low testes	25	10	10	5
Abdominal testes	31	11	12	8
No vessels	5	—	5	—
Transverse testicular ectopia	2	1	1	—

REFERENCES

1. Pare A. In: Keynes G, ed. *The Apology and Treatise of Ambroise Paré.* Chicago: University of Chicago Press; 1952:110.
2. Adams JE. Transition of the testicle into the perineum. *Lancet.* 1871;1:710.
3. Annandale. Congenital malposition of the testicle in the perineum. *Medico-Chirurg Soc Edinburgh.* 1878;1:657.
4. Cruise FR. The utility of the endoscope as an aid in the diagnosis and treatment of disease. *Dublin Q J Med Sci.* 1865;39:329.
5. Jacobaeus HC. Ueber die moglichkeit die zystoskopie bei untersuchung seroser hohlungen anzuwenden. *Munch Med Wochenschr.* 1910;57:2090.
6. Bosch PF. Laparoskopie. *Schweiz Z Krankenhaus Anstaltsw.* 1936;6:62.
7. Palmer R. La celioscopie gynecologique. *Rapport Prof Mocquot Acad Chir.* 1946;72:363.
8. Cortesi N, Bertaglia A, et al. A case of symmetric bilateral agenesis of the uterus (Rokitansky–Kuster's syndrome). *Endoscopy.* 1972;4:43.
9. Cortesi N, Ferrari P, Zambarda E, Manenti A, Baldini A, Pignatti Morano F. Diagnosis of bilateral abdominal

cryptorchidism by laparoscopy. *Endoscopy.* 1976;8:33.
10. Cortesi N. Laparoscopy in routine and emergency surgery. *Am Surg.* 1979;137:647.
11. Uson AC. Re: Laparoscopy for cryptorchidism. *J Urol.* 1982;128:829.
12. Silber SJ, Cohen R. Laparoscopy for cryptorchidism. *J Urol.* 1980;124:928.
13. Scott JES. Laparoscopy as an aid in the diagnosis and management of the impalpable testis. *J Pediatr Surg.* 1982;7:14.
14. Lowe DH, Brock WA, Kaplan GW. Laparoscopy for localization of nonpalpable testes. *J Urol.* 1984;131:728.
15. Malone PS, Guiney EJ. The value of laparoscopy in localizing the impalpable undescended testis. *Br J Urol.* 1984;56:429.
16. Manson PS, Terhune D, et al. Preoperative laparoscopic localization of the nonpalpable testis. *J Urol.* 1985; 134:919.
17. Brothers LR III, Weber CH Jr, Ball TP Jr. Anorchism versus cryptorchidism: The importance of a diligent search for intra-abdominal testes. *J Urol.* 1978;119:707.
18. Bloom DA, Ayers JWT, McGuire EJ. The role of laparoscopy in management of nonpalpable testes. *J Urol.* 1988;94:465.
19. Kogan SJ, Gill B, Bennett B, Smey P, Reda EF, Levitt SB. Human monorchism: A clinicopathological study of unilateral absent testes in 65 boys. *J Urol.* 1986;135:758.
20. Plotzker ED, Rushton HG, Belman AB, Skoog SJ. Laparoscopy for nonpalpable testes in childhood—Is inguinal exploration also necessary when vas and vessels exit the inguinal ring? *J Urol.* 1992;148:635.
21. Harris BH, Webb HW, Wilkinson AH Jr, Steven PS. Protection of the solitary testis. *J Pediatr Surg.* 1982;17:950.
22. Bellinger MF, Abramowitz HB, Brantley S, Marshall G. Orchiopexy: An experimental study of the effect of surgical techniques on testicular histology. *J Urol.* 1989; 142:553.
23. Ehrlich RM. Silicon testicular prosthesis. *Soc Pediatr Urol Newslett.* Oct 23, 1992:31–32.
24. American Academy of Pediatrics, annual meeting, 1992. Informal survey.
25. Reitleman C. Discussion. *J Urol.* 1992;148:643.
26. Jordan GH. Laparoscopic orchidopexy. *J Endourol.* 1992, in press.
27. Hinman F Jr. Survey: Localization and operation for nonpalpable testes. *Urology.* 1987;30:193.
28. Youngson GG, Jones PF. Management of the impalpable testis: Long-term results of the preperitoneal approach. *J Pediatr Surg.* 1992;26:618.
29. Steinhardt GF, Kroovand RL, Perlmutter AD. Orchiopexy: Planned 2-stage technique. *J Urol.* 1985;133: 534.
30. Stephens FD. Fowler–Stephens orchiopexy. *Semin Urol.* 1988;6:103.
31. Silber SJ, Kelly J. Successful autotransplantation of an intra-abdominal testis to the scrotum by microvascular technique. *J Urol.* 1976;115:452.
32. Pascual JA, Villaneuva-Meyer J, Salido E, et al. Recovery of testicular blood flow following ligation of testicular vessels. *J Urol.* 1989;142:549.
33. Salman FT, Fonkalsrud EW. Effects of spermatic division for correction of the high undescended testis on testicular function. *Am J Surg.* 1990;16:506.
34. Bloom DA. Two-step orchiopexy with pelviscopic clip ligation of the spermatic vessels. *J Urol.* 1991;145:1030.
35. Gornall PG, Pender DJ. Crossed testicular ectopia detected by laparoscopy. *Br J Urol.* 1987;59:283.
36. Semm K. *Operative Manual for Endoscopic Abdominal Surgery.* Chicago: Year Book Medical; 1987.
37. Bloom DA, Ehrlich RM. Omental evisceration through small laparoscopy port sites. *J Endourol.* 1993;7:31.

CHAPTER 6

Laparoscopy for the Female Patient

CHRISTOPHER R. MOIR

Gynecologic procedures are arguably the most common indication for operative laparoscopy. Although the laparoscopic techniques have only recently been applied to other abdominal operations,[1] pediatric surgeons and gynecologists have a long history of combining their efforts to achieve the best operative outcome for the female pediatric patient. General or pediatric surgeons should learn the basic techniques of gynecologic laparoscopy and be able to perform some simple but necessary procedures. The female teenager who presents with abdominal pain is an excellent example of a situation in which a surgeon may encounter a gynecologic condition at the time of laparoscopy. With experience, the surgeon may be able to immediately treat a gynecologic emergency without resorting to open laparotomy.

This chapter outlines the specific techniques of gynecologic laparoscopy and reviews the operative diagnosis and treatment of the most common and important pediatric conditions.

TECHNIQUE

Equipment

The basic set of age- and size-appropriate laparoscopes, cannulas and insufflation equipment is identical to that used for other intraabdominal endoscopic operations. All sets should contain large grasping forceps, toothed forceps, and probes. An atraumatic ovarian grasping forceps or basket should be available to stabilize the ovary for operative procedures. Coagulation using hooked cautery, bipolar cautery, laser, or combination instruments may also be used. Suction and irrigation are essential. The technique of aquadissection has been popularized for tubal and ovarian surgery.[2,3] In this technique, pressurized water is used to develop a plane between the ovarian cyst and the parenchyma (Figure 6–1). Finally, intracorporeal suturing is often required for such procedures as oophoropexy or closure of surgical defects. Staplers are rarely used.

Lasers for dissection and coagulation have been popular in gynecologic surgery.[2–5] There are fewer concerns regarding endoscopic coagulation when working in the pelvis, away from other intraabdominal viscera. Special precautions still, however, apply; in particular, when the ovary is being operated on, it should be elevated against a muscular portion of the pelvic wall such that any stray laser coagulation will occur over a muscular surface rather than a portion of the viscera.

Patient Position

Proper positioning depends on the patient's age and physical maturity (Figure 6–2). The uterus of the older, postmenarchal adolescent may block adequate adnexal visualization and is easily manipulated by transvaginal cervical instrumentation. The standard lithotomy position is cumbersome and potentially dangerous to the patient. We prefer an almost level positioning of the patient's thighs with the body, allowing the feet and legs to rest and bear some weight on the lower half of the brace. The legs are wrapped and pressure points padded. The prepubertal child will not require uterine manipulation and may be placed supine on the operating table. Again, the legs should be wrapped to improve venous return as the pelvic viscera are manipulated and the intraabdominal pressure is increased.

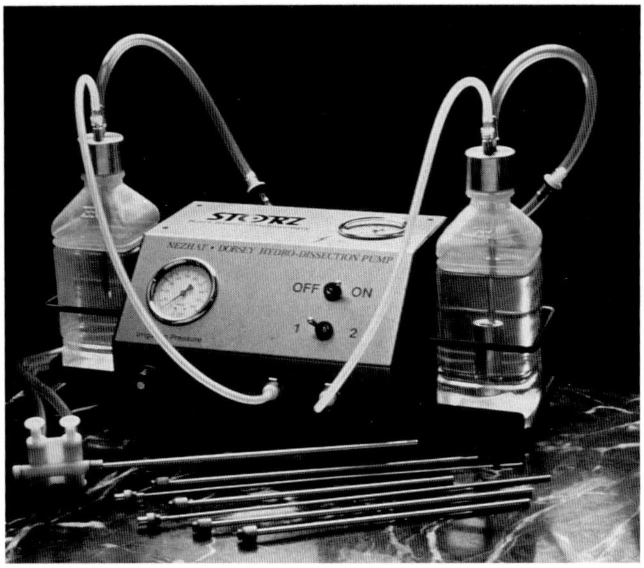

Figure 6–1. The technique of aquadissection has been used for laparoscopic tubal and ovarian surgery. The equipment is combined with suction probes for dissection and operative field cleansing.

Patient Preparation

In addition to the standard placement of a nasogastric tube, Foley catheter, and endotracheal tube, the adolescent is prepared for intraoperative manipulation of the uterus. Following perineal preparation, the cervix is grasped with a tenaculum and the cervical canal intubated with a long-handled trocar (Figure 6–3). The patient is then prepped and draped in a sterile fashion, leaving these instruments available for later use.

As an alternative to the tenaculum and trocar, we have found that a standard Foerster sponge stick placed transvaginally will be adequate for operative manipulation of the cervix. This technique is especially important in patients who are not sexually active. Use of the tenaculum has been associated with postoperative bleeding that can be quite distressing.

Although pediatric surgeons are very aware of their patients' sensitivities regarding gynecologic conditions, one point cannot be overemphasized. What may be routine for surgeons used to operating on adults may be extremely traumatic for the adolescent. Standard procedures should be carefully reviewed and modified as necessary for this age group.

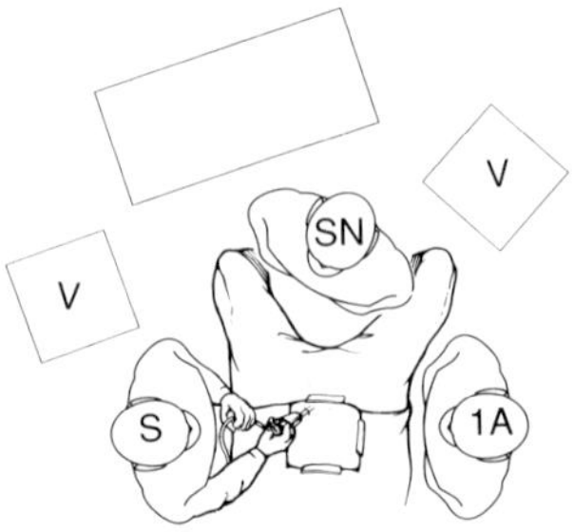

Figure 6–2. Usually, two video monitors are used and are positioned at the foot of the operating table for visualization by the surgeon and assistant. The scrub nurse is often positioned between the patient's legs for gynecologic laparoscopy.

Cannula Placement

The umbilicus is the universal access point for the laparoscope. It provides ideal exposure except in the very young child with a shallow pelvis. To avoid interference with the other operating instruments in young children, the laparoscope may be placed in a supraumbilical location.

At most, two other ports are placed in the suprapubic position (Figure 6–4). Each port is placed just medial or lateral to the inferior epigastric vessels. The line of placement of the two cannulas should closely approximate the position of a Pfannenstiel incision, in case conversion to an open pelvic procedure is neces-

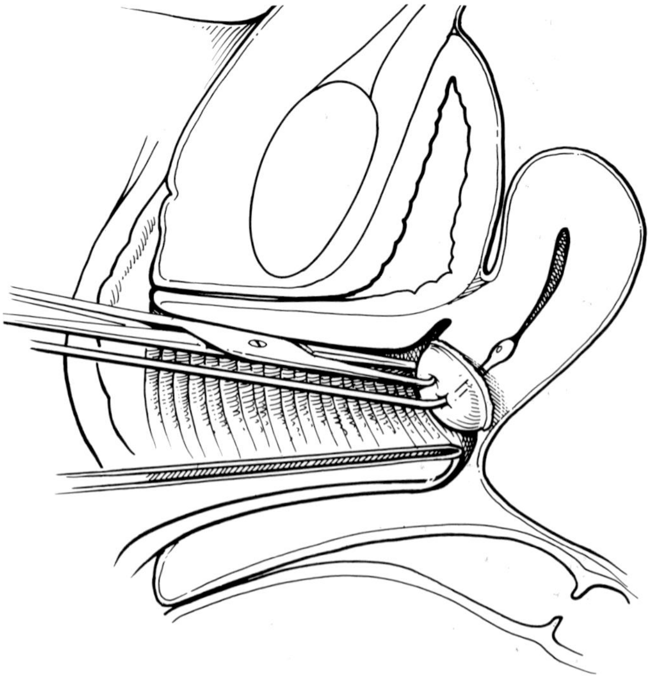

Figure 6–3. Following perineal preparation, the cervix is grasped with a tenaculum and the cervical canal intubated with a long-handled trocar for manipulation during laparoscopy.

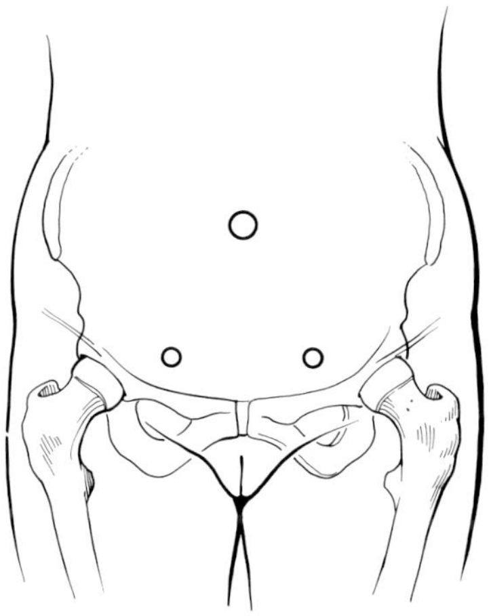

Figure 6–4. Usually, a three-cannula technique is employed for laparoscopy in the female child. Each lower abdominal port is placed just medial or lateral to the inferior epigastric vessels. The line of port placement should closely approximate the position of a Pfannenstiel incision for conversion to an open pelvic procedure if necessary.

sary. The transcervical instrument can be considered a third port.

Intraoperative Positioning

After the cannulas and laparoscope are introduced and the pelvis is visualized, the patient is rotated to a steep Trendelenburg position. The small bowel falls away from the pelvis, providing a clear visual field. A right-handed operating surgeon stands to the patient's left, viewing a video monitor placed to the right of the patient's right leg. The assistant watches a second monitor placed on the patient's left while standing opposite the surgeon. The scrub nurse or technician usually stands between the patient's legs when the lithotomy position is used (*see* Figure 6–2). The operation is easier if the operative field remains between the surgeon and the video monitor. If necessary, the monitors or the surgeon can be moved to retain this relationship.

SPECIFIC PROBLEMS

Abdominal Pain

Surgeons are most likely to encounter a pediatric gynecologic condition when evaluating children who present with acute abdominal pain.[6–8] The increasing utilization of abdominal and pelvic ultrasound has allowed preoperative planning for the surgical treatment of some of these conditions.[9,10] When possible, it is best to work in collaboration with a gynecologist in the management of these pediatric problems.

The limitations of preoperative evaluation and the urgency to proceed with an acute surgical emergency may place the surgeon in the position of discovering pediatric gynecologic conditions at the time of operation. This is particularly true in the evaluation of the female teenager. Statistically this group has the highest percentage of missed preoperative diagnosis, leading to delayed operation or, in hindsight, unnecessary operation.[11] It is this group who may benefit the most from laparoscopic evaluation. Many thoughtful surgeons are chagrined to find that a patient with a normal appendix often requires a larger incision and more visceral manipulation to search for the source of pain than those children with uncomplicated but acutely inflamed appendices. Laparoscopy allows near-total abdominal and pelvic exploration without a large incision.[6,12,13]

The next section reviews the most common pediatric gynecologic conditions that may be discovered at emergency laparoscopy. Once diagnosed, these problems can often be corrected without converting to an open procedure.

Adnexal Torsion

Excluding neonatal patients, the diagnosis of adnexal torsion is rare, with approximately 200 cases described.[14] Despite the reported infrequency of adnexal torsion, the importance of the condition mandates early diagnosis and treatment. The reported average time of 15.5 hours to operative therapy remains far too long to preserve ovarian and tubal function.[15] It is hoped the availability of laparoscopy will shorten this delay.

Usually the affected ovary has been enlarged by a cyst or tumor prior to torsion, but, occasionally, a normal adnexa will twist.[16,17] In a literature review, Mordehai et al noted that 60 of the over 200 reported cases had normal adnexa.[14] In their own series, 6 of 14 patients with torsion had normal fallopian tubes and ovaries. Several theories for torsion include adnexal enlargement from cyst or tumor the innate mobility of the tube and ovary made worse by a long mesentery and adnexal venous congestion around the time of menarche.

Most patients present with lower abdominal pain, lateralizing to the affected side. The pain is usually intense and does not resolve. In many instances, the physical findings of low-grade fever and mild leukocytosis may not correlate with the severity of the pain.[8] This may mislead the evaluating physician into pursuing more conservative treatment. Serial examinations to identify a mass will often confirm the diagnosis too late for operative correction. A pelvic ultrasound may demonstrate a complex mass corresponding to an enlarged edematous tubo-ovarian complex.[18] Color flow doppler ultrasonography usually confirms decreased or absent flow to the ovary.[19,20] The presence of a complex pelvic mass should encourage laparoscopic visualization for diagnosis and treatment.

At laparoscopy, the diagnosis can be made by visual inspection (Figure 6–5). A careful search for ovarian vein thrombosis precedes any attempt at laparoscopic detorsion. If fully necrotic, the torsion should not be corrected; rather, the pedicle may be ligated using an intracorporeal suturing technique. The pedicle is divided between sutures, and the ovary is exteriorized through a secondary incision or after morcellation in a specimen retrieval bag. Histologic examination of the specimen is, however, important to exclude an associated tumor. Therefore, open removal is favored if difficulties occur with removal.

Many torsed adnexa will appear dusky and blue secondary to venous congestion but will not be infarcted. In these patients, laparoscopic reduction is appropriate.[21] Correction is accomplished with probes placed through 5-mm ports. It is best not to grasp the mass. Once the adnexal torsion has been corrected, the ovary should be examined for cysts or tumors. Simple cysts may be aspirated or resected. Occasionally, the ovarian capsule is incised to relieve venous congestion. Bilateral oophoropexy can be performed to prevent further episodes of torsion but this concept remains controversial.

Ovarian Cysts

Simple ovarian cysts are almost universally present in adolescent females. These cysts are usually small and multiple and rarely cause significant symptoms.[9]

In the preovulatory stage of the menstrual cycle, a number of follicles develop to approximately 1 cm in diameter. Usually one of these follicles becomes the dominant graafian follicle, reaching up to 3 cm. At ovulation, this follicle releases the ovum and then forms the corpus luteum, which is usually less than 3 cm. In the absence of pregnancy, the corpus luteum involutes in the latter half of the cycle. These physiologic cysts are all less than 3 cm and are usually multiple.[22,23] Therefore, cysts of this size are rarely the etiology for abdominal pain. If such cysts are seen at diagnostic laparoscopy, the same statement holds true. Once diagnosed, no further therapy is indicated.

Functional retention cysts develop from a follicle or a corpus luteum that has failed to involute. These cysts are usually solitary and cycle with menses. Involution is expected over 4 to 8 weeks. Functional cysts are smooth-walled and sharply demarcated and have few internal echoes on ultrasound.[24,25] Most cysts are over 4 cm, with some reaching 10 cm in diameter. Pain usually begins in the second half of the menstrual cycle and is usually poorly defined, often bilateral and not disabling. At laparoscopy, a follicular or corpus luteum cyst is usually an incidental finding. Diagnosis is confirmed by visualization of the smooth surface of the ovarian capsule, lack of any signs of malignancy in the area, and operative impression of serous fluid

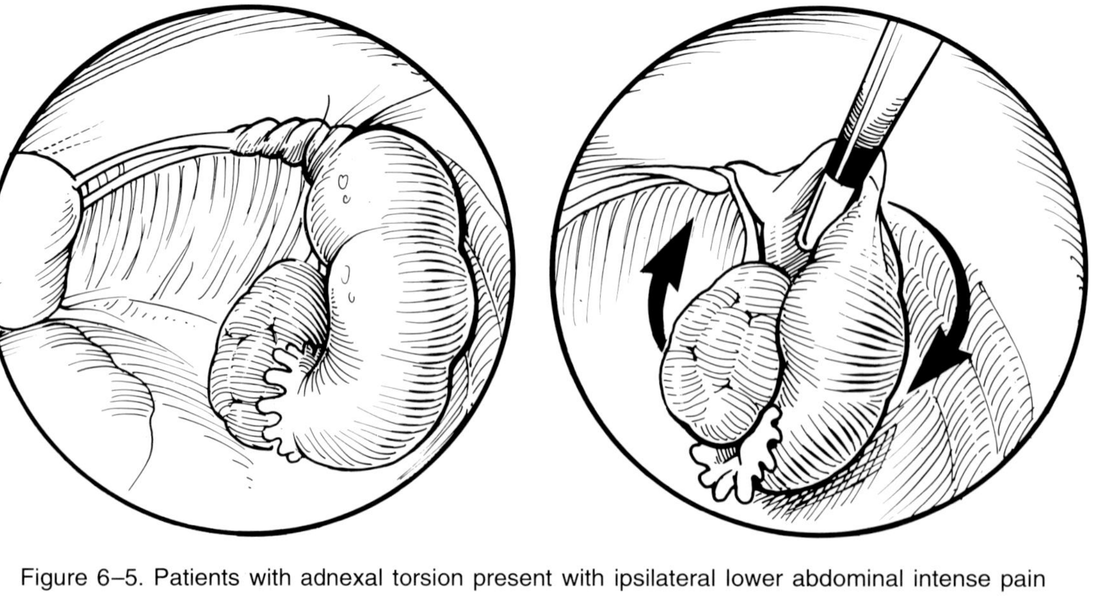

Figure 6–5. Patients with adnexal torsion present with ipsilateral lower abdominal intense pain that does not resolve. Laparoscopy is diagnostic (*left*) and may be therapeutic. Detorsion is accomplished by placing a probe through an ipsilateral 5-mm cannula (*right*).

within the cyst. Occasionally, the cyst may be aspirated by direct placement of a long spinal needle through the anterior abdominal wall under laparoscopic visualization (Figure 6–6). These cysts do not require resection nor should they be marsupialized into the peritoneal cavity. Generally the cysts will resolve over 4 to 8 weeks. If not, ovarian suppression is indicated. Larger cysts may certainly be the cause of the patient's pain and will respond to aspiration either by ultrasound or, if noted at laparoscopy, by direct visualization. Otherwise, these patients can be managed expectantly.[26]

Hemorrhagic Cysts

Functional cysts occasionally bleed, causing acute abdominal pain. These cysts are usually corpus luteum cysts that expand in the second half of the menstrual cycle. Hemorrhage occurs within the cyst and produces rapid adnexal enlargement. Rupture of a hemorrhagic cyst or free bleeding from an open corpus luteum cyst will cause severe pelvic pain that is sudden and dramatic. The pain is initially well localized but soon becomes diffuse. Generally, the adnexa is not palpable but an ultrasound will demonstrate a complex cyst in the adnexal region with good doppler flow in the surrounding vessels.[27,28] Differential diagnoses of complex adnexal masses include adnexal torsion, ectopic pregnancy, and bleeding corpus luteum of pregnancy.[29] Torsion is excluded by color flow doppler.[19] Serum human chorionic gonadotropin (HCG) should be obtained on all postpubertal female teenagers. If the HCG is elevated, an intrauterine pregnancy likely exists and should be evaluated by ultrasound. An intrauterine embryonic sac makes the diagnosis of the complex ovarian mass more likely to be a bleeding corpus luteum, which may be treated expectantly.

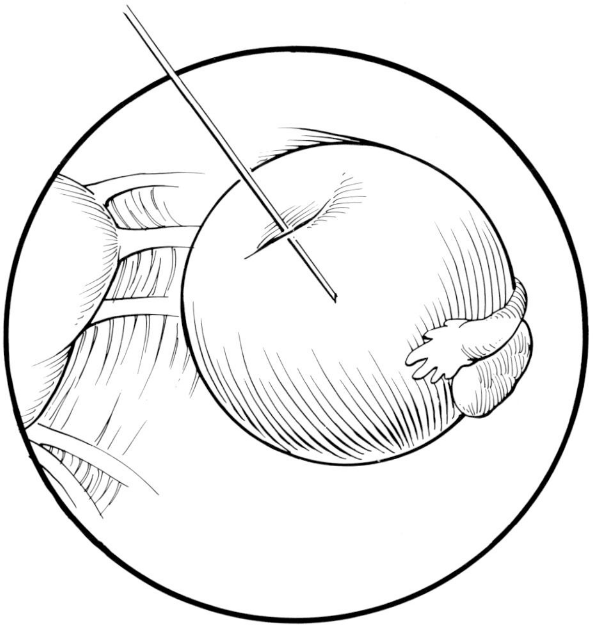

Figure 6–6. Functional ovarian cysts are smooth-walled and sharply demarcated and appear to be filled with serous fluid at laparoscopy. Aspiration of the cyst is usually sufficient treatment. Resection or marsupialization into the peritoneal cavity is not necessary.

A hemorrhagic corpus luteum cyst discovered at operation is generally clearly identified by dark red bleeding on the ovarian surface. The ovary is enlarged, but again shows a smooth white capsule without other evidence of malignancy. Complex ultrasound masses that do not show definite signs of bleeding at laparoscopy are more difficult to diagnose as hemorrhagic corpus luteum cysts. The clinical setting of acute pain in the second half of the menstrual cycle and the laparoscopic visualization of an otherwise normal ovary suggest this diagnosis. If aspiration of the cyst reveals old blood, the diagnosis of a hemorrhagic corpus luteum cyst is confirmed. Again, no further therapy is necessary. The ovary should not be resected, nor should the cyst be opened for drainage. These hemorrhagic cysts will usually resolve in 1 to 2 months.

Ectopic Pregnancies

Over 95% of tubal pregnancies occur in the ampulla. These pregnancies present as localized or diffuse pelvic pain, and further history will elicit menstrual irregularity in most patients, but this may be a common history in normal teenagers. Less than one half of the patients report other subjective symptoms of pregnancy. Prolonged or severe hemorrhage will lead to hypovolemic shock, and maternal death is still reported.[8,30]

Serum HCG levels should be drawn on every female teenager presenting with abdominal pain. Correlation with pelvic ultrasound findings is diagnostic.[31] As previously mentioned, an elevated HCG level indicates pregnancy. If an intrauterine embryonic sac is not found on ultrasound, the diagnosis of a tubal pregnancy can be made with confidence.[32,33]

Laparoscopy is now recommended for the treatment of most patients with ectopic pregnancy.[5] The enlarged ampulla may be easily visualized (Figure 6–7). Management is best accomplished in collaboration with an operative gynecologist. Usually a linear salpingostomy with vascular control of the mesosalpinx is employed. The products of conception are removed using aquadissection and all bleeding points carefully cauterized. The salpingostomy is usually

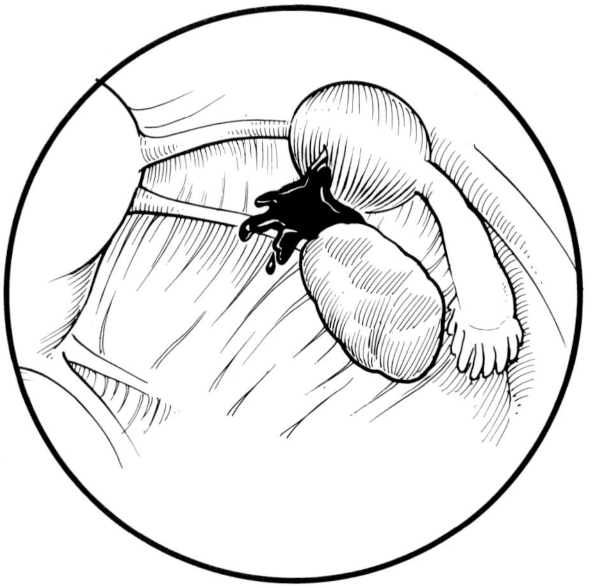

Figure 6–7. A ruptured ectopic pregnancy may be the etiology for intense pelvic pain in older girls. Laparoscopic management can be accomplished, but collaboration with an operative gynecologist may be preferred.

not closed.[34,35] Postoperative HCG levels are monitored until they have returned to normal. If a plateau is reached, it is possible that products of conception have been retained. Newer therapeutic modalities are now being used in these situations.[36,37]

Tubo-ovarian Abscess

Pelvic inflammatory disease is becoming an increasingly important diagnostic consideration in adolescents. The most common organisms remain *Neisseria gonorrhoeae* and *Chlamydia*.[8] Usually diagnosed by history, physical examination, and ultrasound, laparoscopy has been used to confirm the diagnosis and direct treatment.[38] It should be noted that 33% of patients with tubo-ovarian abscesses are afebrile, and 25% have a normal white blood cell count. Extreme pain and tenderness are the most common findings.[38] Sonography will confirm a complex mass, but occasionally, tubo-ovarian abscesses have presented as simple masses without major internal echoes.[7]

Laparoscopic evaluation has been diagnostic, but now it may also be therapeutic.[39,40] The fibrinous purulent exudate associated with the infection is removed and the tubo-ovarian abscess is drained. Proponents of this therapy cite shorter hospital stays and potential preserved fertility as advantages over more prolonged in-hospital medical therapy.[41,42]

ELECTIVE PROCEDURES

Intersex

Laparoscopy may be extremely useful in the identification and localization of the pelvic gonads in intersex patients.[43–47] Streak gonads are easily removed laparoscopically using grasping forceps and bipolar cautery. As these structures are small and in close proximity to the ureter, careful visualization is necessary before proceeding. The most common genetic abnormality requiring laparoscopic gonadectomy is Turner's mosaicism (XO/XY). These patients have streak gonads with a high potential for malignant degeneration during adolescence and early adulthood.[47] Outpatient laparoscopic gonadectomy has been accomplished using the previously described two-cannula technique in two patients.

Ovarian Teratoma

A benign ovarian teratoma is usually easily identified by ultrasound.[25] The most common finding is mural nodularity and acoustic shadowing.[48] Fluid levels are common within the mass,[49] and most masses are conglomerates of solid and cystic structures.[25,50] Patients with ovarian teratomas may present with minimal pelvic pain. Most patients are easily distinguished from those presenting with hemorrhagic corpus luteum cysts, ectopic pregnancies, or adnexal torsion.[25] Teratomas are generally large, with an average diameter of 10 cm. This again helps to distinguish these masses from the smaller functional cysts and torsions.

Laparoscopic removal of teratomas is possible using the techniques of cauterization, aquadissection, and controlled removal[29,51] (Figure 6–8). Tumor markers should be drawn prior to laparoscopic surgery.[2] The surgeon should ensure that the HCG, α-fetoprotein, and CA-125 markers are normal,[42] as a malignant teratoma requires an open exploration.

Ovarian Malignancies

More than 80% of all pediatric gynecologic malignancies arise from the ovary. Approximately 85% of these ovarian tumors arise in teratomas or germinomas.[25] Epithelial or stromal tumors are far less common in the pediatric patient, representing 5 and 10% of ovarian tumors, respectively. The most common patient is a postmenarchal teenager. These tumors are large, averaging 15 cm in diameter, and usually show other signs of malignancy, including capsular invasion, irregularity, enlarged pelvic lymph nodes, ascites, peri-

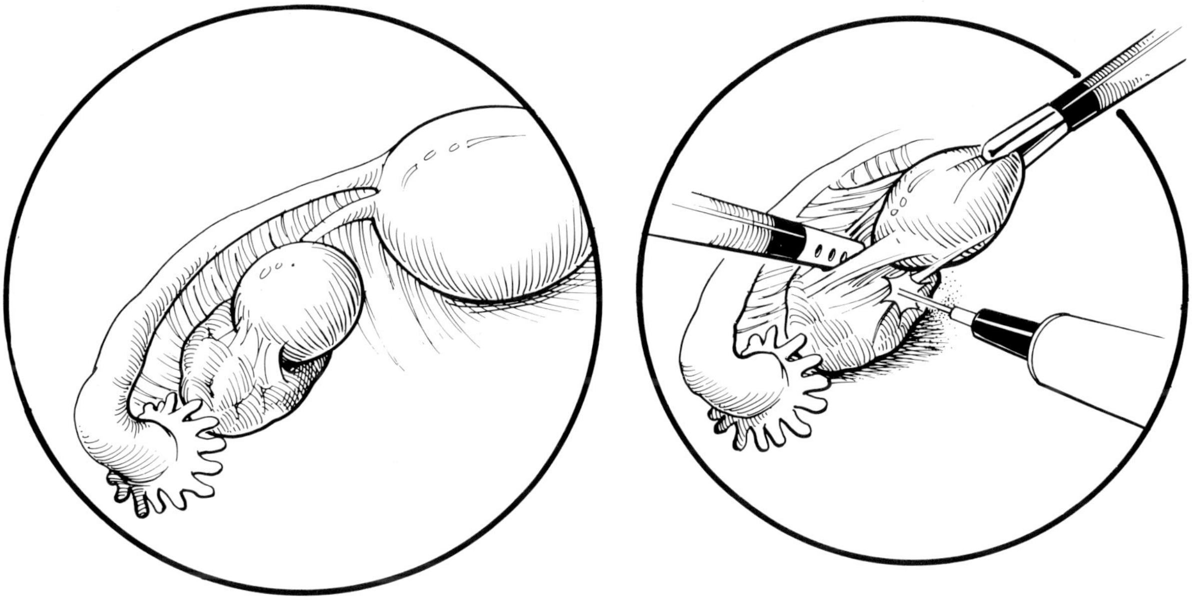

Figure 6–8. In laparoscopic removal of benign cysts and tumors, laser or electrocautery dissection opens the ovarian capsule. Blunt dissection using the "aquadissector" allows for laser or electrocautery coagulation of the remaining strands of vascular tissue.

toneal implantation, and liver metastasis. If any of these signs of malignancy are noted at laparoscopy, the pelvic fluid should be aspirated and sent for cytology and the operation converted to an open procedure.[42,51]

Endometriosis

Although fortunately rare in the adolescent, endometriosis is another cause of cyclical abdominal pain. Laparoscopy is the ideal method of diagnosis. Once visualized, the lesions may be photocoagulated with the laser.[4]

SUMMARY

The majority of pediatric gynecologic conditions are benign, incidental findings seen at laparoscopy. Nevertheless, certain conditions such as adnexal torsion or large functional cysts with hemorrhage may be diagnosed and managed laparoscopically. Operative ovarian procedures are less common and are best accomplished in collaboration with an operative gynecologist. Many cysts and benign tumors may now be removed laparoscopically. Once only a diagnostic tool, gynecologic laparoscopy has expanded to include a large range of operative procedures.

REFERENCES

1. Moir CR, Donohue JH, van Heerden JA. Laparoscopic cholecystectomy in children: Initial experience and recommendations. *J Pediatr Surg.* 1992;27:1066.
2. Sanfilippo JS. Operative laparoscopy in the adolescent. *Obstet Gynecol Clin North Am.* 1992;19(1):163.
3. Rock J. Ectopic pregnancy. In: Liende TE, ed. *Operative Gynecology.* 7th ed. Philadelphia: JB Lippincott; 1991.
4. Sanfilippo J. Endometriosis in adolescents. In: Wilson E, ed. *Endometriosis.* New York: Alan R. Liss; 1987.
5. Cartwright PS, Herbert CM, Maxson WS. Operative laparoscopy for the management of tubal pregnancy. *J Reprod Med.* 1986;31:589.
6. Easter DW, Cuschieri A, Nathanson LK, et al. The utility of diagnostic laparoscopy for abdominal disorders. Audit of 120 patients. *Arch Surg.* 1992;127(4):379.
7. Vercellini P, Fedele L, Arcaini L, et al. Laparoscopy in the diagnosis of chronic pelvic pain in adolescent women. *J Reprod Med.* 1989;34(10):827.
8. Burnett LS. Gynecologic causes of the acute abdomen. *Surg Clin North Am.* 1988;68(2):385.
9. Haller JO, Friedman AP, Schaffer R, et al. The normal and abnormal ovary in childhood and adolescence. *Semin Ultrasound.* 1983;4:206.
10. Graif M, Itzchak Y. Sonographic evaluation of ovarian torsion in childhood and adolescence. *AJR.* 1988;150:647.
11. Berry J Jr, Malt RA. Appendicitis near its centenary. *Ann Surg.* 1984;200:567.
12. Sackier JM. Laparoscopy in pediatric surgery (editorial). *J Pediatr Surg.* 1991;26(10):1145.

13. Waldschmidt J, Schier F. Laparoscopic surgery in neonates and infants. *Eur J Pediatr Surg.* 1991;1(3):145.
14. Mordehai J, Mares AJ, Barki Y, et al. Torsion of uterine adnexa in neonates and children: A report of 20 cases. *J Pediatr Surg.* 1991;26(10):1195.
15. Evans JP. Torsion of normal uterine adnexa in premenarchial girls. *J Pediatr Surg.* 1978;13:195.
16. Farrell TP, Boal DK, Teele RL, et al. Acute torsion of normal uterine adnexa in children, sonographic demonstration. *AJR.* 1982;139:1223.
17. Davis AJ, Feins NR. Subsequent asynchronous torsion of normal adnexa in children. *J Pediatr Surg.* 1990;25(6):687.
18. Helvie MA, Silver TM. Ovarian torsion: Sonographic evaluation. *J Clin Urol.* 1989;17:327.
19. Van-Voorhis BJ, Schwaiger J, Syrop CH, et al. Early diagnosis of ovarian torsion by color doppler ultrasonography. *Fertil Steril.* 1992;58(1):215.
20. Taylor KJW, Burris PN, Wells PNT, et al. Ultrasound doppler flow studies of the ovarian and uterine arteries. *Br J Obstet Gynaecol.* 1985;92:240.
21. Shalev E, Mann S, Romano S, et al. Laparoscopic detorsion of adnexa in childhood: A case report. *J Pediatr Surg.* 1991;26(10):1193.
22. Fleischer AC, Daniell JF, Rodier J, et al. Sonographic monitoring of ovarian follicular development. *J Clin Urol.*1981;9:275.
23. Ritchie WGM. Sonographic evaluation of normal and induced ovulation. *Radiology.* 1986;161:1.
24. Hall DA. Sonographic appearance of the normal ovary, of polycystic ovary disease, and of functional ovarian cysts. *Semin Ultrasound.* 1983;4:149.
25. Surratt JT, Siegel MJ. Imaging of pediatric ovarian masses. *Radiographics.* 1991;11:533.
26. Kullendorff CM. Diagnosis and treatment of ovarian cysts in children. *Ann Chir Gynaecol.* 1991;80(1):65.
27. Baltarowitch OH, Kurtz AB, Pasto ME, et al. The spectrum of sonographic findings in hemorrhagic ovarian cysts. *AJR.* 1987;148:901.
28. Reynolds T, Hill MC, Glassman LM. Sonography of hemorrhagic ovarian cysts. *J Clin Urol.* 1986;14:449.
29. Parker WH. Management of adnexal masses by operative laparoscopy. Selection criteria. *J Reprod Med.* 1992;37(7):603.
30. Weinstein L, Morris MB, Dotters D, et al. Ectopic pregnancy—A new surgical epidemic. *Obstet Gynecol.* 1983;61:698.
31. Taylor KJW, Ramos IM, Feyock AL. Ectopic pregnancy: Duplex doppler evaluation. *Radiology.* 1989;173:93.
32. Nyberg DA, Mack LA, Jeffrey RB Jr, et al. Endovaginal sonographic evaluation of ectopic pregnancy: A prospective study. *AJR.* 1987;149:1181.
33. Fossum G, Davajan V, Kletzky O. Early detection of pregnancy with transvaginal ultrasound. *Fertil Steril.* 1988;49:788.
34. Stangel JJ, Gomel V. Techniques in conservative surgery for tubal gestation. *Clin Obstet Gynecol.* 1980;23:1221.
35. DeCherney A, Romero R, Naftolin F. Surgical management of unruptured ectopic pregnancy. *Fertil Steril.* 1981;35:21.
36. Stovall T, Ling F, Gray L, et al. Methotrexate treatment of unruptured ectopic pregnancy: A report of 100 cases. *Obstet Gynecol.* 1991;77:749.
37. Ammerman M, Shafer MA, Snyder D. Ectopic pregnancy in adolescents: A clinical review for pediatricians. *J Pediatr.* 1990;117:677.
38. Landers DV, Sweet R. Current trends in the diagnosis and treatment of tubo-ovarian abscess. *Am J Obstet Gynecol.* 1985;151:1098.
39. Reich H. Endoscopic management of tuboovarian abscess and pelvic inflammatory disease. In: Sanfilippo J, Levine R, eds. *Operative Gynecologic Endoscopy.* New York: Springer-Verlag; 1989.
40. Reich H, McGlynn F. Laparoscopic treatment of tuboovarian and pelvic abscess. *J Reprod Med.* 1987;32:747.
41. Levine R. Economic impact of pelviscopic surgery. *J Reprod Med.* 1985;30:655.
42. Maiman M, Seltzer V, Boyce J. Laparoscopic excision of ovarian neoplasms subsequently found to be malignant. *Obstet Gynecol.* 1991;77:563.
43. Atlas I, Stone N. Laparoscopy for evaluation of cryptorchid testis. *Urology.* 1992;40(3):256.
44. Heiss KF, Shandling B. Laparoscopy for the impalpable testes. *J Pediatr Surg.* 1992;27(2):175.
45. Wilson-Storey D, MacKinnon AE. The laparoscope and the undescended testis. *J Pediatr Surg.* 1992;27(1):89.
46. Joshi NP, Sotrel G. Diagnostic laparoscopy in apparent uterine agenesis. *J Adolesc Health Care.* 1988;9(5):403.
47. Portuondo JA, Neyro JL, Barral A, et al. Management of phenotypic female patients with an XY karyotype. *J Reprod Med.* 1986;31(7):611.
48. Sisler CL, Siegel MJ. Ovarian teratomas: A comparison of the sonographic appearance in prepubertal and postpubertal girls. *AJR.* 1990;154:139.
49. Nour S, MacKinnon AE, Dickson JAS. Ovarian cysts and tumours in childhood. *J R Coll Surg Edinb.* 1992;37(1):39.
50. Gedeit RG, Jay MS, Ros SP. The role of MRI in evaluation of an adolescent with a pelvic mass. *J Adolesc Health Care.* 1990;11(6):516.
51. Schwobel MG, Stauffer UG. Surgical treatment of ovarian tumors in childhood. *Prog Pediatr Surg.* 1991;26:112.

CHAPTER 7

Laparoscopic Management for Inguinal and Hiatal Hernia (Nissen Fundoplication)

THOM E LOBE • KURT P. SCHROPP • DAVID A. ROGERS

Now well accepted in general surgical practice, minimally invasive techniques appear to be advantageous to the patient because of decreased hospitalization, less postoperative pain, and early return to unrestricted activities. Despite these apparent advantages, several criteria must be met for procedures to be considered better than more conventional operative approaches. The complication rate must be less than or at least as good as that for conventional surgery, and any repair or reconstructive procedure also must have a recurrence rate as low as that of the conventional procedure it proposes to replace. With these caveats in mind, the role of laparoscopy in the management of inguinal and hiatal hernias in children, including Nissen fundoplication, is reviewed.

As detailed elsewhere in this book, the techniques that evolved to make possible the treatment of abdominal hernias in children laparoscopically have only recently been developed. In the explosion of minimally invasive technology, new tools and techniques are being perfected that will most certainly impact on the management of these disorders in the future.

INGUINAL HERNIAS IN CHILDREN

The goals in the diagnosis and repair of inguinal hernias in children are to establish a permanent repair on the symptomatic side and to make an accurate diagnosis of the presence or absence of a hernia on the asymptomatic contralateral side. We have accepted that the asymptomatic contralateral side can be accurately diagnosed using laparoscopy.

The technique we use is as follows: In small infants, the bladder is emptied by a Credé maneuver and the stomach is emptied with an orogastric tube before the abdomen is insufflated. Although it may be possible to ventilate the child by mask, we prefer endotracheal intubation and believe this is safer. After the abdomen is prepped and draped, the infant is placed in a mild Trendelenburg position and a standard Veress needle is inserted through a stab wound in the inferior rim of the umbilical ring. The abdomen is then insufflated to a pressure of 8 to 10 torr with carbon dioxide. It is helpful to elevate the abdominal wall during these maneuvers to avoid visceral injury. A 3-mm cannula is then inserted through the umbilical stab wound and a 2-mm 0-degree telescope is passed through this cannula to observe the internal inguinal rings from the inside of the abdomen (Figures 7–1 and 7–2).

When a hernia is present it is usually obvious. A small hernia may be indicated by the presence of a funnel-shaped configuration, the bottom of which cannot be clearly seen. A veil of peritoneum may also cover a patent process vaginalis or small hernia opening. In inspection of the internal inguinal ring from the perspective of the umbilicus, it is apparent how a hernia could be missed if it was evaluated from the symptomatic side by passing the telescope through an opened hernia sac. The veil of peritoneum is often subtle and cannot be seen well when viewed from

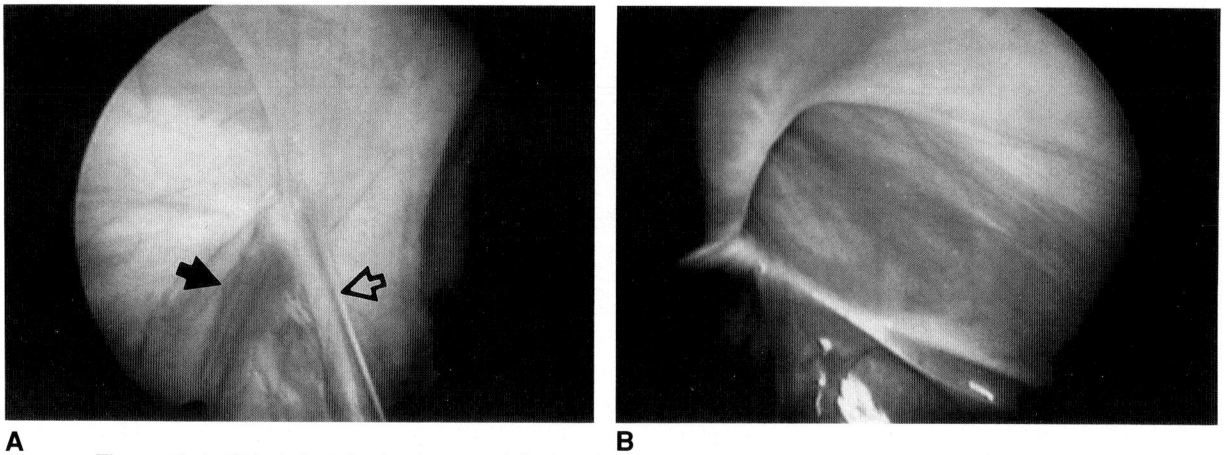

Figure 7–1. This infant had a known right inguinal hernia **(B)**. At laparoscopy, there was not a contralateral left patent processus vaginalis **(A)** and left inguinal exploration was avoided. The vas deferens (*open arrow*) and testicular vessels (*solid arrow*) are identified on the left side.

medial to lateral, at least not nearly so well as it can be seen from lateral to medial.

It is also apparent when inspecting hernias in this fashion why the simple instillation of carbon dioxide into the abdomen to create a pneumoperitoneum as proposed by several authors does not always document a hernia.[1] The veil of peritoneum covers the opening to the hernia sac similarly to the way the septum primum covers the foramen ovale in the heart. Thus, the simple establishment of a pneumoperitoneum is not adequate for diagnosis in all cases and may result in false-negative observations.

When we observe a contralateral patent processus vaginalis at laparoscopy in infants and children, we call that a positive inguinal examination and explore and repair that side in a conventional fashion. When we do not see a patent processus, we call that a negative inguinal exploration and do not explore that side. In our experience of 100 inguinal explorations, no postoperative hernias have been discovered after a negative laparoscopic inguinal exploration. Also, each time we identified a hernia, there was a hernia or a patent process vaginalis present at exploration.

Since 1991, surgeons have been performing laparoscopic herniorrhaphy for direct and indirect inguinal herniorrhaphy in adult patients.[2–7] The essentials of the techniques are as follows: The laparoscope is inserted through an umbilical cannula, and two additional cannulas are inserted lateral to the rectus muscle on either side, at or just below the level of the umbilicus. A transverse peritoneal incision is first made above the hernia defect moving from medial to lateral. The peritoneum is dissected from the cord structures until the hernia sac is free from the cord structures and can be excised (Figure 7–3). Depending on the technique used, a roll of polypropylene mesh

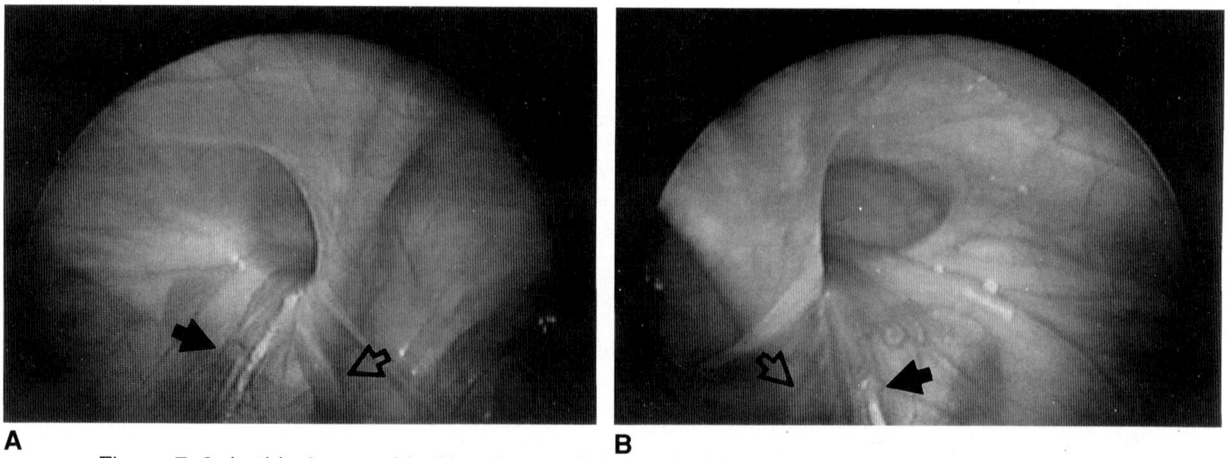

Figure 7–2. In this 3-year-old with a known right inguinal hernia **(B)**, a contralateral left patent processus vaginalis **(A)** is also seen. Again, note the vas deferens (*open arrow*) and testicular vessels (*solid arrow*).

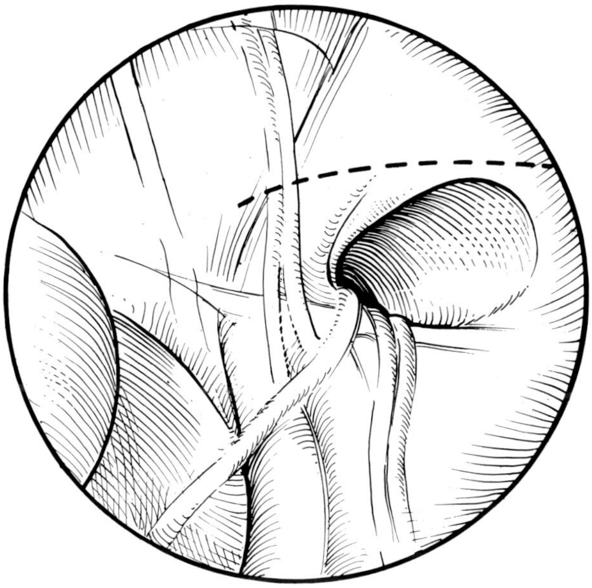

Figure 7–3. For laparoscopic herniorrhaphy, a transverse peritoneal incision is made above the internal opening. The operator should proceed medial to lateral when making this incision.

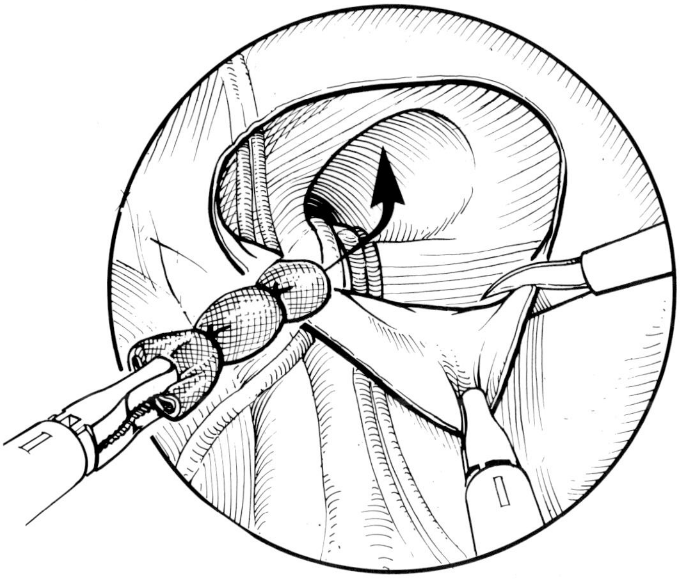

Figure 7–4. A roll of polypropylene mesh can be inserted into the inguinal canal when an indirect hernia is noted.

can be inserted into the exposed inguinal canal in cases of indirect inguinal hernias or this step can be omitted (Figure 7–4).[8,9] A section of polypropylene mesh is then fashioned to cover the hernia defect. This is notched to accommodate the epigastric vessels and is then secured using a hernia stapler to fasten the mesh to the posterior abdominal wall fascia (Figure 7–5). The area is reperitonealized using the stapler to approximate the edges of the cut peritoneum. Although this technique has now been used many times in adults, its long-term results have not been prospectively compared with those of conventional herniorrhaphy.

The advantages of this approach are similar to those of other operations performed laparoscopically. Specifically, there is decreased pain and early return to unrestricted activities. When one questions adults who have experienced repairs accomplished by both approaches, they uniformly comment that the laparoscopic repair is easier to tolerate and allows them to return to work and strenuous activity more quickly

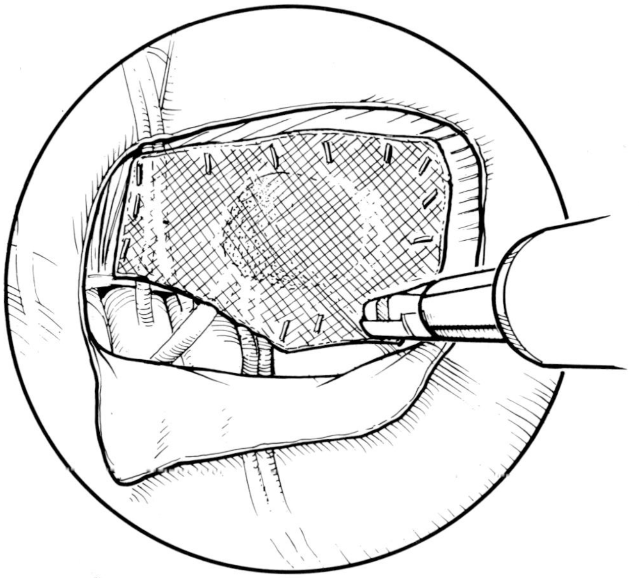

Figure 7–5. A piece of mesh is fashioned and placed over the internal opening. The mesh is secured to the posterior abdominal wall using a hernia stapler.

than the conventional approach. If the repair stands the test of time and the recurrence rate is less than or no greater than the result with the conventional approach, then there is no question it will be quickly adopted by the majority of the surgical community.

One disadvantage of this technique is that general anesthesia is required for laparoscopy, whereas regional or spinal anesthesia can be used to complete an inguinal herniorrhaphy in the standard fashion. Another disadvantage is that a prosthetic mesh is used. Although prosthetic materials are used in other hernia repairs, they are usually reserved for recurrent hernias and difficult or large hernias.

Because conventional inguinal herniorrhaphy and inguinal exploration in infants and small children are so easily tolerated, it is hard to justify the laparoscopic repair for routine cases. In older children and adolescents, however, the laparoscopic approach may be reasonable, particularly if one is dealing with a young athlete who wants to return almost immediately to his or her unrestricted activity or sport.

The technique we prefer for laparoscopic herniorrhaphy in older children and adolescents is a modification of the procedure described earlier for adults. The access is similar, using three trocars. The peritoneum above the hernia is incised and the hernia sac is everted as it is dissected free from the cord structures. It is then excised. The hernia defect, which is usually small compared with those in adults, is closed primarily with interrupted nonabsorbable sutures of an appropriate size (2-O or O), rather than employing a piece of polypropylene mesh. These sutures can be placed using laparoscopic techniques in such a way as to avoid injuring the cord structures (Figure 7–6). After the repair is completed, the cut edge of the peritoneum can be reapproximated using a running suture technique or a hernia stapler, depending on the preference of the surgeon.

We have not performed enough of these procedures to be able to report the durability of this repair. Because it is a sutured repair, however, and the principles of the repair are similar to those of an open inguinal exploration (the only difference being the surgical approach), we believe that it will likely stand the test of time.

Potential complications of the laparoscopic approach to herniorrhaphy are obvious and include transection of the spermatic vessels or vas deferens, injury to the epigastric or femoral vessels, and potential injury to the bladder. It is common after these procedures to see ecchymosis or a hematoma develop in the inguinal canal or scrotum, but this does not usually present any significant difficulty.

This same laparoscopic approach can be used to repair direct or indirect hernias and is certainly an approach to be considered for abdominal wall hernias that are residual or recurrent after open repair of abdominal wall defects or after failed inguinal herniorrhaphy. Another group of patients for whom the laparoscopic repair with mesh might be suitable are those patients with ascites in whom hernia recurrences are frequent.

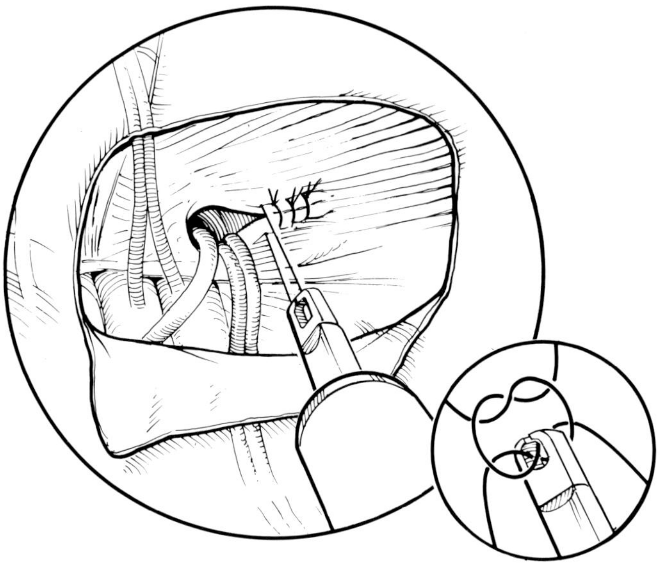

Figure 7–6. Our preferred technique is laparoscopic closure of the defect with interrupted nonabsorbable sutures. A knot-pusher is used to secure the knot.

HIATAL HERNIAS AND ANTIREFLUX SURGERY

The same video technology and endoscopic instrumentation previously described allow reconstructive procedures such as Nissen fundoplication to be performed laparoscopically.

The laparoscopic approach to Nissen fundoplication is not new. Dallemagne et al first performed a laparoscopic Nissen fundoplication at the Clinique Saint Joseph in Liege, Belgium, in January 1991.[10] Later that year, Geagea performed a similar procedure in Nova Scotia.[11]

Cuschieri and colleagues began performing laparoscopic antireflux surgery in 1989 and have described their technique in eight elderly patients, ranging from 60 to 79 years, with a mean follow-up of 11 months.[12]

Dallemagne et al has performed over three dozen procedures in patients ranging from 29 to 69 years of age. Their mean operative time varies between 1.5 to 2 hours. Most of their patients ate and drank on the first postoperative day and were discharged from the hospital on the second postoperative day. Their long-term results are similar to those achieved by laparotomy.

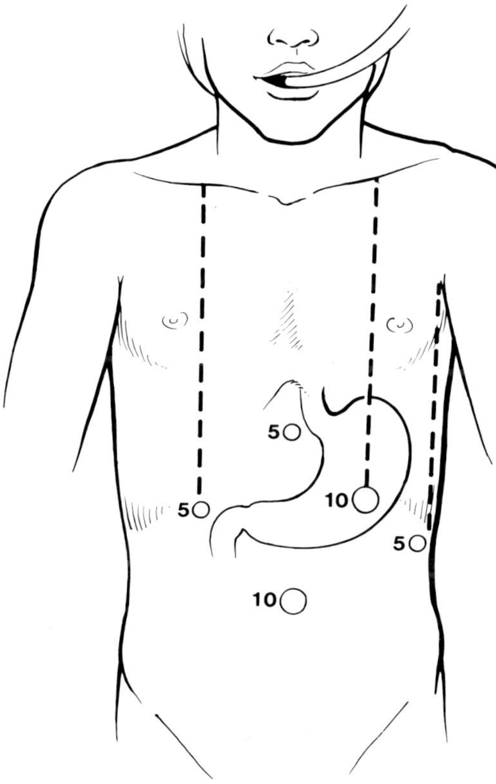

Figure 7–7. A five-port technique is employed for laparoscopic fundoplication.

Although some patients have some early, transient dysphagia, their postoperative course is described as benign and uneventful.

The indications for performing a laparoscopic antireflux procedure for gastroesophageal reflux in children are the same as those for the open approach. The theoretical advantages of the laparoscopic approach are related to the absence of an abdominal incision. In obese patients an incision is more likely to develop a wound complication and it may impair postoperative pulmonary function. In the debilitated child, particularly those with severe mental retardation or those who cannot follow instructions, the incision may impair pulmonary function and predispose the patient to atelectasis or pneumonia.

It has also been suggested by many that the laparoscopic approach minimizes the risks of developing adhesions. As adhesive bowel obstructions, wound complications, and postoperative pulmonary complications constitute the greatest risks of antireflux surgery in children, the laparoscopic approach is likely to minimize these complications. It is too early in our experience to be certain whether or not all these arguments will prove correct.

The technique we use involves insertion of five cannulas into the abdomen: one for viewing with the telescope, one for retracting the liver, two for tissue manipulation, and one for suturing. The operation is identical to the procedure we perform at laparotomy: the liver is retracted away from the esophageal hiatus, the esophagus is mobilized, the diaphragmatic crura are approximated with sutures, the short gastric vessels are divided as necessary, a 360-degree fundoplication wrap is sutured into position, and a gastrostomy is placed if needed.

The details of the procedure are as follows: Under general endotracheal anesthesia, the bladder is catheterized and a nasogastric tube is passed to empty the bladder and the stomach. Using sterile technique, a carbon dioxide pneumoperitoneum is established and maintained, and a 5- or 10-mm 0-degree laparoscope is passed via an umbilical cannula. A 5-mm cannula is placed below the right costal margin in the midclavicular line, and another is placed in the epigastrium. A 10-mm cannula is placed in the left midclavicular line below the costal margin, and a 5-mm cannula is placed in the left anterior axillary line below the costal margin (Figure 7–7). The liver is retracted via the epigastric cannula to expose the esophageal hiatus. The short gastric vessels are divided between surgical clips as necessary (Figure 7–8). The esophagus with as large a bougie in place as it will accommodate is mobilized and retracted using a short segment of umbilical tape. After the posterior margin of the esophagus is clearly identified, the retroesophageal space can be exposed more easily if the bougie is temporarily removed. The exposed diaphragmatic crura are approximated to close the hiatus using interrupted 2-O silk sutures (Fig-

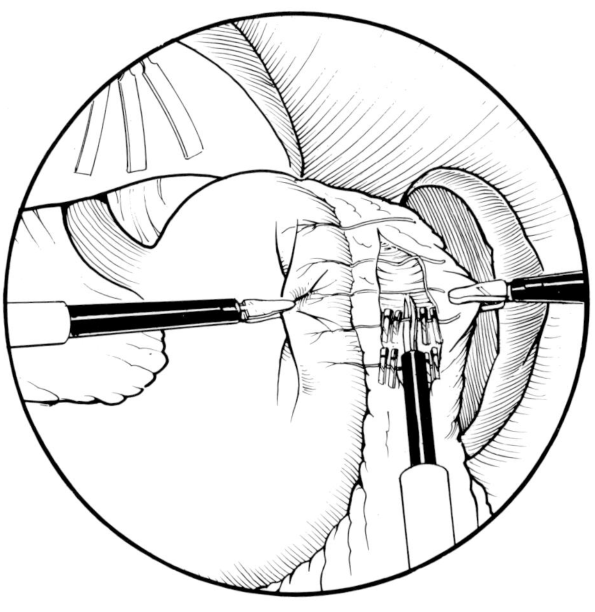

Figure 7–8. The short gastric vessels are divided between surgical clips or ligatures to free the greater curvature of the stomach. Note the fan retractor, which is placed through the 5-mm epigastric trocar, retracting the liver for exposure.

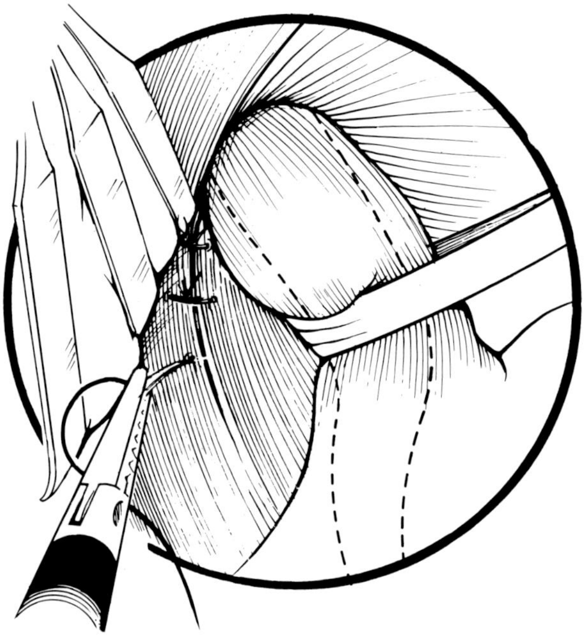

Figure 7–9. The exposed diaphragmatic crura are approximated to close the esophageal hiatus using interrupted 2-O silk sutures. Note the umbilical tape around the intraabdominal esophagus, which is used to retract and manipulate the esophagus.

ure 7–9) after the bougie is replaced. We find extracorporeal knot-tying techniques are the easiest to use to secure the square knots in the standard fashion. The intracorporeal technique can also be used. The stomach is passed behind the esophagus and a 3- to 5-cm wrap is secured using interrupted 2-O silk sutures, as is our practice for the open procedure (Figures 7–10 and 7–11). The esophageal bougie and the cannulas are then removed.

All incisions are closed with subcuticular sutures and dressed with a transparent occlusive dressing. The procedure now takes us between 1 and 2 hours to complete. A TransDerm Scope patch (CIBA Pharmaceuticals, Edison, NJ) is applied behind the patient's ear to minimize nausea and metoclopramide is prescribed for the same reason.

Of our first 12 laparoscopic Nissen fundoplications, 2 were female and the rest were male. Their ages ranged from 3 months to 11 years and their weight from 2.5 to 53 kg. Our first three attempted procedures were converted to open procedures because the proper instruments were not available (one case), a patient was discovered to have portal hypertension and the procedure was aborted (one case), and an opening was made in the posterior esophagus that we preferred to repair using open techniques (one case). Since these initial cases, none of the operations have required conversion to an open laparotomy.

Gastrostomies were placed in all but one patient.

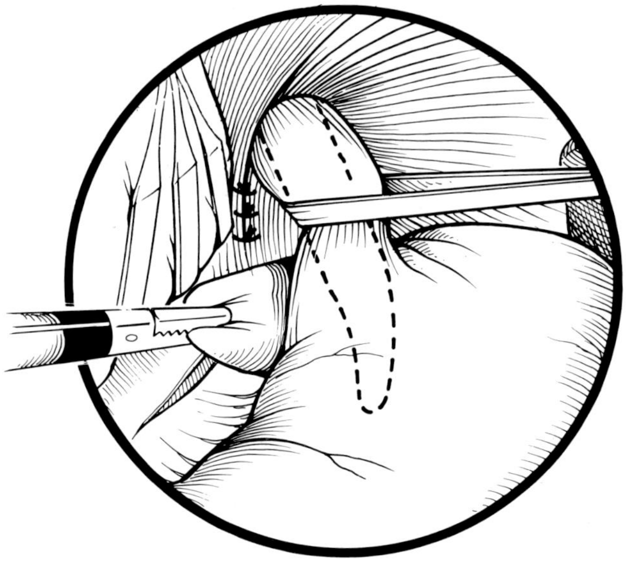

Figure 7–10. The greater curvature of the stomach is passed behind the esophagus. Note the esophageal bougie, which has been inserted into the stomach.

Initially, we used a percutaneous endoscopic technique while observing the stomach with the laparoscope (Figure 7–12). Now we use the laparoscope to determine the optimal position of the gastrostomy; we grasp the correct spot on the anterior gastric wall and externalize the stomach through the subcostal midclavicular line trocar site. The gastrostomy is secured after the fundoplication is completed.

Because of a lack of suitably small instruments,

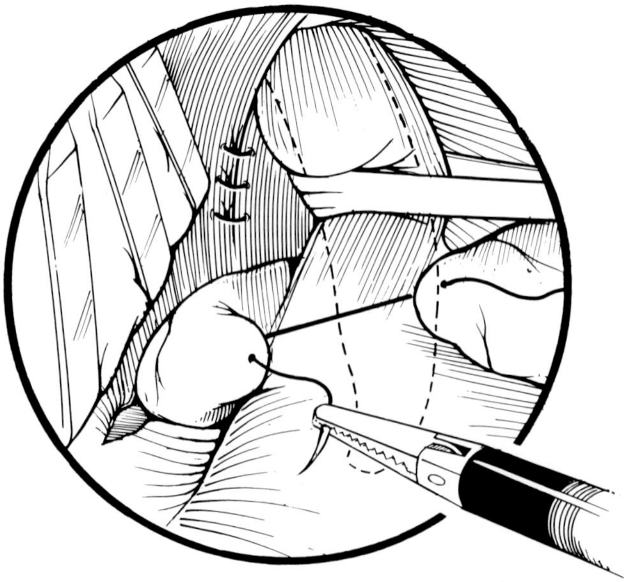

Figure 7–11. A 3- to 5-cm fundoplication is secured using interrupted 2-O silk sutures, as is our practice for open procedures.

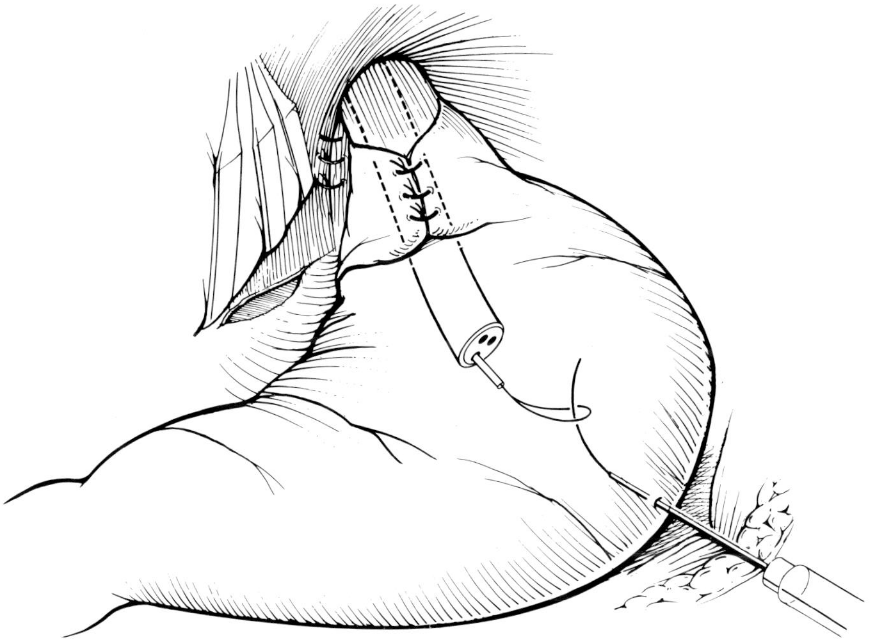

Figure 7–12. Following fundoplication, the esophageal bougie is removed and an endoscope can be inserted for percutaneous endoscopic gastrostomy.

the procedure is more difficult in infants weighing less than 3 kg and we prefer the conventional approach in these patients.

Postoperatively, patients are given liquids on the evening of their surgery and are on full diet (by tube or by mouth) the following day. They are generally discharged between 36 and 48 hours after surgery, at which time they can return to unrestricted activities as before the surgery. Other than those initial cases that require conversion to an open procedure, we have had no complications. Follow-up to 18 months shows all patients to be asymptomatic for gastroesophageal reflux.

When considering reconstructive surgery such as a laparoscopic fundoplication, it is important to remember that the operative technique should vary little from the open operative approach. If the procedure is significantly different then it should be considered a different operation altogether instead of simply the laparoscopic variant of the operation. For example, some surgeons prefer to use hernia staplers to approximate the diaphragmatic crura and to secure the wrap for their laparoscopic fundoplications. This converts the procedure to a different operation because few surgeons would consider using staples for an open fundoplication. The current hernia staplers take shallow bites of tissue and appear more likely to dislodge from tissues that are in constant motion like the diaphragm or the stomach. If the surgeon relies solely on the staplers, then the operation may be less durable. If such a reconstruction fails, the failure may be due to the use of staples to hold the tissue, not the laparoscopic approach.

The major benefits to this laparoscopic approach appear to be shorter hospitalization, earlier return to eating and unrestricted activities, and decreased pulmonary and wound complications. We see no reason why a laparoscopic fundoplication would not equal the long-term results of an open fundoplication except for access. The operation is essentially the same. The postoperative benefits appear to outweigh any potential risks and we believe that laparoscopic fundoplication is the operation of choice in infants weighing more than 3 kg requiring fundoplication for symptomatic gastroesophageal reflux.

REFERENCES

1. Lobe TE, Schropp KP, Gilchrist BF. Inguinal hernias in pediatrics: Initial experience with laparoscopic inguinal exploration of the asymptomatic contralateral side. *Laparoendosc Surg.* 1992;2(3):135.
2. Spaw AT, Ennis BW, Spaw LP. Laparoscopic hernia repair: The anatomic basis. *Laparoendosc Surg.* 1991; 1(5):269.
3. Seid AS, Deutsch H, Jacobson A. Laparoscopic herniorrhaphy. *Surg Laparosc Endosc.* 1992;2(1):59.
4. Gazayerli MM. Anatomical laparoscopic hernia repair of direct or indirect inguinal hernias using the transversalis fascia and iliopubic tract. *Surg Laparosc Endosc.* 1991; 2(1):49.
5. Arregui ME, et al. Laparoscopic mesh repair of inguinal hernia using a preperitoneal approach: A preliminary report. *Surg Laparosc Endosc.* 1992;2(1):53.
6. Nyhus LM. Laparoscopic hernia repair: A point of view. *Arch Surg.* 1992;127(1):137.

7. Ger R, et al. Management of indirect inguinal hernias by laparoscopic closure of the neck of the sac. *Am J Surg.* 1990;159(1):370.
8. Arregui ME, et al. Laparoscopic mesh repair of inguinal hernia using a preperitoneal approach: A preliminary report. *Surg Laparosc Endosc.* 1992;2(1):53.
9. Shulman AG, Lichtenstein IL, Amid PK. The 'plug' repair of 1402 recurrent inguinal hernias. *Arch Surg.* 1990;125(1):265.
10. Dallemagne B, et al. Laparoscopic Nissen fundoplication: Preliminary report. *Surg Laparosc Endosc.* 1991; 1(3):138.
11. Geagea T. Laparoscopic Nissen's fundoplication is feasible (letter). *Can J Surg.* 1991;34(4):313.
12. Cuschieri A, Shimi S, Nathanson LK. Laparoscopic reduction, crural repair, and fundoplication of large hiatal hernia. *Am J Surg.* 1992;163:425.

CHAPTER 8

Laparoscopic Procedures in Neonates and Infants

JÜRGEN WALDSCHMIDT • FELIX SCHIER

Laparoscopy allows inspection of the organs of the abdomen, pelvis, and retroperitoneal space caudal to the kidneys at low risk, even in neonates. Control biopsies can be obtained from the liver, spleen, intestinal wall, mesentery, omentum, gonads, lymph nodes, and tumors. In addition, various surgical procedures can be performed with minimal tissue trauma.

Prior to the procedure, the child must be evaluated as an anesthetic candidate. Laparoscopy cannot be performed in the presence of cardiac or pulmonary decompensation, liver insufficiency, or severe coagulation disturbances. In addition, diaphragmatic hernia must be excluded as a diagnosis; however, peritonitis and functional or mechanical ileus do not represent contraindications to the procedure. Following induction of anesthesia, the stomach, rectum, and bladder must be decompressed. In newborns and infants, laparoscopy should be performed using general anesthesia with muscle relaxation.

TECHNIQUE

We use the Storz pediatric laparoscope with a 0-degree telescope. The pneumoperitoneum is established with carbon dioxide and intraabdominal pressure is maintained at a maximum of 15 mm Hg. All procedures are displayed on video monitors. In this way, everyone in the operating theater can follow and assist appropriately. The patient is prepped and draped to ensure immediate conversion to an open procedure if necessary.

For laparoscopic surgery, the instrument set is supplemented with various forceps, monopolar and bipolar diathermy units, needle holders, clip applicators, and the "Roeder sling" (pretied ligature). The laser is advantageous in neonates and small children. We use the neodymium:YAG (Nd:YAG) laser and a "bare fiber" with a diameter of 0.4 mm. Usually, 10 to 25 watts (W) suffices with an impulse length of 0.5 second and intervals of 0.3 second (0.5 second/0.3 second). Resections are performed in the contact mode and bleeding is controlled in the noncontact mode. The interstitial mode, which is used rarely in laparoscopy, requires energies of 4 to 6 W in continuous waves. The "bare fiber" is introduced through a regular cannula and air leaks around the fiber can be sealed with bone wax.

In older children, the technique is essentially the same as in adults; however, a number of specific differences need to be considered in newborns and small children. Instruments are smaller and telescopes narrower; therefore less light is available. Sufficient light for video and photographic documentation is only provided with short telescopes and thick light cables.

The thin fatty layer of the abdominal wall in infants and children is a disadvantage, as the cannulas are seldom airtight and are difficult to seal. Therefore, we secure the cannula to the abdominal wall with a suture to prevent loss of pneumoperitoneum.

The insertion sites for the Veress needle, telescope, and ports must be individualized. The small abdominal cavity of newborns and infants necessitates short working distances. Puncture of the quadrant diagonal and contralateral to the organ involved is preferable (right upper abdominal quadrant for access to left pelvis and vice versa). Periumbilical access is discouraged because of the wide umbilical ring in newborns, the frequent remnants of the umbilical cord, and the fragility and vulnerability of umbilical vessels. In addition, the apex of the bladder may extend near the umbilicus. Therefore, it is best to select "Munro's point" for the first puncture (Figure 8–1). In newborns, the greater omentum can be very troublesome as it contains little fat. Also, it floats within the abdominal

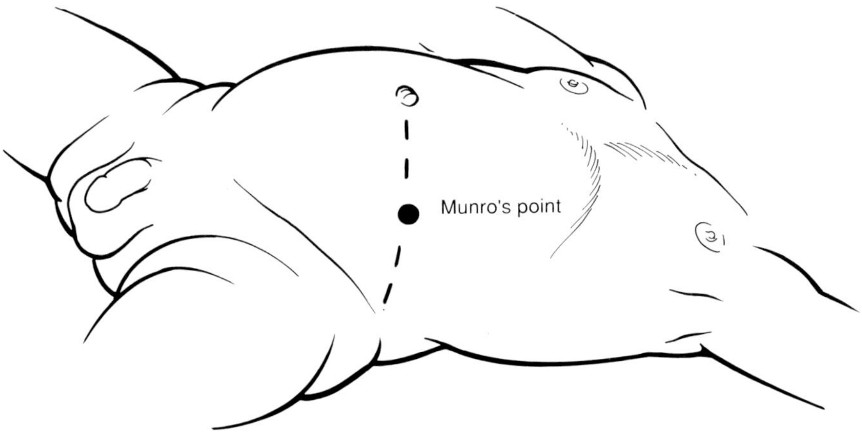

Figure 8–1. Munro's point is often selected for insertion of the first cannula in newborns and infants. This site is at the lateral edge of the rectus abdominis muscle, between the umbilicus and the anterior superior iliac spine.

cavity and frequently covers the telescope and cannulas. A useful maneuver is to retract the omentum with a cannula. One other problem may be difficulty in removing tissue through ports measuring only 5 mm in diameter. Therefore, it may be necessary to reduce the tissue to smaller pieces.

INDICATIONS

Specific indications for laparoscopy in newborns and infants include evaluation for an abdominal testis, management of embryonic remnants of the omphaloenteric duct and vitelline vessels, Meckel's diverticulectomy, and evaluation of the internal genitalia in females.[1–6] This latter indication encompasses evaluation of children for intersex anomalies, management of ovarian cysts, management of complications of the cyst, and drainage of abscesses.[7] Laparoscopy for abdominal testes is discussed in Chapter 5 and intersex anomalies in Chapter 10. Other specific indications in newborns include adhesiolysis, organopexy, laparoscopic cholecystocholangiography, and percutaneous endoscopic gastrostomy.[8–10] Pyloromyotomy has been

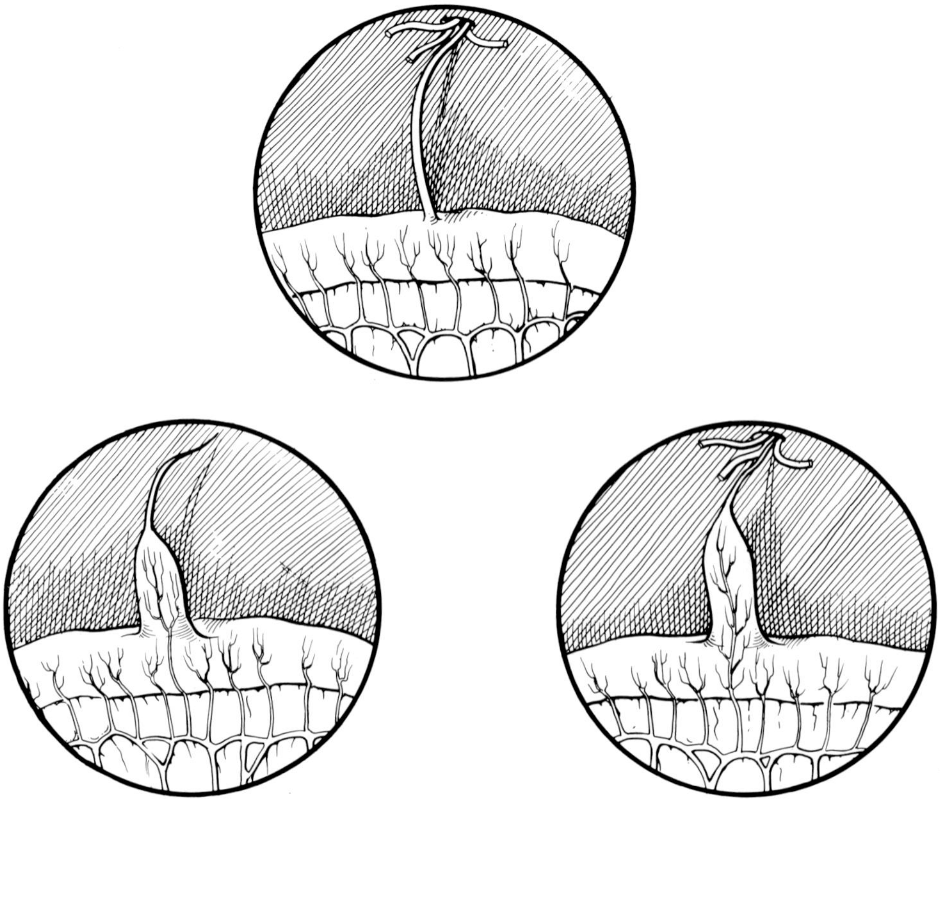

Figure 8–2. Embryonic remnants of the vitelline duct and vessels may cause symptoms such as persistent umbilical drainage, if communication to the ileum is present, or small bowel obstruction around persistent embryonic ligaments.

reported laparoscopically,[11] but we do not have personal experience with this procedure.

Embryonic Remnants

Intraabdominal embryonic remnants of the vitelline duct and vessels present in various ways (Figure 8–2). Remnants of the vitelline duct include a persistent omphaloenteric duct, Meckel's diverticulum, Roser cyst and umbilical sinus, allantoic duct, and tissue heterotopia in the small bowel. Remnants of the vitelline artery include a mesoenteric ligament, omphaloenteric ligament, filum terminale, and ligamentum terminale.

For evaluation of these remnants, the telescope is inserted at Munro's point. Associated anomalies at the cecum and appendix make simultaneous appendectomy appear sensible and indicated. Also, abnormal ligaments originating from the ileum and colon and concomitant malformations of the vitelline vein may be transected (Figure 8–3). Because of the abundance of blood vessels, ligatures or laser coagulation is indicated. A preduodenal portal vein can be ignored as it usually does not cause duodenal obstruction.

Indications for laparoscopy for suspected remnants of the vitelline duct or vessels include an umbilical fistula, scintigraphic documentation of a Meckel's diverticulum, recurrent abdominal pain, recurring small bowel obstruction, and intestinal bleeding.

Meckel's Diverticulum

Resection of a Meckel's diverticulum or an omphaloenteric duct is technically similar to appendectomy. In newborns, a 5-mm telescope and cannula and a 2-mm working cannula are inserted as is a Roeder sling. In addition, the laser is also used. The diverticular artery and vein are transected together using diathermy or laser. The tip of the diverticulum is grasped and elevated with a forceps. The diverticulum is stretched and ligated along its base with a Roeder sling. Mucosa at the stump is destroyed with the laser, which results in a small pinpoint scar (Figure 8–4). In older children a Meckel's diverticulum can be resected using the endostapler. Exteriorization of the diverticulum as described by Attwood et al for adults is not necessary in children.[12] In addition to a Meckel's diverticulum, other associated remnants may be resected as well and may be followed by appendectomy. Chronic inflammatory adhesions can be dissected cautiously using the Nd:YAG laser.

Female Internal Genitalia

All parts of the internal genitalia are easily accessible for laparoscopic inspection. As a result of the magnification effect, very small details can be appreciated to an extent not possible to the naked eye.

Diagnostic and surgical laparoscopy is indicated primarily in older girls for genital malformations, endometriosis, primary amenorrhea, polycystic ovary in the Stein–Leventhal syndrome, chronic pelvic pain, adhesiolysis, Fitz–Hugh–Curtis syndrome, and drainage of abscesses. In newborns and infants, laparoscopy can be used for intersex anomalies, persistent ovarian cysts, adnexal torsion, and complications from the cysts and from peritonitis.

The newborn is placed in Trendelenburg position. The 5-mm telescope and cannula and 2-mm working cannula are inserted in the diagonal quadrant. In older girls, the usual umbilical approach may be chosen for the telescope. The laser is used for precise dissection technique as well as vascular control and allows good

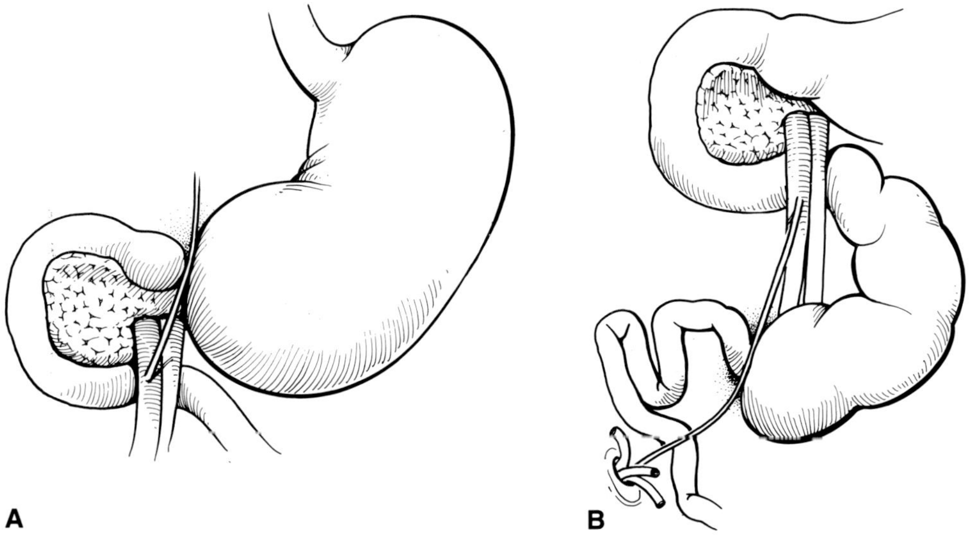

Figure 8–3. Persistent embryonic remnants of the vitelline vein may cause either gastric **(A)** or intestinal **(B)** obstruction. These remnants can be ligated and divided laparoscopically.

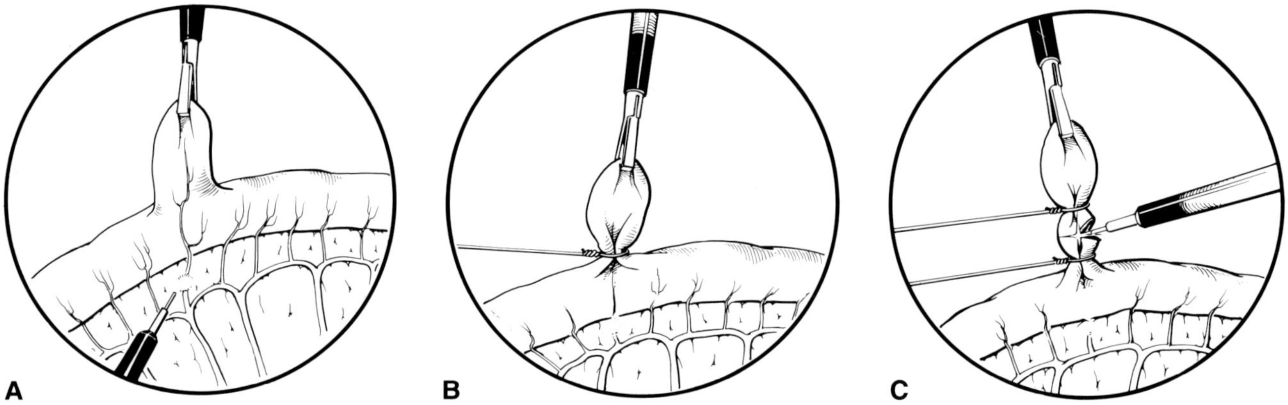

Figure 8–4. Resection of a Meckel's diverticulum is technically similar to appendectomy. **A.** The diverticular artery and vein are transsected using cautery or laser. **B.** The diverticulum is stretched and ligated with a Roeder sling. **C.** Mucosa at the stump is destroyed with the laser, resulting in a small pinpoint scar.

visualization. We prefer the Nd:YAG laser, the "bare fiber" at 15 W, and intervals of 0.2 to 0.3 second.

Gonadectomy

Puncture of the diagonal quadrant for unilateral gonadectomy or midline for bilateral gonadectomy is followed by dissection of the ligamentum suspensorium ovarii, including the ovarian propria vessels. This is best achieved with the laser. The gonad is elevated from the mesosalpinx with a forceps and resected along the mesovarium with the laser. Finally, the gonad can be removed through the working port. With this technique, the fallopian tube is preserved (Figure 8–5).

Ovarian Cysts

Functional cysts of newborns contain a serous liquid. They may be multilocular and, in many cases, are diagnosed prenatally by ultrasound. Most cysts regress spontaneously. Clinical and sonographic examinations at 10- to 14-day intervals are necessary for continued evaluation of spontaneous regression of the cyst. Laparoscopy should be performed only with significant increase in size or with the onset of clinical symptoms such as irritability, vomiting, and pain (Figure 8–6). Sonography will demonstrate internal echoes together with an edematous cyst wall and intraperitoneal fluid collection.

Large functional cysts in newborns with a diameter greater than 3 cm often do not regress spontaneously or regression is so slow that complications develop. Bleeding or rupture may occur, but these complications are not as severe as torsion of an appendage and involvement with a sister organ, the omentum, or intestine. Secondary agonadism and ileus may result.

Management of the cysts will depend on the findings at laparoscopy. For smaller cysts, puncture and decompression of the cyst will be sufficient. A sample is drawn for cytology and for estradiol and progesterone determinations. Following puncture and cyst reduction, it is best to destroy the epithelial lining with a laser (7 W continuous wave for 8 to 10 seconds).

For larger multiloculated cysts, puncture alone will often be insufficient. The cyst may encompass the entire ovary, with the stroma becoming part of the

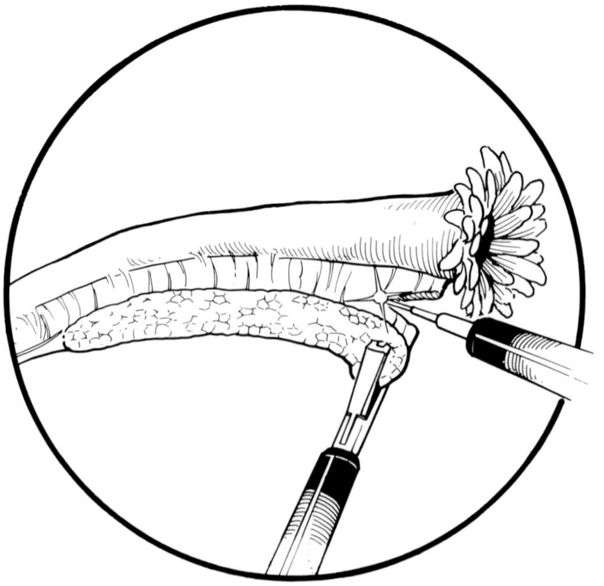

Figure 8–5. For gonadectomy, the gonad is elevated from the mesosalpinx with a grasping forceps and resected along the mesovarium using the laser. The fallopian tube is preserved with this technique.

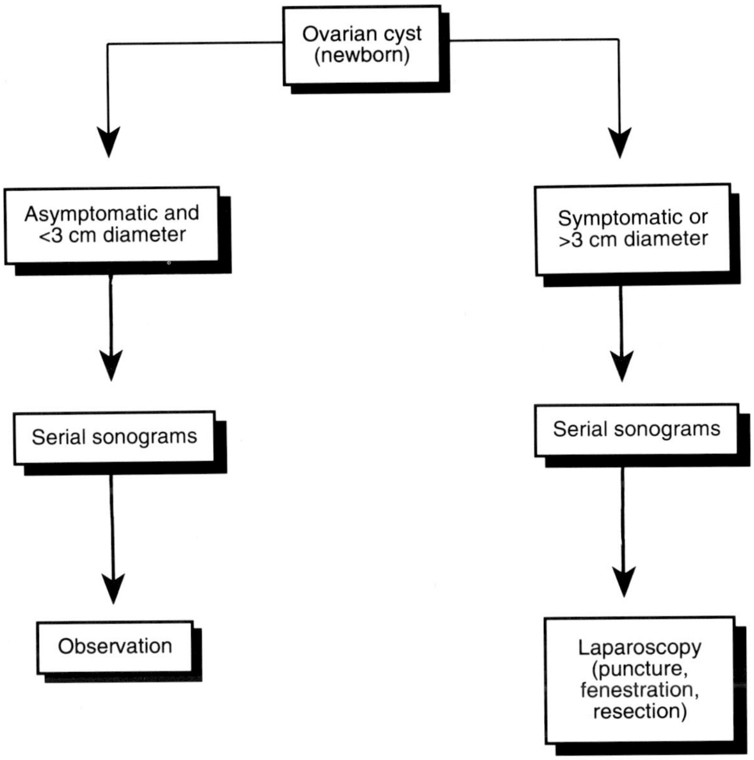

Figure 8–6. This algorithm describes management for ovarian cysts in the newborn. Laparoscopy should be performed only with significant increase in size of the cyst or with the onset of clinical symptoms. Management of the cyst will depend on the endoscopic findings.

cyst capsule. Cystectomy would mean removal of all the normal ovarian tissue. Therefore, fenestration of the cyst with vaporization of the inner surface with the laser (20 W, 0.5/0.3-second intervals) is the best management (Figures 8–7A and 8–7B). Thereafter, the cyst will subsequently shrink and form a new gonad. Thus, the whole organ can be preserved along with the ovarian stroma within the cyst wall.

Should necrosis of the cyst occur following torsion or adhesion develop with another intraabdominal

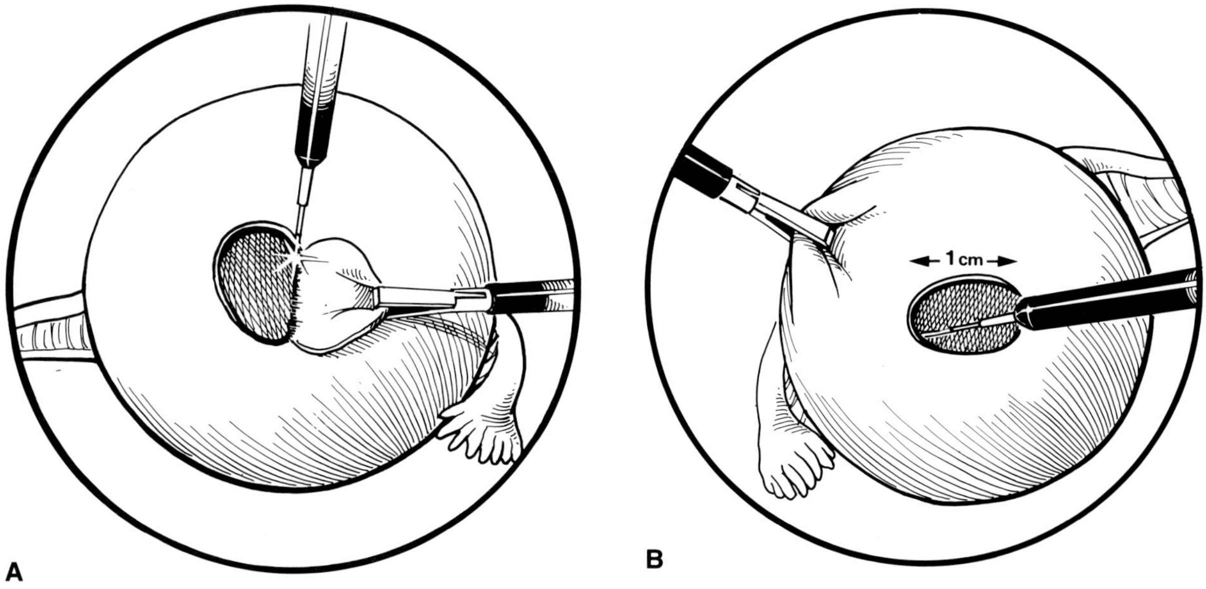

Figure 8–7. **A.** With large, multiloculated cysts, puncture alone will often be insufficient. Therefore, fenestration of the cyst should be employed. **B.** Following fenestration, the inner surface is vaporized with the laser, inducing shrinkage of the cyst and formation of a new gonad. Ovarian cystectomy would mean removal of all normal ovarian tissue that is encapsulated within the cyst.

organ, the cyst should be aspirated and the lining removed. Bleeding is controlled by ligating the torqued base of the cyst with a Roeder sling. The procedure is identical for cysts with solid segments in the capsule as these require histologic examination (Figure 8–8).

Spontaneous adnexal torsion is rare but may involve the tube or ovary alone or in combination. Symptoms of torsion include irritability, abdominal pain, and vomiting. Sonography reveals an enlarged and edematous organ with venous congestion. Detorsion is possible at emergency laparoscopy. In newborns the torqued structures recover quickly following reduction; however, a necrotic adnexa must be excised and this is analogous to cyst resection. After the stalk is ligated with a Roeder sling, the torqued organ is removed with the laser (Figure 8–9).

A final problem with internal genitalia in female infants is inflammatory adnexal pseudotumors. Infected cysts originating either from Gartner's duct or the wolffian duct (paraovarian cysts) or confluent processes are extraperitoneally drained by laparoscopy. It may also be necessary to perform adhesiolysis with neighboring bowel loops or the greater omentum. Laparoscopy may be repeated as required.

Lysis of Adhesions

Adhesions rarely cause symptoms in newborns and older children. When encountered, they are either congenital or acquired. Congenital adhesions may be found in the ileocecal region as a pathologic ileoparietale ligament (Figure 8–10). This has also been called the mesoileum ventrale. In addition, congenital adhesions may be found along the colon as a ligamentum coloparietal, Jackson's membrane, or Ladd's band. In addition, they may be found in the right upper abdomen as a persisting ligamentum cystoduodenale, cystocolicum, or hepatoduodenale dextrum.

In most cases, coloparietale ligaments and adhesions in the right upper abdomen do not cause clinical problems. They may regress spontaneously in early childhood. Ladd's bands, however, can be massive enough to obstruct the duodenum. Occasionally, the gallbladder neck or Hartmann's pouch can be so distorted from persisting ligaments that cholestasis results from compression of the common duct or the

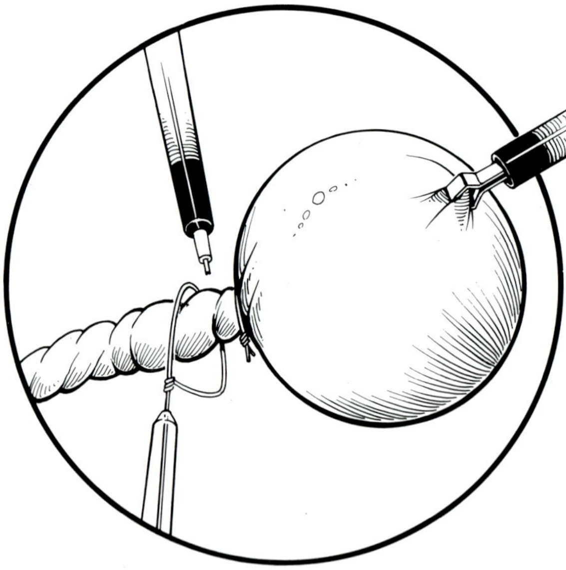

Figure 8–8. For cysts with solid components that require histologic examination or for a necrotic adnexa following torsion, excision is indicated. A Roeder sling is placed around the base of the cyst and the stalk divided with the laser.

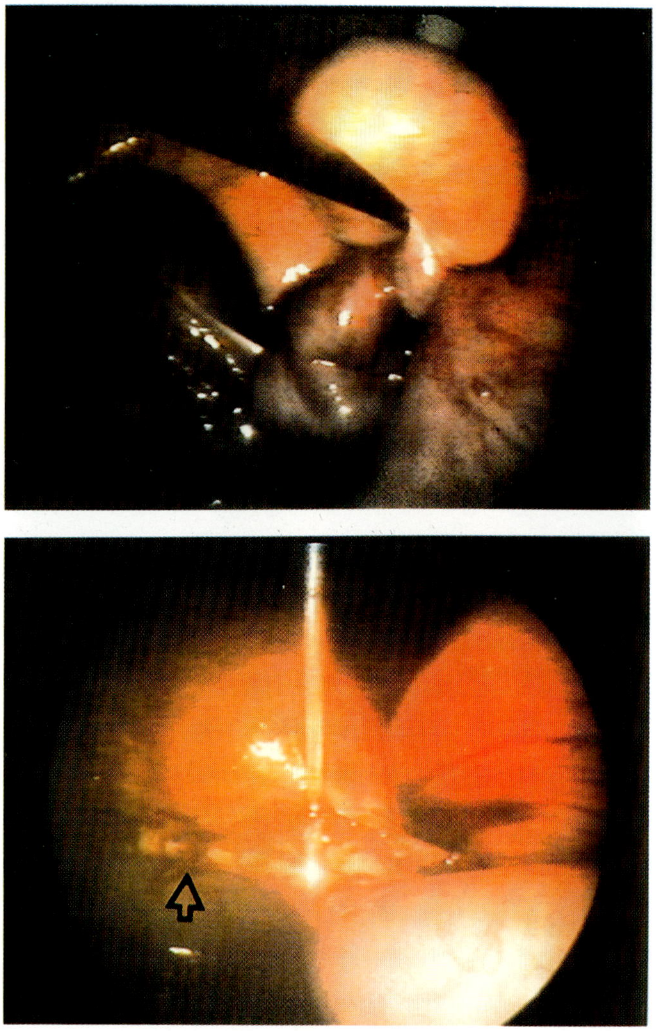

Figure 8–9. Spontaneous torsion of the right adnexa has occurred in this newborn as a result of a large ovarian cyst (*top*). Following reduction, the adnexa remained ischemic and resection was indicated. Following application of a Roeder sling (*arrow*) the stalk is divided with the laser (*bottom*).

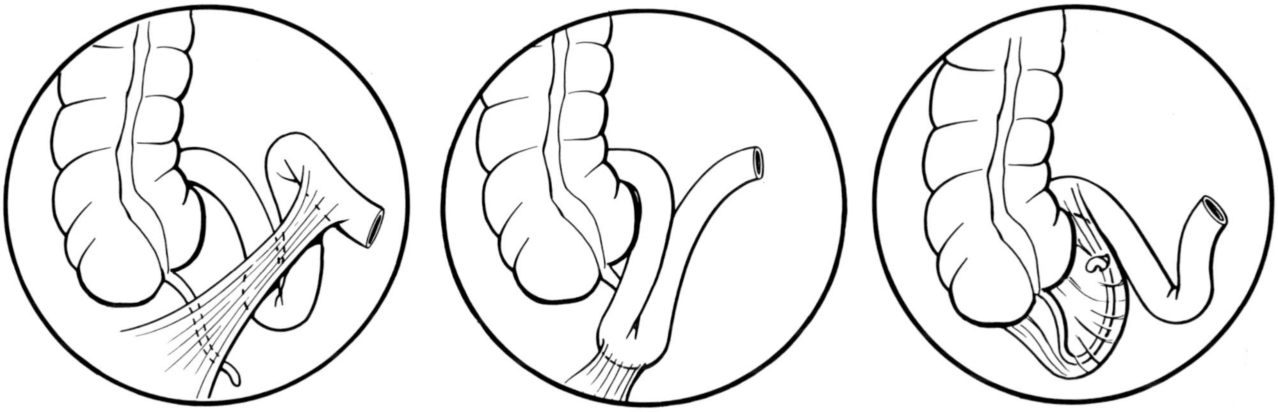

Figure 8–10. Congenital adhesions are occasionally found in the ileocecal region as pathologic ileoparietale bands. Lysis of symptomatic adhesions can be performed laparoscopically.

hepatic bifurcation, mimicking Mirizzi syndrome (Figure 8–11).

Acquired adhesions occur in early childhood and are most frequently encountered at the ileum and in the omentum and, in girls, in the adnexal region (Figure 8–12). The most frequent causes are small bowel perforation, hematogenous peritonitis, migration peritonitis, adnexitis, necrotizing enterocolitis, and previous surgery. Omental adhesions may be found following peritonitis, herniotomy, and other surgery.

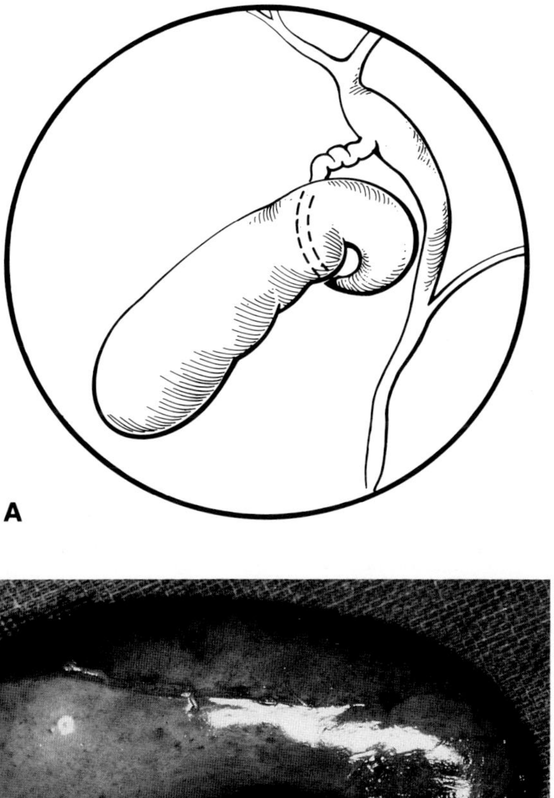

A

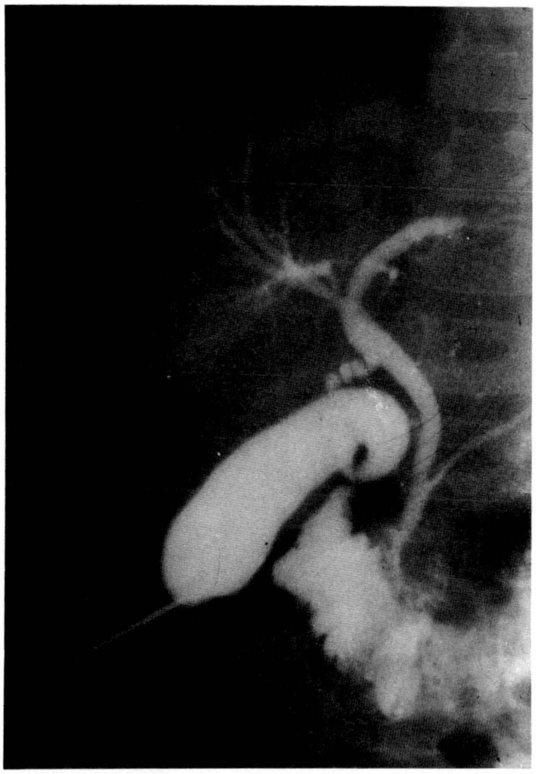

B

C

Figure 8–11. **A.** In this newborn, the gallbladder infundibulum was distorted by persisting congenital ligaments, resulting in cholestasis. **B.** A cholangiogram showed distortion of the infundibulum with flow into the duodenum. **C.** The gallbladder was removed because of the symptomatic cholestasis.

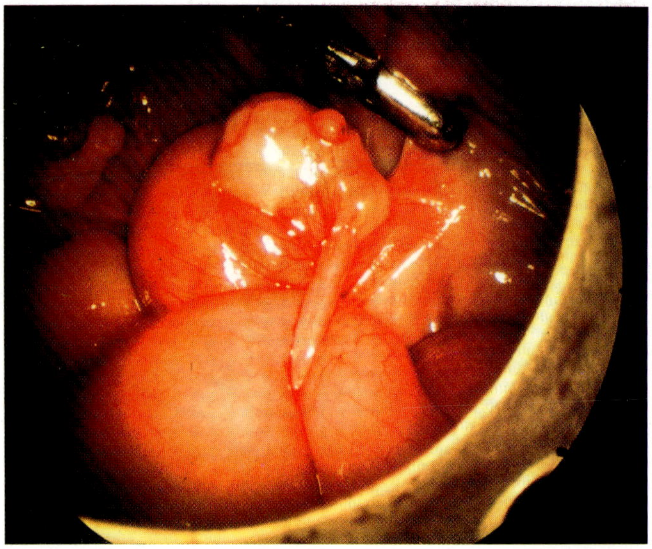

Figure 8–12. This inflammatory adhesion developed between the mesentery and a Meckel's diverticulum, causing distal small bowel obstruction.

The adhesions can be transected by laser, cautery, or laparoscopic scissors (Figure 8–13). Bleeding stumps are controlled with a clip or ligature. Continuous bleeding may produce new adhesions, and the technique that best preserves tissue is again the laser. Bleeding and fibrinous exudate are reduced to a minimum, and the dissected areas shrink. Rapid reperitonealization may prevent formation of new adhesions.

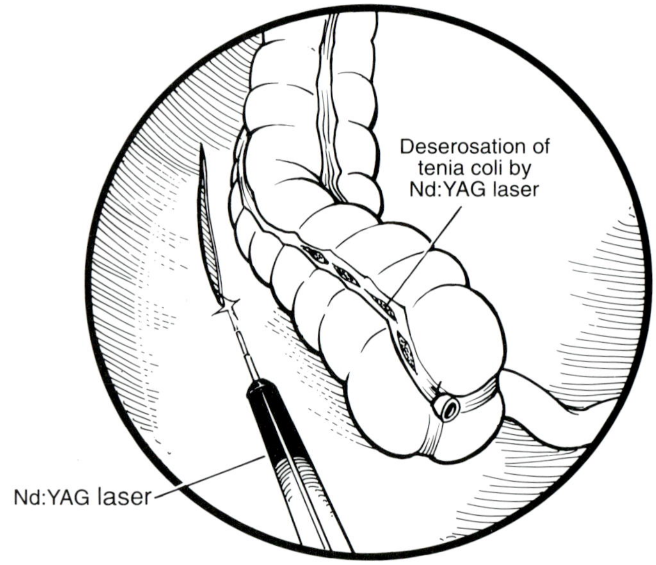

Figure 8–14. For colopexy, an extended deserosalized area is created along the taenia coli and peritoneum and transverse fascia. Fibrin glue is used for organopexy.

Organopexy

Combined with the laser and human fibrin glue, laparoscopic pexis represents an efficient and safe method for cecopexy for the mobile cecum and colopexy for mesoileocolicum commune. Other indications include right-sided pexis of the transverse colon in coloptosis type B (long gastrocolic ligament without gastropto-

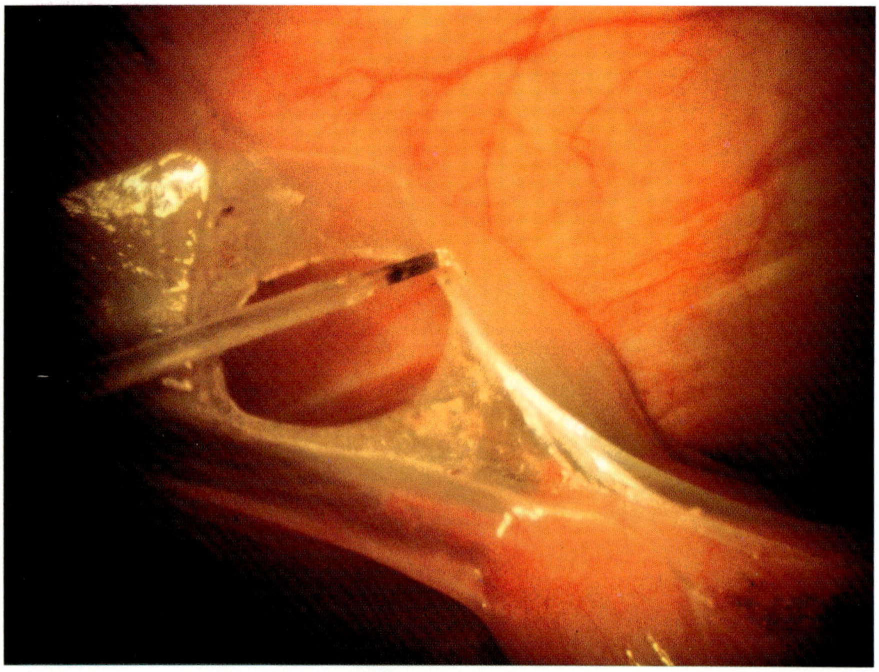

Figure 8–13. Acquired adhesions may occur as a result of peritonitis or previous surgery. In this infant, small bowel obstruction developed from acquired adhesions following medical management for necrotizing enterocolitis. The adhesions are being divided with the Nd:YAG laser.

sis) and hepatopexy in Chilaiditi syndrome (type B, anterior interposition). A final indication is splenopexy for the wandering spleen.

The technique of organopexy includes creation of an extended deserosalized area between the parietal peritoneum and the organ involved, which is best achieved with the laser (15 W, 0.5/0.3-second intervals) (Figure 8–14). In addition, this area should be covered with fibrin glue. The intraabdominal pressure is then reduced and the organ approximated to the abdominal wall with forceps. In colopexy, the deserosalization of the parietal peritoneum alone will not suffice. The transverse fascia must be exposed as well. Otherwise, the peritoneum will lift like a mesentery and the pathologic mobility will recur with torsions, kinking, and strangulation.

Cysts

The most frequent intraabdominal cysts in newborns are ovarian cysts. They can have long stalks and can be encountered in all parts of the abdomen. Moreover, they may be interposed between other organs such as between the liver and transverse colon. In such cases, the stalk may be long and too thin to be noticed on ultrasound. Also, the boundaries to the neighboring organs may not be well defined and differentiation from other cysts may not be possible.

Included in the differential diagnosis of cystic abdominal masses are mesenteric, omental, duplication, choledochal, liver, and pancreatic cysts. The laparoscopic technique for excising these cysts is identical to the technique used for management of ovarian cysts.

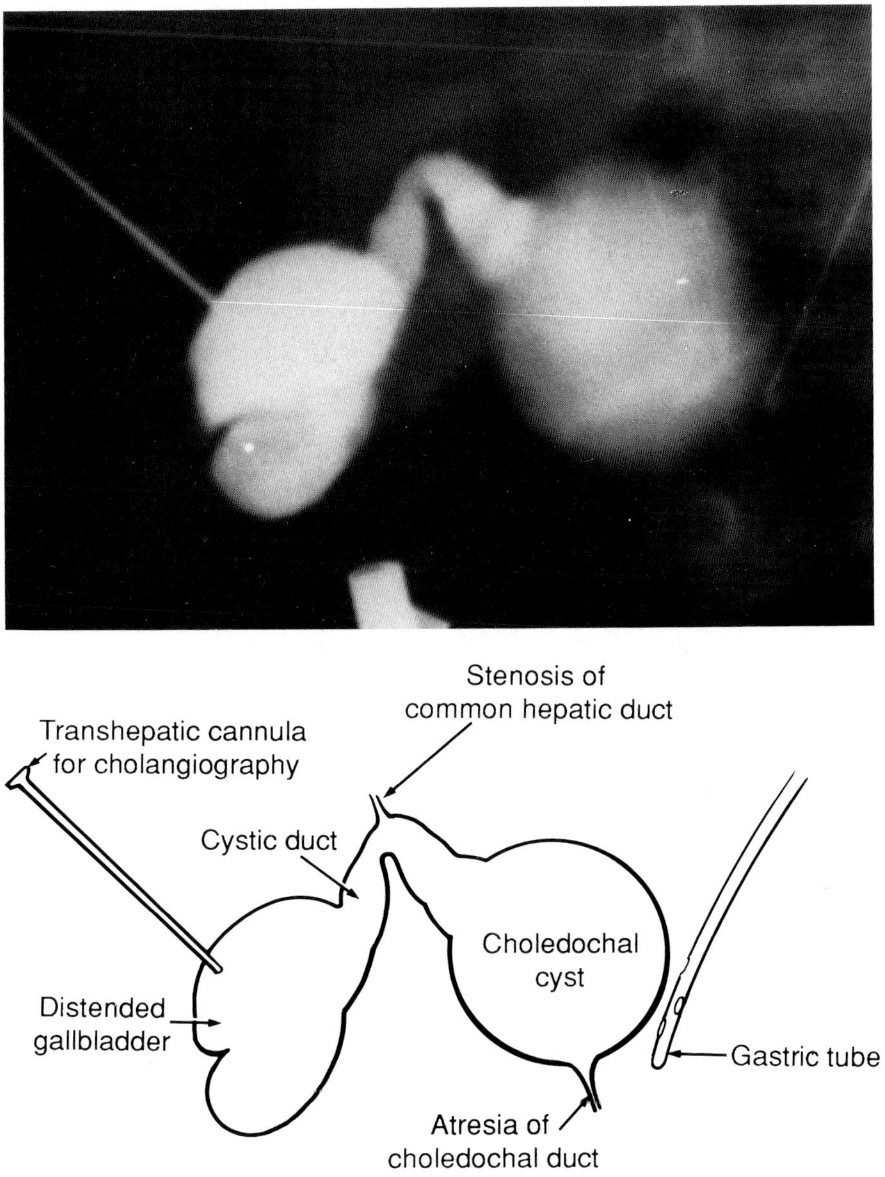

Figure 8–15. A 5-week-old infant presented with obstructive jaundice. Laparoscopy and cholecystocholangiography were performed through a distended gallbladder. The needle for cholangiography was placed transhepatically. A choledochal cyst was identified. Laparotomy and choledochocystectomy were then performed.

Cysts of the mesentery, omentum, or liver can be fenestrated or extirpated with the laser. For choledochal cysts, spherical duplications, pancreatic cysts, and lymphangioma, laparoscopy remains diagnostic and should usually be followed by laparotomy (Figure 8–15); however, for spherical duplications, laparoscopic fenestration and mucosectomy could be considered.

REFERENCES

1. Frangenheim H. Indikationen und Technik der Laparoskopie in der Chirurgie. *Chir Praxis.* 1979;25:257.
2. Gans SL, Berci G. Advances in endoscopy of infants and children. *J Pediatr Surg.* 1971;6:199.
3. Karamehmedovic O, Dangel P, Hirsig J, et al. Laparoscopy in childhood. *J Pediatr Surg.* 1977;12:76.
4. Leape LL, Ramenofsky ML. Laparoscopy in infants and children. *J Pediatr Surg.* 1977;12:929.
5. Scott ES. Laparoscopy as an aid in the diagnosis and management of the impalpable testis. *J Pediatr Surg.* 1982;17:14.
6. Waldschmidt J, Schier F. Surgical correction of abdominal testes after Fowler–Stephens using neodymium YAG laser for preliminary vessel dissection. *Eur J Pediatr Surg.* 1990;1:54.
7. Shalev E, Mann S, Romano S, et al. Laparoscopic detorsion of adnexa in childhood: A case report. *J Pediatr Surg.* 1991;26:1193.
8. Murphy C, Rosemurgy AS, Albrink MH, et al. A simple technique for laparoscopic gastrostomy. *Surg Gynecol Obstet.* 1992;174:424.
9. Neufang T, Köhler H, Bukhari W, et al. Die perkutane laparoskopische gastrotomie (PLG). *Min Invas Chir.* 1992;1:31.
10. Waldschmidt J, El Dessouky M, Charissis G, et al. Validity of endoscopy in the diagnostics of biliary atresia. *Z Kinderchir.* 1988;43(suppl I):57.
11. Alain JL, Grousseau D, Terrier G. Extramucosal pylorotomy by laparoscopy. *J Pediatr Surg.* 1991;26:1191.
12. Attwood SEA, McGrath J, Hill ADK, et al. Laparoscopic approach to Meckel's diverticulectomy. *Br J Surg.* 1992;79:211.

CHAPTER 9

Laparoscopic Gastrostomy

KEITH E. GEORGESON

Surgical techniques to enhance nutrition have been successfully employed for over 100 years.[1–6] The first feeding gastrostomy associated with survival of the patient is attributed to Jones in 1875.[1,5,6] Verneuil (1876), Trendelenburg (1878), and Staton (1880) reported successful placement of feeding gastrostomies in children with esophageal lye strictures.[2–4,6] Few surgical procedures have stimulated more creativity in surgeons than the formation of a gastrostomy. Feeding gastrostomies now rank among the most common procedures performed in children. At the Children's Hospital of Alabama in 1992, gastrostomies were the fourth most common procedure performed by pediatric surgeons.

Indications for placement of a feeding gastrostomy in infants and children continue to expand, with the more common indications listed in Table 9–1. Cerebral palsy is currently the most common indication for a feeding gastrostomy in children. The number of neurologically impaired children is increasing as a result of the increased survival of severely affected infants in neonatal and pediatric intensive care units. Neurologic impairment is associated with prematurity, hypoxic brain injury, birth defects, and traumatic brain injuries. The most common presenting symptoms in these unfortunate children include severe swallowing difficulties and frequent vomiting, resulting in failure to thrive; primary and secondary aspiration, leading to chronic bronchitis and pneumonia; and difficulty with oral feeding procedures, leading to overwhelming time demands on the caretakers.

Neurologically normal infants and children considered for feeding gastrostomy include medically fragile children with failure to thrive and children with chronic lung or heart disease with inadequate weight gain. Children with swallowing disorders, including esophageal lye strictures, muscular dystrophy, esophageal atresia, and cleft palate, are sometimes considered for gastrostomy tube placement if long-term feeding difficulties are anticipated. Children with short-gut syndrome usually need a feeding gastrostomy for progressive advancement of enteral feedings.

The preoperative assessment of any child considered for a feeding gastrostomy should include careful evaluation for gastroesophageal (GE) reflux. The most frequently used studies for evaluating patients for GE reflux are listed in Table 9–2.[7] The studies listed in Table 9–3 are used selectively for evaluation of GE reflux when the initial study is not conclusive. Patients who have demonstrated significant GE reflux should be considered for fundoplication in addition to gastrostomy.

The surgeon should also assess gastric emptying in patients under consideration for a gastrostomy.[8] Radionuclide gastric emptying is commonly employed for this purpose. Children with very slow gastric emptying will tolerate intragastric feedings poorly. A gastric outlet procedure should be performed in conjunction with feeding gastrostomy if gastric emptying is delayed.

TREATMENT OPTIONS

Medical therapy should always be attempted before surgical intervention is considered in children with failure to thrive. Calorie and protein supplementation of oral intake may improve the nutritional status in some of these patients.[9,10] Nasoenteric alimentation is useful in patients with temporary feeding difficulties and is also helpful in optimizing the nutritional status of children with profound failure to thrive prior to operative gastrostomy. Therapy to improve the acceptance of oral feeding by the patient and to increase oral motor skills is sometimes beneficial in these children. Those patients who do not respond to medical therapy or who require nasogastric tube feedings for 3 months or longer should be considered for feeding gastrostomy. Gastrostomy feeding

TABLE 9–1. INDICATIONS FOR GASTROSTOMY

Neurologic impairment
Gastroesophageal reflux
Swallowing disorders
Chronic lung disease
Congenital heart disease
Short-gut syndrome

has been shown to induce weight gain and growth and to improve development in many patients with failure to thrive.[9,11,12]

A gastrostomy may be either temporary or permanent. Temporary gastrostomies lack apposition of the gastric mucosa to the skin and will often close spontaneously if the tube is removed. Operative Stamm gastrostomy and the percutaneous endoscopic gastrostomy (PEG) are the most commonly employed temporary gastrostomies. Permanent gastrostomies use gastric mucosal approximation to the skin. Patency of the gastrostomy is maintained when the tube is removed. The most commonly employed permanent gastrostomy is the Janeway gastrostomy. It has been used less frequently in the last few years because of problems with leakage of gastric contents onto the skin and because of the development and broad usage of gastrostomy buttons to maintain the patency of temporary gastrostomies. The operative Stamm gastrostomy remains the most popular technique in children.[13] It has been largely replaced by the PEG in adults.[6,14,15]

The PEG technique is popular in adults because it can be performed with local anesthesia and sedation. In children, most surgeons use general anesthesia to perform this endoscopic procedure because of the lack of patient cooperation and because of the precarious status of the child's airway; however, both the PEG and Stamm gastrostomies have been shown to induce gastroesophageal reflux.[15–19] The cause for this postgastrostomy reflux seems to be related to shortening of the intraabdominal esophagus and widening of the angle of His.[19–24]

Stringel and Seekri and co-workers have recently demonstrated in separate studies that placement of the gastrostomy tube in the lesser curvature of the stomach diminishes postgastrostomy GE reflux[25,26] (Figure 9–1). Lesser-curvature gastrostomy can be performed by open technique or laparoscopically. Lesser-curvature gastrostomy has not been described using the PEG technique. Attempting to perform a lesser curvature procedure endoscopically would increase the difficulty of the procedure and also the potential for complications such as injury to the liver. Laparoscopic lesser-curvature gastrostomy is an attractive alternative in children to both the operative Stamm procedure and the PEG technique. Further clinical studies are needed to determine conclusively whether lesser-curvature gastrostomy decreases the incidence of postgastrostomy GE reflux when compared with the Stamm gastrostomy and PEG.

TABLE 9–2. THREE COMMONLY USED INITIAL TESTS TO EVALUATE FOR GASTROESOPHAGEAL REFLUX

Upper gastrointestinal series
24-hour esophageal pH monitoring
Radionuclide study for reflux and gastric emptying

TABLE 9–3. OTHER MEASURES TO EVALUATE FOR GASTROESOPHAGEAL REFLUX

Esophagoscopy with biopsy
Bronchoscopy with washings for lipid-laden macrophages
Esophageal manometry
Computerized gammagraphy

A discussion of feeding gastrostomy would not be complete without considering the appropriateness of prophylactic fundoplication in all children undergoing gastrostomy. There is a high incidence of gastroesophageal reflux in the population of patients with failure to thrive who are being considered for a feeding gastrostomy.[16,20,27] Moreover, as mentioned previously, gastrostomy induces GE reflux. Bolus feedings into the stomach may also make the patient more susceptible to reflux.[21] The literature is replete with articles describing both sides of the controversy regarding prophylactic fundoplication.[23,28–30]

The author's current approach is to carefully evaluate all candidates for gastrostomy for GE reflux using the commonly employed radiographic studies. Moreover, selective other studies are also employed when necessary (see Table 9–3). In children with significant reflux, or in those who are unable to protect their airway, feeding gastrostomy and fundoplication are performed laparoscopically. If the children do not demonstrate reflux and have effective laryngeal reflexes, a laparoscopic lesser-curvature gastrostomy is performed without prophylactic fundoplication. Children with delayed gastric emptying are treated with an appropriate gastric outlet drainage procedure.

LAPAROSCOPIC GASTROSTOMY

Following creation of the pneumoperitoneum, three 5-mm ports are placed (Figure 9–2). The cannula on the right side should be located well below the liver margin and away from the epigastric vessels. The cannula on the left side is placed in a mirror image to the right-sided port. The liver is retracted using grasping forceps placed through the right port. A second for-

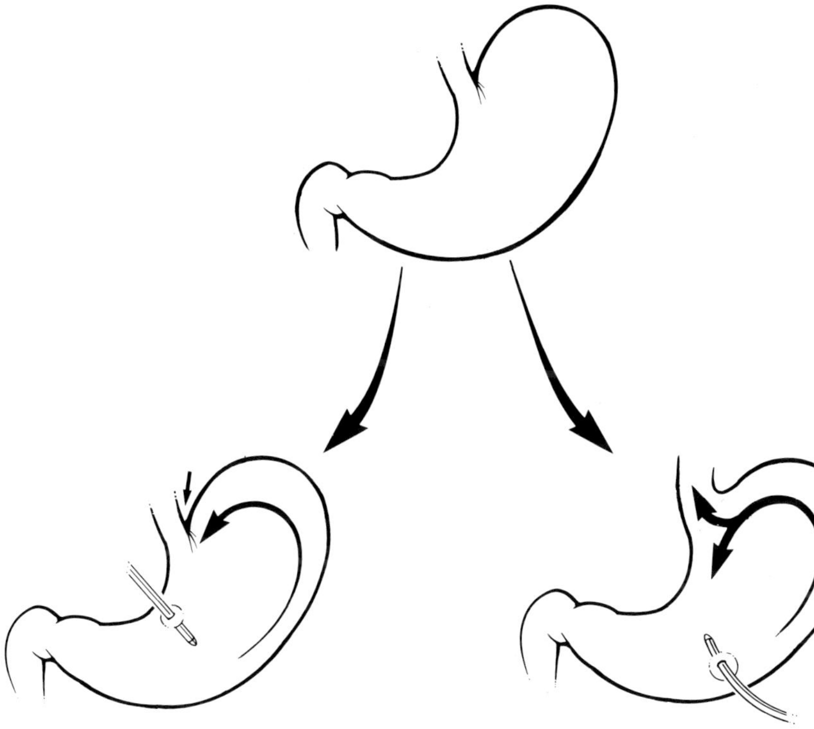

Figure 9–1. The angle of His is important in preventing gastroesophageal reflux. With greater-curvature gastrostomy, the angle may be increased, thereby promoting reflux. With lesser-curvature gastrostomy, however, the intraabdominal esophagus may be lengthened and the angle of His decreased, which may protect against reflux.

ceps is passed through the left cannula and the stomach is grasped near the lesser curvature above the incisura. The stomach should be grasped at a point that will cause a snug but not tight pull on the lesser curvature when the gastrostomy is completed.

When deciding where to exteriorize the gastrostomy tube, allowance should be made for the anterior displacement of the abdominal wall by the pneumoperitoneum. The pneumoperitoneum can be released momentarily to allow a more accurate assess-

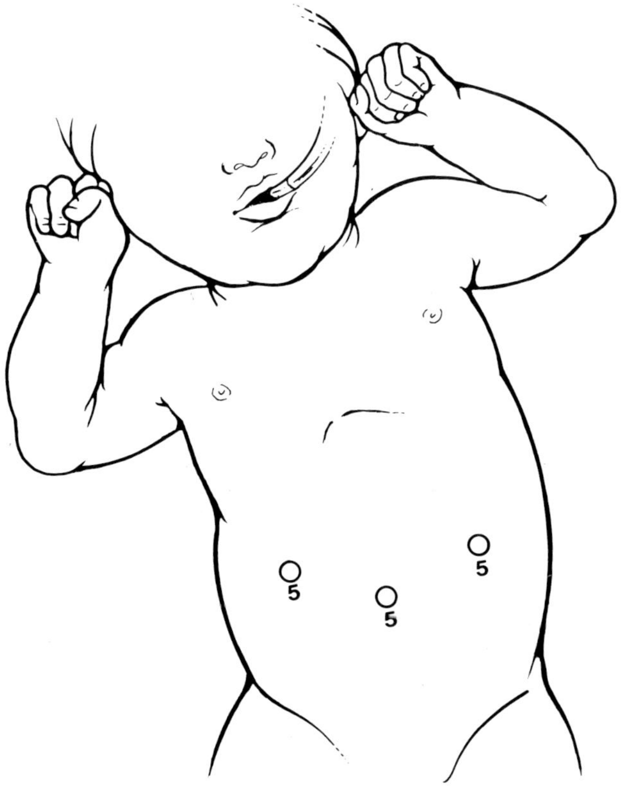

Figure 9–2. Three 5-mm cannulas are placed for laparoscopic gastrostomy.

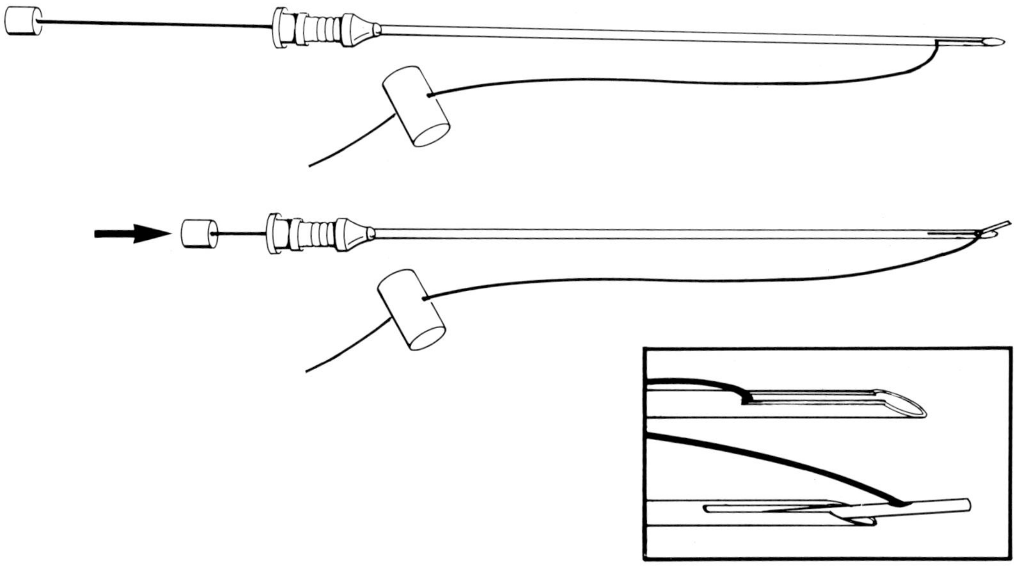

Figure 9–3. T-fasteners are used to secure the stomach to the anterior abdominal wall. The T-fastener is initially placed into a slotted needle. The needle penetrates the anterior gastric wall, and the T-fastener is then discharged into the gastric lumen. After four T-fasteners are placed, the anterior gastric wall is elevated to the anterior abdominal wall.

ment for the appropriate site of exteriorization on the abdominal wall. The right grasping forceps is used to apply countertraction to the lesser curvature of the stomach. Four Brown-Mueller T-fasteners (Flexiflo Gastrostomy kit, Ross Laboratories, Columbus, OH) are introduced through the abdominal wall, forming a square (Figure 9–3). The T-fasteners are inserted into the lesser curvature of the stomach as the gastric wall is kept taut between the two graspers (Figure 9–4). Once the T-fasteners are situated, they are pulled upward, bringing the stomach near the anterior abdominal wall. A needle is inserted through the center of the square created by the four T-fasteners and advanced into the gastric lumen (Figure 9–5). A guidewire is inserted through the needle into the stomach. Following removal of the needle, a dilator is inserted over the

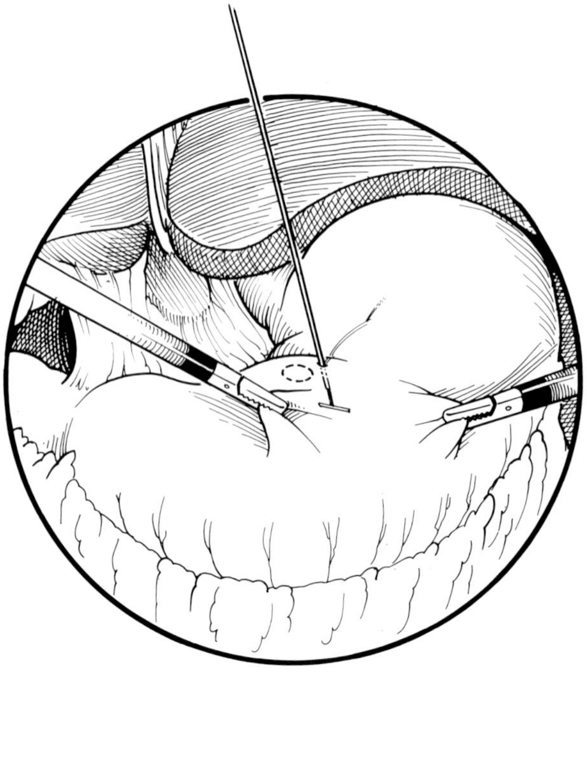

Figure 9–4. Grasping forceps are introduced through the lateral 5-mm ports and hold the stomach taut for insertion of the T-fasteners. The initial T-fastener has been placed in this diagram.

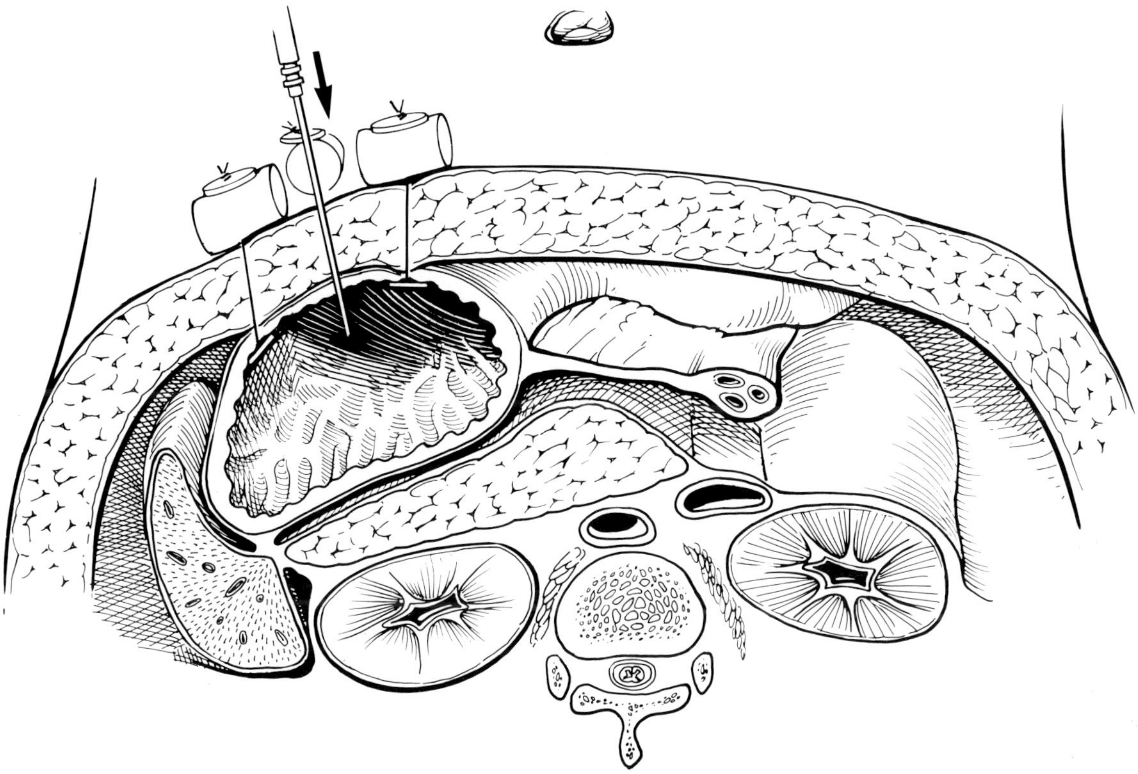

Figure 9–5. Following placement of all four T-fasteners, a needle is inserted into the stomach in the center of the square created by the T-fasteners.

guidewire, and the abdominal wall and stomach are dilated appropriately to accept the Foley catheter selected for use as the gastrostomy tube (Figure 9–6). A needle is introduced through the tip of the Foley catheter and the guidewire is passed in a retrograde direction through the needle and advanced through the catheter (Figure 9–7). The Foley catheter is then advanced over the guidewire through the abdominal wall into the stomach (Figure 9–8). The lesser curvature of the stomach should be pulled snugly against the abdominal wall at all times during this procedure. The guidewire is withdrawn and the Foley balloon is

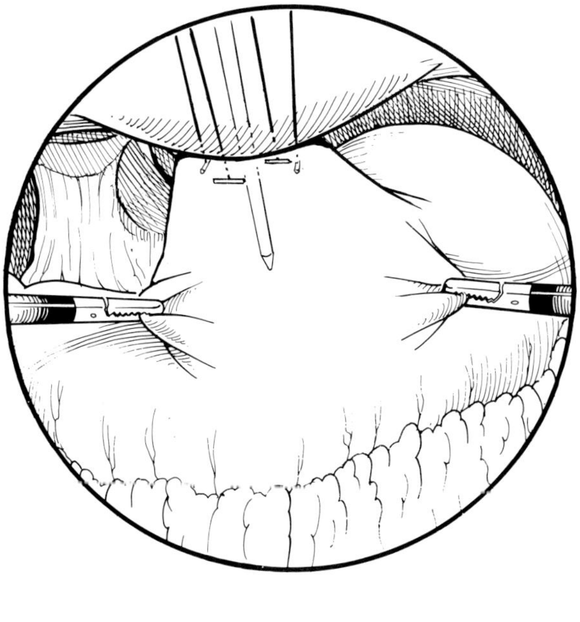

Figure 9–6. The stomach is held taut against the anterior abdominal wall, and a dilator is introduced over the guidewire to dilate the tract.

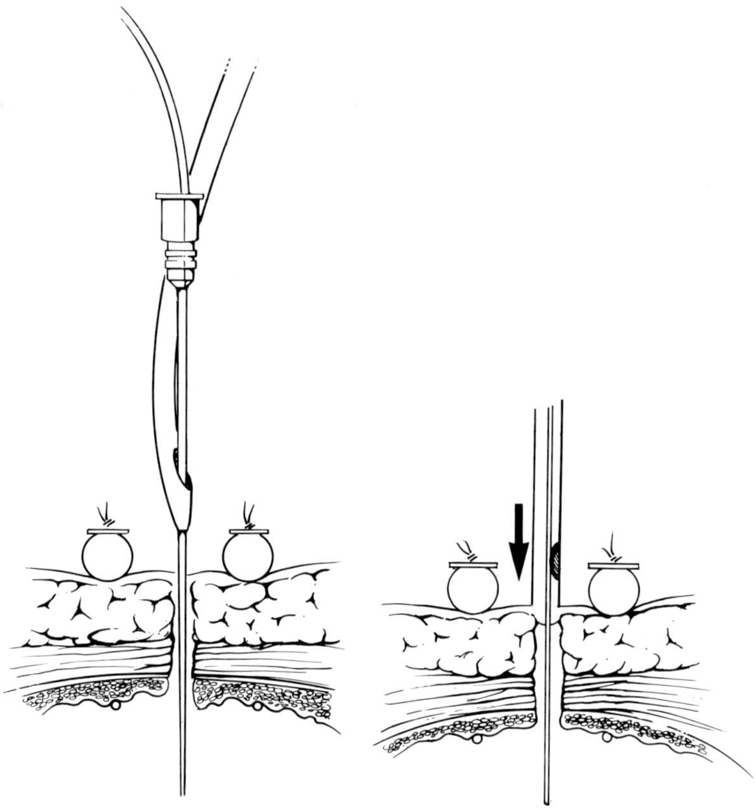

Figure 9–7. The dilator is removed and the wire is threaded in a retrograde direction up a Foley catheter. The wire is initially threaded through the tip of a needle inserted in the side port of the catheter and the needle removed. The wire is reinserted into the catheter and exteriorized through the open end of the Foley catheter. The catheter is then introduced into the stomach over the wire.

inflated (Figure 9–9). The T-fasteners are secured to each other over a bolster, and the gastrostomy tube is secured to the skin of the abdominal wall with a silk suture.

Complications can be avoided with careful attention to details. No attempt should be made to pass a T-fastener into the stomach without first lifting the lesser curvature anteriorly, creating a space within the stomach to accept the T-fastener. If this space is not created in the stomach, there is the possibility that the T-fastener will go through both the anterior and posterior walls of the stomach. If a T-fastener is dropped outside of the stomach, one of the forceps can be used to retrieve it. Alternately, the crossbar of the T-fastener can be left. It is also important not to dilate the opening in the stomach excessively. Too large a gastrostomy is prone to leakage of gastric contents.

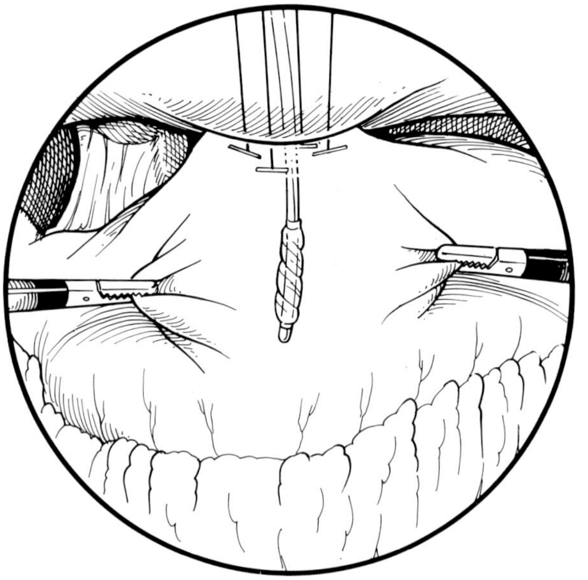

Figure 9–8. The Foley catheter is inserted into the gastric lumen over the wire.

GASTRIC OUTLET PROCEDURES

The author's current practice is to perform a pyloroplasty in those patients with severely delayed gastric emptying. Pyloromyotomy is employed for children with moderately delayed gastric emptying. A gastric drainage procedure is not performed if gastric emptying is normal.

Pyloromyotomy can also be performed laparoscopically. T-fasteners are inserted in the duodenum just distal to the pylorus. These T-fasteners are positioned 1 to 2 cm apart and provide traction on the

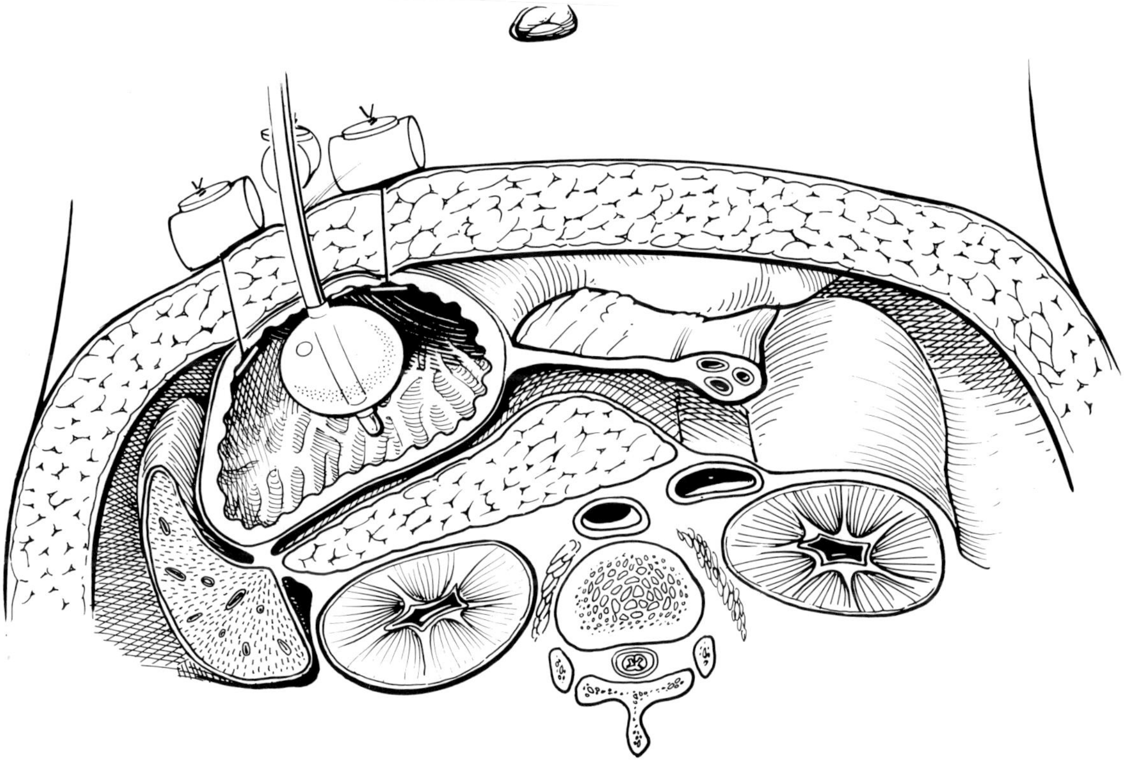

Figure 9–9. Following placement of the Foley catheter, the balloon is inflated and it is pulled taut against the anterior wall.

pylorus. The pyloric muscle is then divided with electrocautery and opened with a spreading laparoscopic clamp. A pyloromyotomy of 2 to 3 cm is sufficient.

Pyloroplasty is most easily performed by enlarging the right upper quadrant port to 3 cm. The pylorus is delivered into the wound and the pyloroplasty is performed in the standard open fashion. The pyloroplasty may also be performed laparoscopically by dividing the duodenum and distal stomach linearly and closing it transversely. The middle suture is placed using 2-O silk. The remainder of the pyloroplasty can be closed with a hernia stapling device. Special attention is given to elevating the stapler and the anterior wall of the pylorus and duodenum as they are approximated so that the posterior wall of the duodenum is not incorporated into the staples.

Postoperatively, children who have had only a laparoscopic gastrostomy can be fed within 6 hours, either through the gastrostomy tube or by mouth. Most patients who have had laparoscopic fundoplication and an outlet procedure are not fed for 12 hours. Oral or gastrostomy feedings are then initiated and advanced to full feedings in 24 to 36 hours. Discharge may occur at 48 hours if adequate gastrostomy training and support mechanisms are available to aid the family during the first few days of home care following discharge.

THE UNIVERSITY OF ALABAMA EXPERIENCE

Forty laparoscopic gastrostomies were performed between June 1991 and December 1992. Twenty-six were placed on the greater curvature of the stomach because they were performed in association with a laparoscopic fundoplication. Fifteen gastric outlet procedures were also performed in this group of 40 patients, with 11 pyloromyotomies and 4 pyloroplasties. Fourteen children were treated with a lesser-curvature gastrostomy alone. Weight gain has been noted in all children.

Complications have been similar to those noted with the open procedure. One child developed GE reflux 16 months after placement of a lesser-curvature gastrostomy and underwent laparoscopic fundoplication. One of the patients suffered a small tear in the esophagus, and another patient developed a small tear in the left hemidiaphragm during the dissection for laparoscopic fundoplication. Both tears were repaired laparoscopically with 2-O silk suture and did not cause further problems.

Postoperative retching has occurred sporadically in some of the neurologically impaired patients. This symptom has been managed medically. One patient developed leakage around the gastrostomy because of incorrect placement of the T-fasteners in the stomach. The leak was repaired by open Stamm gastrostomy. One severely impaired girl died 3 months postoperatively of apparent pharyngeal aspiration.

Six children had an attempt at fundoplication that was converted to an open procedure because of technical difficulties. None of these six patients are included in the series of 40 patients undergoing successful laparoscopic fundoplication and/or gastrostomy.

Early in this experience, discharge was delayed until the fifth postoperative day. The last 10 patients with fundoplication and gastrostomy were discharged within 3 days postoperatively. Home support services were used both for teaching feeding techniques and gastrostomy care and for troubleshooting problems after discharge.

SUMMARY

Laparoscopic lesser-curvature gastrostomy has been performed in 14 patients, with development of clinically apparent GE reflux in only one of the 14 patients. In another 26 children, laparoscopic fundoplication was performed in addition to the laparoscopic gastrostomy. None of these 26 patients have developed clinically detectable reflux postoperatively. Most of the 40 patients have shown excellent weight gain. Discharge from the hospital, return to a full feeding program, and full recovery appear to be faster in patients managed laparoscopically than in those having open gastrostomy and fundoplication.

REFERENCES

1. Jones S. Gastrostomy for stricture (cancerous) of esophagus: Death from bronchitis forty days after operation. *Lancet.* 1875;1:678.
2. Verneuil OO. Observation de gastrostomie practiquee avec succes pour un retrecissement cicatricial infranchissable de l'oesophage. *Bull Acad Med (Paris).* 1876;5:1023.
3. Trendelenburg F. Ueber einen fall von gastrostomie bei oesophagusstrictur. *Arch Klen Chir.* 1878;22:227.
4. Walker LGJ. L. L. Staton, M.D., and the first successful gastrostomy in America. *Surg Gynecol Obstet.* 1984;158:387.
5. Thorek M. The history and development of gastrostomy. *J Int Coll Surg.* 1943;6:295.
6. Gauderer MWL, Stellato TA. Gastrostomies: Evolution, techniques, indications, and complications. *Curr Probl Surg.* 1986;26:661.
7. Wesley JR, Coran AG, Sarahan TM, et al. The need for evaluation of gastroesophageal reflux in brain-damaged children referred for feeding gastrostomy. *J Pediatr Surg.* 1982;16:866.
8. Jolley SG, Tunell WP, Leonard JC, et al. Gastric emptying in children with gastroesophageal reflux. II. The relationship to retching symptoms following antireflux surgery. *J Pediatr Surg.* 1987;22:927.
9. Sullivan PB. Gastrostomy and the disabled child. *Dev Med Child Neurol.* 1992;34:547.
10. Gisel EG, Patrick J. Identification of children with cerebral palsy unable to maintain a normal nutritional state. *Lancet.* 1988;1:283.
11. Shapiro BK, Green P, Krick J, et al. Growth of severely impaired children: Neurological versus nutritional factors. *Dev Med Child Neurol.* 1986;28:729.
12. Rempel GR, Colwell SO, Nelson RP. Growth in children with cerebral palsy fed via gastrostomy. *Pediatrics.* 1988;82:857.
13. Stamm M. Gastrostomy: A new method. *Med News.* 1894;65:324.
14. Thatcher BS, Ferguson DR, Paradis K. Percutaneous endoscopic gastrostomy: A preferred method of feeding tube gastrostomy. *Am J Gastroenterol.* 1984;79:748.
15. Gauderer MWL. Percutaneous endoscopic gastrostomy: A 10 year experience with 220 children. *J Pediatr Surg.* 1991;26:288.
16. Tunell WP. Gastroesophageal reflux in childhood. *Ann Pediatr.* 1989;18:192.
17. Mollitt DL, Golladay S, Seibert JJ. Symptomatic gastroesophageal reflux following gastrostomy in neurologically impaired patients. *Pediatrics.* 1985;75:1124.
18. Langer JC, Wesson DE, Ein SH, et al. Feeding gastrostomy in neurologically impaired children: Is an antireflux procedure necessary? *J Pediatr Gastroenterol Nutr.* 1988;7:837.
19. Hassett JM, Sunby C, Flint LM. No elimination of aspiration pneumonia in neurologically disabled patients with feeding gastrostomy. *Surg Gynecol Obstet.* 1988;167:383.
20. Wheatley MJ, Wesley JR, Tkach DM, et al. Long-term follow-up of brain-damaged children requiring feeding gastrostomy: Should an antireflux procedure always be performed? *J Pediatr Surg.* 1991;26:301.
21. Berezin S, Schwarz S, Halata MS, et al. Gastroesophageal reflux secondary to gastrostomy tube placement. *Am J Dis Child.* 1986;140:699.
22. Canal DF, Vane DW, Goto S, et al. Changes in lower esophageal sphincter pressure (LES) after Stamm gastrostomy. *J Surg Res.* 1987;42:570.
23. Papaila JG, Vane DW, Colville C, et al. The effect of various types of gastrostomy on the lower esophageal sphincter. *J Pediatr Surg.* 1987;22:1198.
24. Jolley SG, Tunell WP, Hoelzer DJ, et al. Lower esophageal pressure changes with tube gastrostomy: A causative factor of gastroesophageal reflux in children? *J Pediatr Surg.* 1986;21:624.
25. Stringel G. Gastrostomy with antireflux properties. *J Pediatr Surg.* 1990;25:1019.
26. Seekri IK, Rescorla FJ, Canal DF, et al. Lesser curvature

gastrostomy reduces the incidence of postoperative gastroesophageal reflux. *J Pediatr Surg.* 1991;26:982.
27. Cogen R, Wernryb J. Aspiration pneumonia in nursing home patients fed via gastrostomy tubes. *Am J Gastroenterol.* 1989;84:1509.
28. Heij HA, Seldenrijk, Vos A. Anterior gastropexy prevents gastrostomy-induced gastroesophageal reflux: An experimental study in piglets. *J Pediatr Surg.* 1991;26:557.
29. Black TL, Fernandes ET, Ellis DG, et al. The effect of tube gastrostomy on gastroesophageal reflux in patients with esophageal atresia. *J Pediatr Surg.* 1991;26:168.
30. Gauderer MWL. Feeding gastrostomy or feeding gastrostomy plus antireflux procedure? *J Pediatr Gastroenterol Nutr.* 1988;7:795.

CHAPTER 10

Laparoscopy for Intersex Abnormalities

DAVID M. POWELL • KURT D. NEWMAN

Recent years have witnessed significant advances in understanding the basic science of sexual differentiation. Despite breakthroughs exposing the underlying molecular and biochemical basis of intersex abnormalities, clinicians must still rely on relatively empiric means when faced with the urgent difficulties of gender assignment and expeditious surgical reconstruction in children with ambiguous genitalia. Although the evaluation and management of each child and family are individualized, adherence to a few general guidelines is useful. The approach to diagnosis and management is now aided by technical advances that permit endoscopy, laparoscopy, and minimal access surgery in infants and smaller children. These techniques permit more straightforward surgical treatment and more confident answers to the troubled parents when they ask, "Is it a boy or a girl?"

CLINICAL PRESENTATION

A complex series of events must occur in a particular order for the embryo to undergo proper sexual differentiation. Stated simply, these events, and the errors that lead to intersex anomalies, can be divided into two parts. First, the presence or absence of the Y chromosome initially determines whether the undifferentiated fetal gonad will develop into an ovary or a testis. Developmental errors that interfere with the appropriate genetic differentiation of the gonad lead to either *true hermaphroditism*, the coexistence of both ovarian and testicular tissue, or the *dysgenetic gonad syndrome*, limited or absent normal gonadal tissue. In these cases, the abnormal gonad does not adequately direct the development of either a phenotypically correct male or phenotypically correct female.

Second, either male or female internal and external genitalia develop when the appropriate physiologic milieu is provided by the testis or ovary. For example, the testis secretes müllerian inhibiting substance (MIS), responsible for the regression of the fetal müllerian ducts which otherwise develop into the fallopian tubes, uterus, and upper vagina in the female. The testis also secretes testosterone, a steroid hormone, that when converted to dihydrotestosterone binds with a specific intracellular receptor, directing development of male external genitalia including lengthening of the fetal phallus into a penis, fusion of the labioscrotal folds over the urogenital sinus to form the penile urethra and scrotum, and inguinal and scrotal testicular descent. Errors that prevent otherwise normal gonads from effecting successful genital development fall in the group of diagnoses termed *pseudohermaphroditism*. Male pseudohermaphroditism results when the presence of a Y chromosome leads to development of the undifferentiated gonad into the testis, but biochemical abnormalities prevent testosterone from directing development of the male external genitalia (eg, testicular feminization). Conversely, female pseudohermaphroditism results when an excess of circulating androgen resulting from an error in steroid hormone synthesis (congenital adrenal hyperplasia/adrenogenital syndrome) causes the external genitalia to become masculinized, despite the presence of normal ovaries.

DIAGNOSIS

Early and accurate gender assignment is crucial. The diagnostic evaluation should commence as soon as the child is born and an abnormality detected. Although often considered to be a complex set of abnormalities, infants born with ambiguous genitalia usually can be rapidly assigned to one of four diagnostic categories using two basic criteria: the patient's sex chromosomes and the anatomic symmetry of the gonads (Table 10–1).

The laboratory capability exists in most hospitals to quickly determine whether a patient's chromosomal complement is XX or XY based on either rapid fluorescence labeling of the long arm of the Y chromosome or the presence of a Barr body representing the inactive, duplicated X chromosome. These specimens can be obtained from a buccal smear and the results of testing should be available almost immediately. The XX karyotype is present in those patients who are chromosomal females: female pseudohermaphrodites and most true hermaphrodites. Alternatively, the XY karyotype predominates in male pseudohermaphrodites and patients with gonadal dysgenesis.

Evaluation of the gonads, including symmetry, has traditionally relied on physical examination. Recently, minimal access surgery has provided a major contribution for this evaluation. Laparoscopy provides a more complete characterization of the gonads. Both sides of the abdomen can be evaluated for the presence of intraabdominal gonads. The gonads can be inspected visually, biopsied, or even removed if necessary. If the gonads themselves have developed abnormally (true hermaphroditism and gonadal dysgenesis) and are responsible for the defect, their descent into the groin will usually have been asymmetric, as the amount of testicular tissue present is rarely equal on both sides. Alternatively, if a diffuse, global process has prevented the gonads from effecting genital development (pseudohermaphroditism) and was responsible for the incompleteness of sexual differentiation, gonadal descent should remain unaffected and both gonads will be either above (ovaries) or below (testes) the inguinal ring.

Two additional caveats exist that may be helpful during the initial hectic evaluation and may assist the team in determining the gender assignment of the newborn. Every attempt should be made to raise chromosomal females as females, regardless of the amount of masculinization. In chromosomal males, however, gender assignment should be based primarily on the size of the phallus. In a patient with a phallus that measures less than 1.5 to 2 cm long or less than 0.7 cm wide, female gender assignment is strongly encouraged, especially if associated with dysgenetic gonads or testicular feminization.

The complete evaluation of a child with an intersex abnormality is summarized in Table 10–2. A complete family and maternal history should be obtained with special consideration to fetal exposure to progestational agents, androgens, or anticonvulsant medications. During the physical examination special attention is paid to the symmetry and position of the gonads, the size of the phallus, the meatal position, the development of the labioscrotal folds, and the presence of a uterus as identified on rectal exam (Figure 10–1). It is often helpful to review the findings of the infant's examination with the parents in attendance, as this may assist in their understanding of the specific aspects of genital development and eventual reconstruction.

In addition to a buccal smear to determine whether the karyotype is XX or XY, blood should be collected for serum electrolytes. Salt wasting can accompany certain types of the adrenogenital syndrome and may be life-threatening. Leukocytes for tissue culture and complete karyotype analysis should also be obtained. Measurement of specific steroid hormones, precursors, and metabolites can indicate a specific enzymatic defect in female pseudohermaphrodites with the adrenogenital syndrome. Before measuring testosterone in the newborn, exogenous human chorionic gonadotropin (HCG) must be administered to stimulate testosterone secretion from the testis. Alternatively, the baseline MIS level is elevated in the normal male infant and its presence on a random blood screen provides evidence for a functioning testis without requiring the cumbersome HCG stimulation test.[1]

Radiographic studies are used as an extension of the physical examination to delineate the internal anatomy. A retrograde cystourethrogram is performed to determine the presence and extent of a urethrovaginal fistula (Figure 10–2). The fistula's location relative to the urinary sphincter is critical to subsequent surgical reconstruction. A blunt "Christmas tree" adapter is placed against the urogenital sinus opening, rather than being injected through an indwelling catheter, so that a distal fistula is not missed. Although sometimes difficult to interpret in the infant, ultrasound can be

TABLE 10–1. CLASSIFICATION OF INTERSEX ABNORMALITIES

Type	Cause	Karyotype	Gonads
True hermaphroditism	Ovarian and testicular tissue present	Usually 46,XX	Asymmetric
Dysgenetic gonads	Abnormal gonadal development	Usually 46,XY	Asymmetric
Pseudohermaphroditism			
Female	Excess androgen	46,XX	Symmetric
Male	Unsuccessful masculinization	46,XY	Symmetric

TABLE 10–2. DIAGNOSTIC WORKUP FOR THE CHILD WITH AMBIGUOUS GENITALIA

Clinical	Laboratory	Radiographic	Surgical
History	Buccal smear (XX or XY)	Retrograde cystourethrogram	Cystoscopy
Physical exam	Serum electrolytes	Pelvic ultrasound	Laparoscopy
	Serum and urine steroid levels	Magnetic resonance imaging	Gonadal biopsy
	Chromosomal analysis		Genital skin biopsy (androgen receptors)
	Serum testosterone and gonadotropin levels (HCG stimulation test)		
	Serum MIS level		

employed to identify the uterus, the location of intraabdominal gonads, and the presence of adrenal enlargement. More recently, magnetic resonance imaging has been beneficial in delineating pelvic anatomy in complex cases.

The final assessment of urogenital sinus anatomy, however, is made at cystoscopy. The infant cystoscope is used under full water flow, making identification of the external sphincter easier. The vaginal opening is then identified as entering either proximal or distal to this important landmark. If the vagina enters below (caudad) the sphincter, a "cutback" vaginoplasty can be employed to exteriorize the introitus without fear of damaging the sphincter musculature. This procedure can then be performed at any time but is usually accomplished between 3 and 6 months of age, or earlier if social pressures demand it. Conversely, if the vaginal opening is identified above (cephalad) the sphincter, a more complex "pull-through" vaginoplasty is done, usually at an older age (sometime after 6 months).

Gonadal biopsy is frequently required in patients

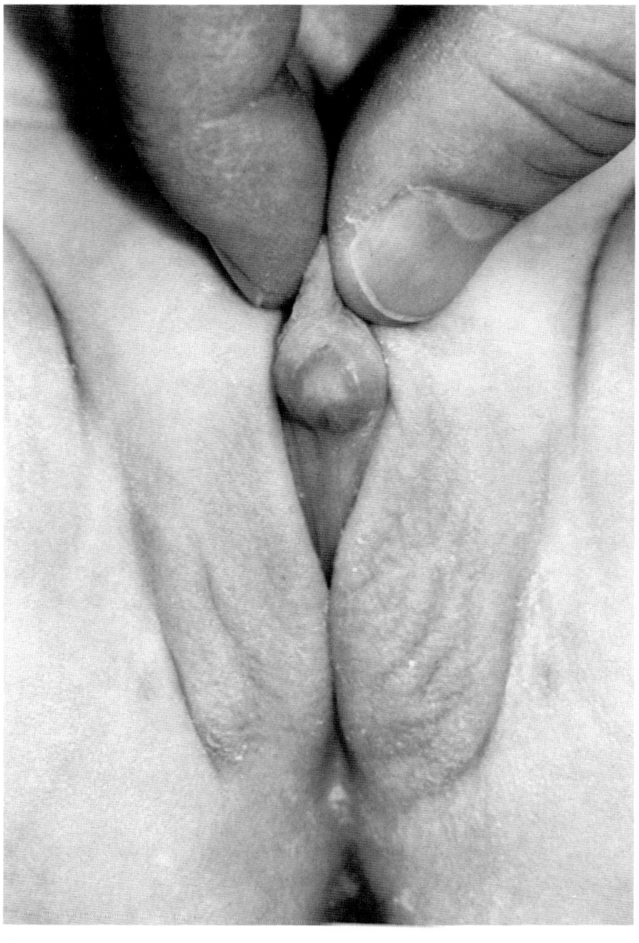

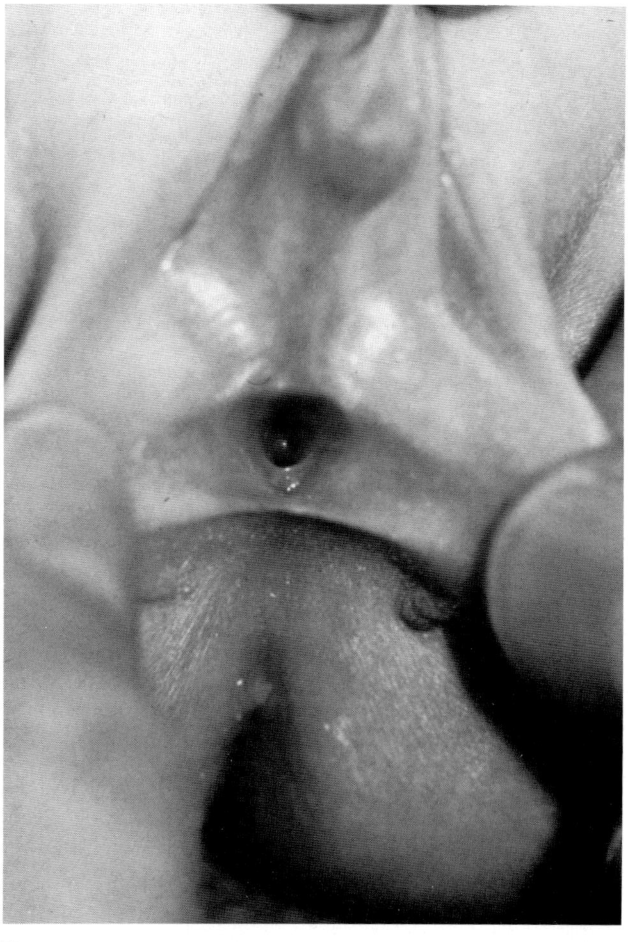

A **B**

Figure 10–1. Perineum of a child with congenital adrenal hyperplasia. Note the enlarged phallus/clitoris **(A)** and urogenital sinus **(B)**.

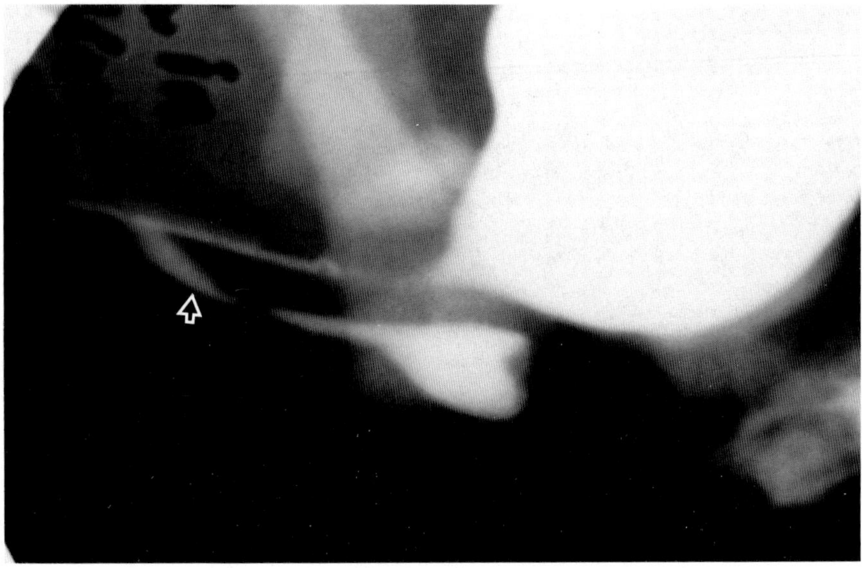

Figure 10–2. Retrograde cystourethrogram demonstrating a vaginal fistula (*open arrow*) coming from a distal urogenital sinus and the proximal "dimple" of cervix at the apex of the vagina.

with either true hermaphroditism or dysgenetic gonads. This procedure, as well as therapeutic gonadectomy, can be performed laparoscopically using infraumbilical and bilateral lower quadrant ports. Atraumatic clamps can be inserted through the cannulas to grasp and mobilize the gonads. The biopsy should be taken longitudinally (parallel to the long axis of the gonad) and include both poles and the center of the gonad. This is important because ovarian tissue is most commonly present in the poles, whereas testicular tissue is usually found near the center of the gonad. In the patient with asymmetric gonads, both gonads should be biopsied. Additionally, the dysgenetic gonad may deteriorate over time, requiring serial biopsies to confirm the diagnosis and to monitor for malignant degeneration in those rare dysgenetic gonad patients in whom gonadectomy has not been performed. At diagnostic laparoscopy in children with intersex anomalies, the entire abdomen, pelvis, and retroperitoneal structures should be completely visualized. The location, descent, and appearance of the gonads are evaluated. Although quite small in the infant, müllerian duct derivatives (fallopian tubes and uterus) should be identifiable. It may, however, be difficult to differentiate the total absence of these structures from severe hypoplasia. A vaginal or uterine remnant may subsequently be identified on cystoscopy or urethrogram.[2]

In patients with male pseudohermaphroditism, a genital skin biopsy provides tissue for assay of 5α-reductase (the enzyme responsible for converting testosterone into the more biologically active dihydrotestosterone [DHT]) or androgen receptor binding abnormalities.

CLINICAL MANAGEMENT

Male Pseudohermaphroditism

Male pseudohermaphroditism occurs in patients who have a 46,XY chromosomal complement but exhibit incomplete masculinization of the external genitalia. This results from a defect in either testosterone production, conversion of testosterone to DHT, or binding of the ligand to the androgen receptor. Masculinization is therefore variable. Patients may display severe penoscrotal hypospadias with microphallus, a blind vaginal pouch coming off the posterior urethra identified at cystoscopy, and otherwise normal internal and testicular anatomy. The effects of MIS persist, however, and these patients will not have müllerian duct structures (fallopian tubes, uterus, and upper vagina). An analogous group of disorders, the retained müllerian duct syndrome, results from either production of abnormal MIS or MIS receptor malfunction. These patients usually present later in childhood with cryptorchidism and uterus inguinali (failure of regression of müllerian structures). Laparoscopy is useful to confirm the presence of and occasionally to resect these müllerian remnants.

Gender assignment and subsequent surgical management of children with male pseudohermaphroditism are determined by the prognosis for later masculinization. This decision is based on knowledge of the specific defect involved and the size of the infant phallus. If the phallus is small, clitoroplasty, labioscrotal reduction, orchiectomy, and vaginoplasty are performed. Children with complete absence of a vagina should undergo vaginal reconstruction. Although a technique employing laparoscopy and chronic traction on the perineum has been described,[3] we prefer vaginal reconstruction with a segment of ascending colon, a procedure that may be assisted by laparoscopy. If the phallus is large enough and androgen receptor binding is demonstrated, exogenous testosterone therapy is initiated. Repair of chordee and hypospadias and correction of a prepenile scrotum are undertaken appropriately. Patients who are raised as females because of receptor abnormalities should undergo orchiectomy to prevent the possibility of malignant degeneration. The appropriate timing of this procedure remains controversial.

Female Pseudohermaphroditism

Female pseudohermaphrodites have a 46,XX karyotype but, because of excess androgen exposure in utero, have become masculinized. Frequently this is due to an error in steroid synthesis that results in overproduction of endogenous androgen. Although the internal organs are normal, the external genitalia are masculinized and the vagina fails to reach the perineum. The vagina ends in a fistula to the urethra, causing a urogenital sinus. Depending on the specific enzymatic defect, life-threatening hyponatremia and hyperkalemia may result and necessitate frequent monitoring after birth. Therefore, adequate steroid and electrolyte replacement is a critical element of early management.

All of these patients should be raised as females and subsequently undergo clitoroplasty and vaginoplasty. Clitoroplasty can be done shortly after birth or at several months of age, but the timing and nature of vaginal reconstruction are dictated by the findings at cystoscopy, as indicated earlier. Recently, with the use of prenatal diagnosis and treatment of the female fetus with congenital adrenal hyperplasia, several investigators have administered steroids to the fetus in an effort to prevent in utero masculinization.[4] In the future, fetoscopy may be useful in following the external genital development of the fetal patient and the response to therapy.

Gonadal Dysgenesis

Children with gonadal dysgenesis are typified by the presence of abnormal gonads, which have the potential for early malignancy.[5] These patients usually have retained müllerian ducts. The appearance of the gonads is extremely variable and is reflected in mosaic karyotypes and asymmetry of descent and genital appearance. Gonadoblastoma has been identified in patients with dysgenetic gonads as early as the newborn period, although dysgerminomas tend to develop in streak gonads later in life.

When identified in infancy, patients should undergo gonadectomy and be raised and reconstructed as females with estrogen and progesterone replacement. Gonadectomy is a relatively simple laparoscopic procedure, as the gonads are small and easy to manipulate.[6,7] An older child who has already received a male gender assignment should still undergo gonadectomy, but receive hypospadias repair, laparoscopic removal of müllerian remnants, and subsequent placement of testicular prostheses and androgen replacement.

A related group of patients, children with Turner's syndrome and mosaic karyotype, have a similar risk of developing gonadal malignancy. Again, laparoscopic removal of streak gonads is easily accomplished (Figure 10–3) and eliminates this risk in later life.

In older children and adolescents, virilizing ovarian tumors often present with hirsutism, voice changes, and clitoromegaly. Following identification with ultrasound and thorough endocrine evaluation, pelvic laparoscopy can be beneficial. Unfortunately, many of these tumors are quite large at the time of presentation. Often, associated torsion requires celiotomy for tumor excision. Unilateral oophorectomy is usually curative for these lesions, which are usually benign. Once the tumor is removed, the virilizing signs and symptoms resolve.

True Hermaphroditism

True hermaphroditism occurs with extreme rarity in the United States, although it may be more frequent in other countries. These children have both histologically normal testicular and ovarian tissue present in the same gonad. In general, when identified early, these patients too should be raised as females.[8] With a laparoscopic approach, testicular tissue is identified and removed and ovarian tissue preserved. It is important to realize that ovarian tissue tends to be present at the ends of the gonad, with testicular tissue located centrally. Serum MIS levels can be used to determine the success with which testicular tissue is completely removed when partial gonadectomy is performed.

SUMMARY

The technical advances of laparoscopic surgery and the expanding applications to children and infants

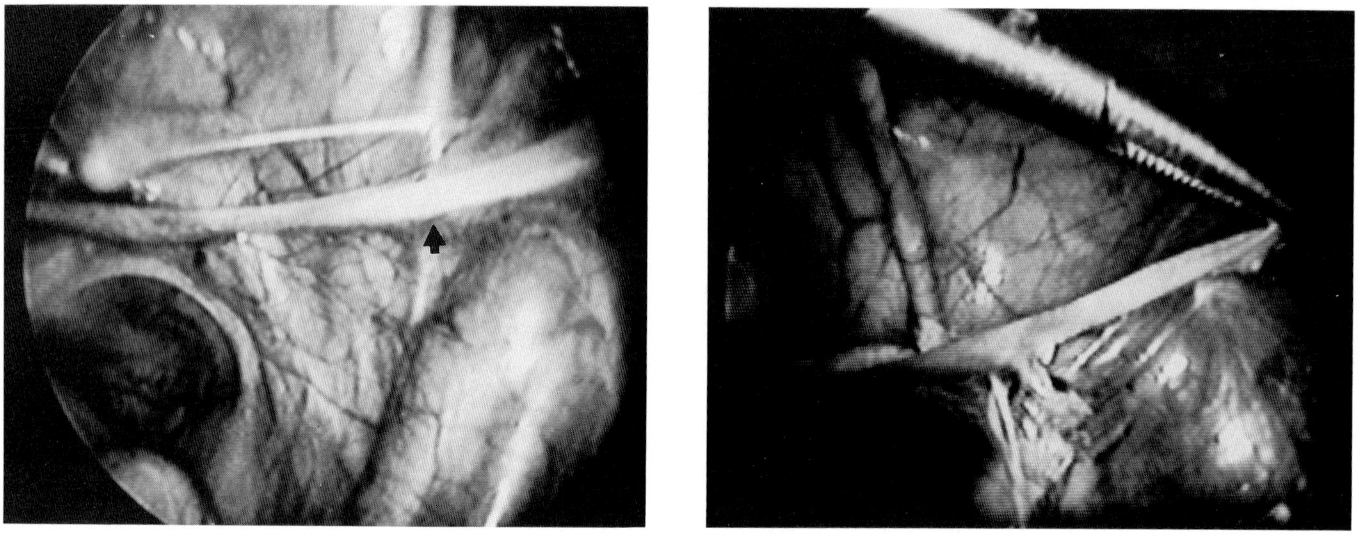

A B

Figure 10–3. Left streak ovary (*arrow*) identified at laparoscopy in a patient with mosaic karyotype Turner's syndrome **(A)**. The bladder and small uterus are identified medially. The gonad was easily resected with cautery **(B)**.

have enhanced the capabilities of the pediatric surgeon in the care of patients with intersex abnormalities. The procedures are safe and are associated with rapid recovery and minimal scarring. The ability to expeditiously identify and visualize intraabdominal gonads, coupled with the ability to biopsy and remove abnormal gonads, is a welcome addition to the surgeon's armamentarium. The further integration of surgical advances and molecular understanding will lead to improved care in future decades for children with these complex problems.

REFERENCES

1. Hudson PL, Dougas I, Donahoe PK, et al. An immunoassay to detect human mullerian inhibiting substance in males and females during normal development. *J Clin Endocrinol Metab.* 1990;70:16.
2. Joshi NP, Sotrel G. Diagnostic laparoscopy in apparent uterine agenesis. *J Adolesc Health Care.* 1988;9:403.
3. Popp LW, Ghirardini G. Creation of a neovagina by pelviscopy. *J Laparoendosc Surg.* 1992;2:165.
4. Pang S, Pollack MS, Marshall RN, et al. Prenatal treatment of congenital adrenal hyperplasia due to 21-hydroxylase deficiency. *N Engl J Med.* 1990;105:799.
5. Robboy SJ, Miller T, Donahoe PK, et al. Dysgenesis of testicular and streak gonads in the syndrome of mixed gonadal dysgenesis. *Hum Pathol.* 1982;13:700.
6. Droesch K, Droesch J, et al. Laparoscopic gonadectomy for gonadal dysgenesis. *Fertil Steril.* 1990;53:360.
7. Wilson EE, Vuitch F, et al. Laparoscopic removal of dysgenetic gonads containing a gonadoblastoma in a patient with Swyer syndrome. *Obstet Gynecol.* 1992;79:842.
8. Donahoe PK, Crawford JD, et al. True hermaphroditism: A clinical description and a proposed function for the long arm of the Y chromosome. *J Pediatr Surg.* 1978;13:293.

Further Reading

Donahoe PK, Powell DM, Lee ML. Clinical management of intersex abnormalities. *Curr Probl Surg.* 1991;28:August.

Newman K, Randolph J, Anderson K. The surgical management of infants and children with ambiguous genitalia. *Ann Surg.* 1992;215(6):664.

CHAPTER 11

Laparoscopic Nephrectomy

KURT KERBL • RALPH V. CLAYMAN • LOUIS R. KAVOUSSI

Although laparoscopic techniques have been used by gynecologists for decades, the utilization of this technique by urologists has been recent. Initially laparoscopy was used in urology for diagnostic procedures, specifically to explore the abdomen for a cryptorchid testicle.[1–13] Over the last 4 years, with the introduction of laparoscopic varicocelectomy[14–17] and pelvic lymphadenectomy,[18–20] the transition from diagnostic to therapeutic laparoscopy has occurred. A further advance in therapeutic laparoscopy was the recent development of an organ removal system (Lapsac, Cook Urological, Inc, Spencer, IN) in combination with a high-speed tissue morcellator (Cook OB/GYN/Cook Urology).[21] With these instruments, removal of solid organs (such as the kidney with/without the ureter) could be accomplished via the same incision used to introduce a 12-mm trocar.[22–27] With continuing advances in stapling and clipping devices, the creation of a laparoscopic probe for the argon beam coagulator, and improvements in intracorporeal suturing, laparoscopic surgery is moving beyond *ablative* therapy and into the realm of *reconstructive* surgery: partial nephrectomy, ureteral reimplantation, and pyeloplasty [28–30] (also W. W. Schuessler and G. Preminger, personal communication, 1992). This is the final phase necessary to complete the transition from open minimally invasive surgery to endoscopic minimally invasive surgery.

The impact of these advances in adult urology on the specialty of pediatric urology is being assessed presently. In this chapter, the technique for performing a laparoscopic nephrectomy in a child and our experience with the procedure are reviewed.

INDICATIONS

The indications for laparoscopic nephrectomy and laparoscopic nephroureterectomy are listed in Table 11–1. In general, laparoscopic nephrectomy is being performed currently in children for benign renal disease. The removal of a tumor-bearing kidney has not yet been reported, as there are significant (and as yet unanswered) concerns regarding the possibility of tumor spread during the laparoscopic procedure.

PRELIMINARY PROCEDURES

In older children prior to laparoscopic nephrectomy, cystoscopy may be performed for placement of a 7-French ureteral occlusion balloon catheter (stiffened with a 0.035-in. Amplatz superstiff guidewire) or a 3-French floppy-tip guidewire into the ureter to facilitate identification and dissection.

Similarly, prior to a laparoscopic nephroureterectomy, cystoscopy can be performed and the ureteral tunnel incised over a 5-mm ureteral balloon dilating catheter. This maneuver will displace the ureteral orifice from the trigone to the level of the ureterovesical junction. In the child, this procedure can be accomplished best using a short 12.5-French ureteroscope with an insulated tip and a 3-French electrode. After removal of the ureteral dilating balloon, dependent on the size of the ureter, a 7-French, 11.5-mm occlusion balloon catheter, stiffened by an 0.035-in. Amplatz superstiff guidewire, or a 3-French floppy-tip guidewire can be inserted to aid in the dissection of the ureter.

TECHNIQUE

Laparoscopic Nephrectomy

Pneumoperitoneum is accomplished using the Veress needle technique as described in Chapter 2. Either a 5- or 12-mm (dependent on the child's size) umbilical trocar and cannula are inserted and diagnostic laparoscopy performed. The intraabdominal organs are inspected for any abnormalities, and any bleeding or injury from insertion of the Veress needle or the trocar

TABLE 11–1. INDICATIONS IN CHILDREN

■ LAPAROSCOPIC NEPHRECTOMY
Symptomatic, hypoplastic, or atrophic kidney
Multicystic dysplastic kidney (controversial)
Recurrent infections in a poorly functioning kidney
End-stage kidney failure
Renal hypertension
■ LAPAROSCOPIC NEPHROURETERECTOMY
An ectopic ureter or refluxing ureter in the presence of a poorly functioning kidney

is noted. After systematic examination of the abdomen, two secondary ports are placed under direct optical control: a 12-mm subcostal port along the midclavicular line (MCL) and a 5-mm port 3 cm below the umbilicus in the MCL. After the patient is turned to a flank position, two other cannulas are placed: a 5-mm port in the anterior axillary line (AAL) at the tip of the 12th rib and a 5-mm port in the AAL at the level of the umbilicus (Figure 11–1).

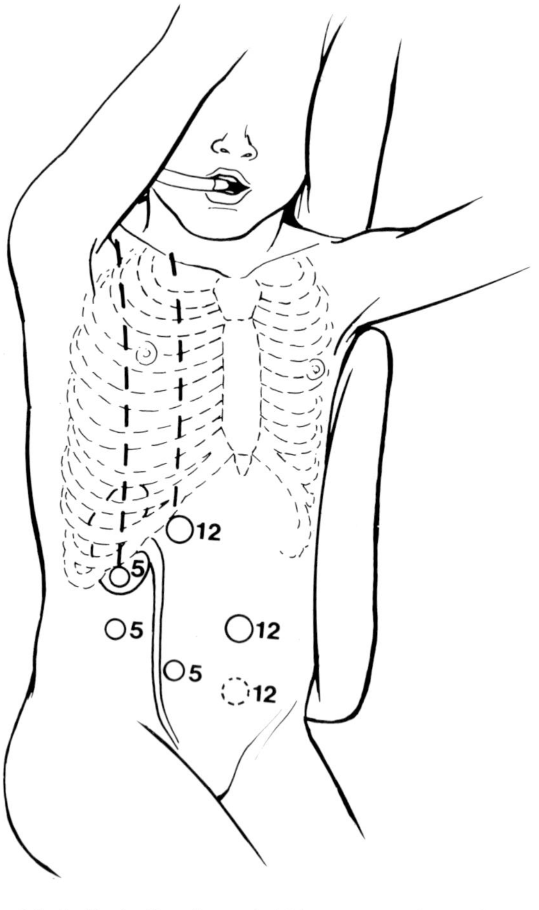

Figure 11–1. Port sites for a right laparoscopic nephrectomy or nephroureterectomy. The sixth port needed for nephroureterectomy is indicated by the dotted circle between the umbilical cannula and symphysis pubis.

For laparoscopic nephroureterectomy, six cannulas are usually placed. The additional port is 12 mm and is positioned in the midline midway between the umbilicus and the symphysis pubis while the patient is in the supine position. All other ports are placed as described for laparoscopic nephrectomy.

In smaller children, the location and number of ports may vary. In our 6-month-old patient who underwent laparoscopic nephrectomy for a multicystic dysplastic kidney, only four cannulas were used: a 10-mm umbilical port and three 5-mm ports in the MCL.

The surgeon usually works through the two MCL ports while the assistant retracts tissue laterally via one or both of the AAL ports. The camera assistant operates the laparoscope via the umbilical port. There are eight steps to performing a laparoscopic nephrectomy (Table 11–2).

After placement of the cannulas, the peritoneal reflection of the colon is incised, thereby mobilizing the colon medially and exposing the retroperitoneal space. This is done on the right side from the cecum up and around the hepatic flexure. On the left the entire descending colon and splenic flexure of the transverse colon are mobilized.

Next, the catheter or guidewire in the ureter is manipulated at the urethral meatus. The ureter is identified and dissected to the level of the renal pelvis. In dissecting the ureter, the gonadal vein is encountered as it crosses the ureter. This vein can be carefully dissected and secured with two pairs of 9-mm titanium clips from the 10-mm clip applier passed via the upper MCL port. At this point, the surgeon can pass a 4-in. piece of umbilical tape into the abdomen and wrap it around the ureter. The ends of the tape can then be approximated with a 9-mm titanium clip passed via the upper MCL port. This tag makes it quite easy for the assistant to use a grasping forceps to manipulate the ureter atraumatically.

Gerota's fascia is sharply incised. The lower pole and lateral surfaces of the kidney are then dissected; the upper pole of the kidney is separated from the adrenal gland (Figure 11–2). The renal pedicle is then dissected. Two atraumatic graspers are passed via the

TABLE 11–2. OPERATIVE STEPS FOR LAPAROSCOPIC NEPHRECTOMY

1. Incise colonic peritoneal reflection
2. Secure ureter
3. Dissect lateral and polar surfaces of the kidney
4. Secure and transect renal vessels
5. Transect the ureter
6. Entrap the kidney in a sack
7. Fragment the kidney and remove renal fragments and sack
8. Exit the abdomen

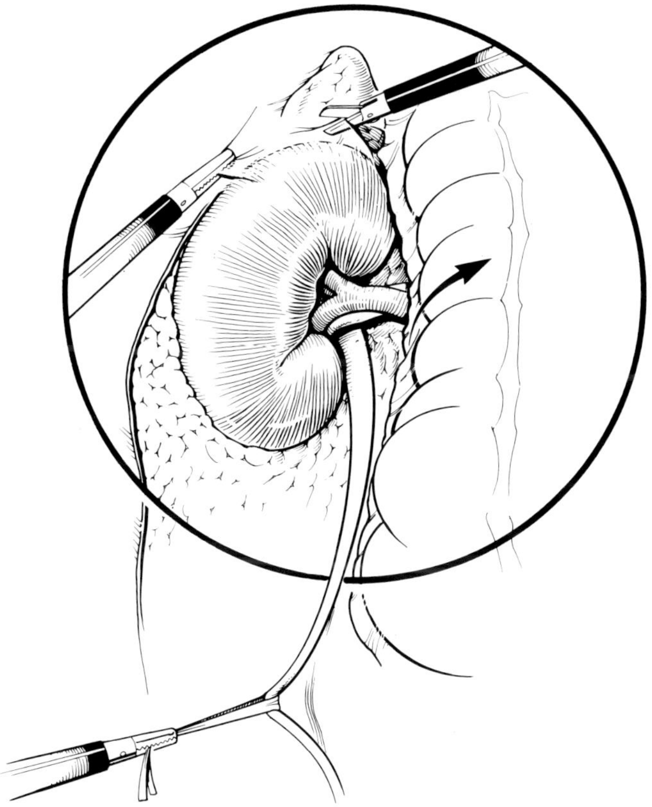

Figure 11–2. The peritoneal reflection of the right colon has been incised and the colon mobilized medially. A 4-in. umbilical tape has been wrapped around the dissected ureter. The tape can then be secured with a grasper (as shown here) or with a 9-mm clip. The lower pole has been exposed and the operator is separating the upper pole from the adrenal gland.

upper and lower AAL ports, and placed over the anterior surface of the upper and lower poles of the kidney respectively. The assistant is now able to retract the kidney laterally, thereby exerting mild traction on the renal hilum. The renal artery and renal vein are separately dissected and ligated with 9-mm titanium clips (three clips on the proximal "stump" end and two clips on the distal "specimen" end) and cut. The dissection of the vessels is again done with the surgeon working with a grasper and electrosurgical scissors passed through the MCL cannulas. Curved grasping forceps can be extremely helpful in clearing the vessels of surrounding tissue. In the child less than 10 years old, the renal vein as well as the renal artery can usually be secured individually with 9-mm clips (Figure 11–3). In the older child, however, a 12-mm laparoscopic vascular stapler (Endo-GIA 30 tissue stapler, U.S. Surgical Corporation, Norwalk, CT) may be needed to occlude and divide the broad renal vein.

Next, the catheter or guidewire is removed from the ureter and the ureter is secured with two clips and cut. The cut ureter is grasped at the ureteropelvic junction (UPJ) with a 5-mm locking traumatic grasper passed via the upper AAL port. The kidney is displaced into the upper abdomen (Figure 11–4).

An impermeable nylon Lapsac is introduced through the 12-mm MCL cannula. The sack is pulled into the abdomen with two atraumatic graspers passed via the lower AAL and lower MCL ports (Figure 11–5). Then the laparoscope is moved to the upper MCL port. Three 5-mm traumatic locking grasping forceps are passed via the umbilical, lower MCL, and lower AAL ports. A grasper is placed onto each of the three tabs on the neck of the sack, which allows the first assistant and surgeon to triangulate open the mouth of the sack. The laparoscope is then passed into the sack and moved in ever-widening circles to open the sack wider. The first assistant uses the upper AAL

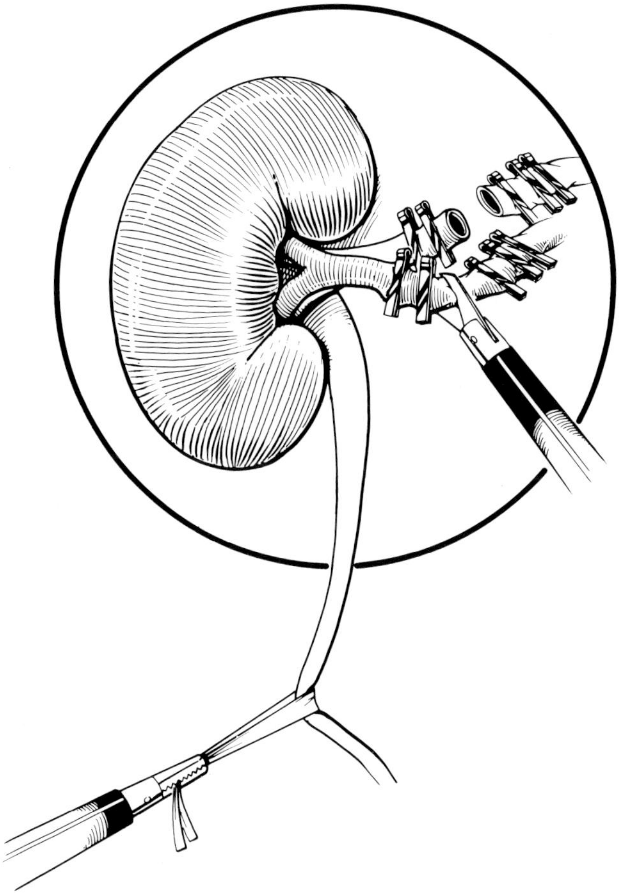

Figure 11–3. The renal artery has been secured with five 9-mm titanium clips and transected so that three clips remain on the stump of the renal artery. The renal vein is also secured with five, 9-mm titanium clips. If the vein is too broad for the 9-mm clips, then a vascular stapler can be used to occlude and transect the renal vein.

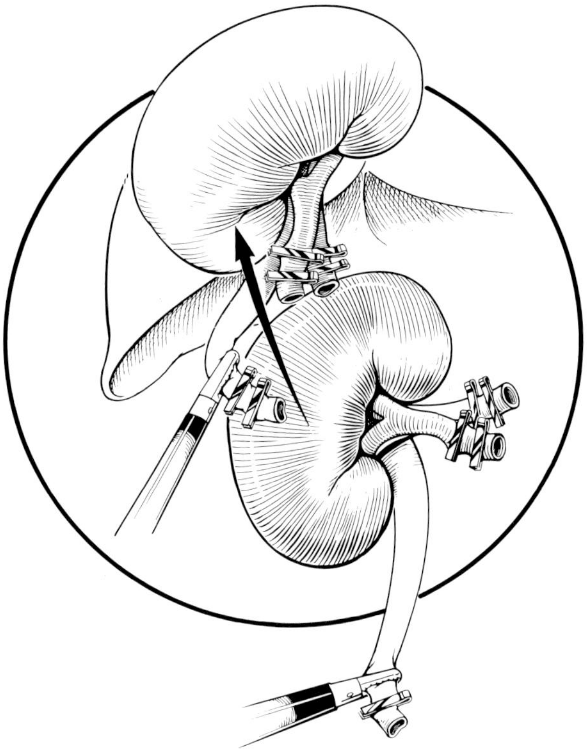

Figure 11–4. The ureteral catheter has been removed and the middle portion of the ureter has been clipped and transected. A traumatic locking grasping forceps has been passed via the upper anterior axillary line port, and the proximal ureter has been grasped and secured. In this case, the right kidney is now transported cephalad until it lies on the anterior surface of the liver.

traumatic grasper, which is still locked onto the proximal ureter, to move the kidney into the open sack (Figure 11–6). With the kidney in the sack, the locking forceps is released and withdrawn from the UPJ. The drawstrings of the sack are delivered into but not through the 12-mm umbilical port using the grasper, thereby closing the sack on the kidney.

The intraabdominal pressure is lowered to 5 mm Hg, and the operative bed and the renal vascular pedicle are carefully examined for hemostasis. Special at-

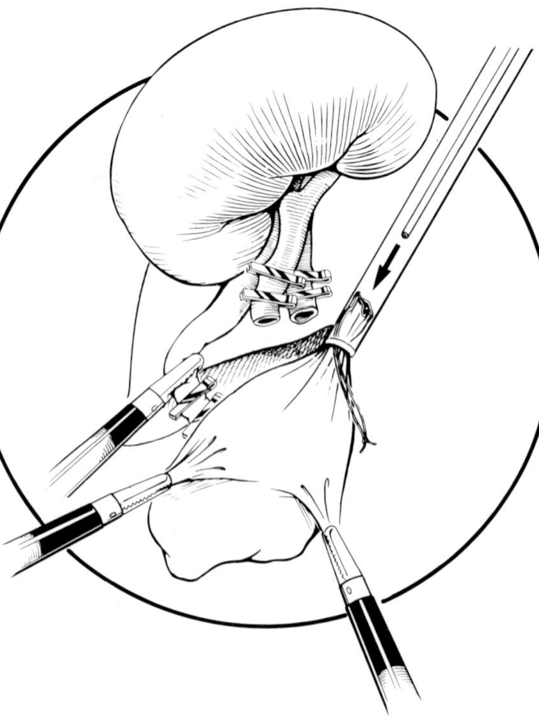

Figure 11–5. A 5 × 8-in. entrapment sack (Lapsac) is introduced via the upper 12-mm midclavicular line port. It is pulled into the abdomen using *atraumatic* grasping forceps.

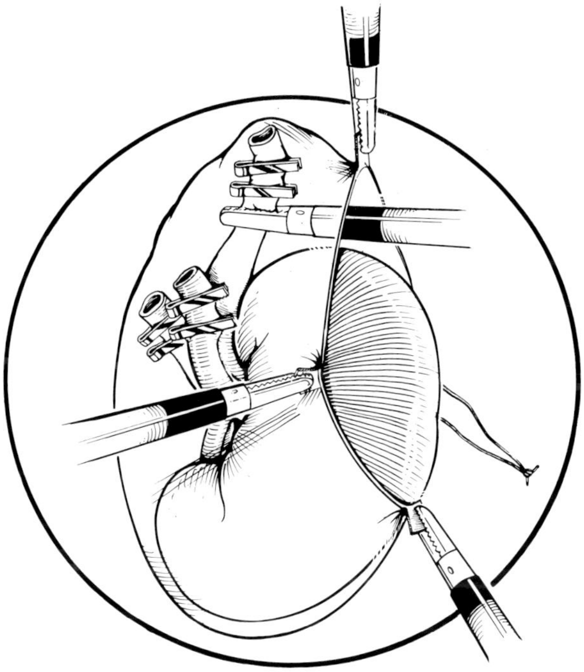

Figure 11–6. A 5-mm *traumatic*, locking grasping forceps is passed via the umbilical, lower midclavicular, and lower anterior axillary line ports. These three graspers are used to secure each of the three tabs on the sack so the mouth of the sack can be triangulated open. The kidney is then manipulated into the open sack, using the locking, traumatic grasper attached to the proximal ureter to lead the kidney into the sack.

tention is directed to the area of the adrenal gland to ensure that there is no bleeding from the edge of the gland.

Next, the patient is returned to a supine position. The drawstrings are pulled through the 12-mm umbilical cannula and the cannula is then removed (Figure 11–7). The drawstrings should now lie on the abdominal wall and the drawstrings are pulled upward, thereby delivering the neck of the sack onto the abdominal wall. The surgeon and first assistant now hold the neck of the sack and lift the sack firmly so the kidney is trapped against the anterior peritoneum. There should not be any folds in the sack when viewed with the laparoscope. The barrel of the 10-mm electri-

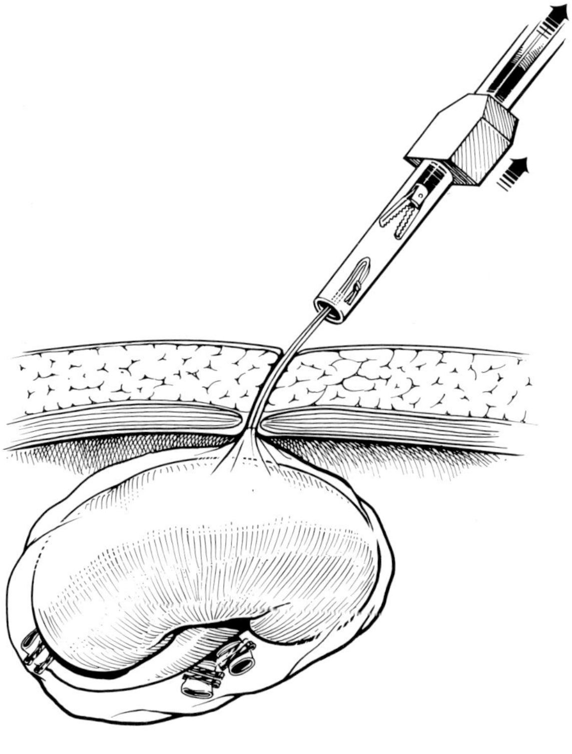

Figure 11–7. The drawstrings on the sack are delivered via the grasper passed through the umbilical port. The umbilical sheath is then withdrawn from the abdomen, and the drawstrings are grasped by the surgeon and pulled further through the abdominal wall until the neck of the sack is delivered through the incision. The kidney is now ready to be fragmented within the sack.

cal tissue morcellator is introduced into the sack and pushed firmly into the renal tissue. Wall suction is applied to the handle, and the surgeon activates the recessed rotary blade by using the foot pedal. Throughout the morcellation process, the morcellator is moved back and forth through the renal tissue, with each advance of the morcellator being in a different direction. If a high-speed electrical tissue morcellator is not available, the entrapped kidney can be fragmented and removed using a ring forceps. The sack, when emptied of the renal tissue, is then withdrawn from the abdomen.

The entire abdomen is again carefully inspected for bowel injury and the intraabdominal pressure is lowered to 5 mm Hg to assess hemostasis. A 5-mm laparoscope is introduced into one of the 5-mm ports. The 12-mm ports and the two 5-mm ports are removed under endoscopic visualization to search for any port-site bleeding. The final 5-mm port is pulled backward onto the shaft of the 5-mm laparoscope. The laparoscope is slowly withdrawn from the abdomen while inspecting the tissues of the abdominal wall for bleeding. All cannula sites are closed with fascial absorbable sutures; the skin is approximated using adhesive skin strips. The 12-mm port sites are also closed with a subcuticular 4-O absorbable suture.

Laparoscopic Nephroureterectomy

In performing a nephroureterectomy, the surgeon follows the same steps as for laparoscopic nephrectomy. The only difference is that the middle portion of the ureter is not incised, as the entire ureter must be dissected to the level of the bladder. For this reason, a sixth port is placed: a 12-mm midline, suprapubic can-

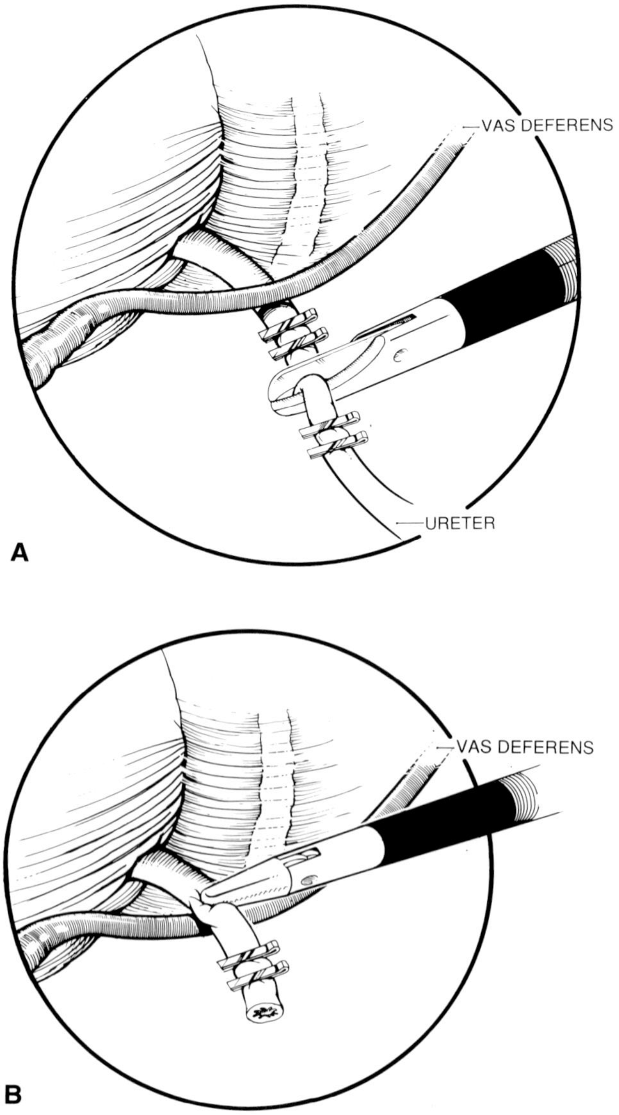

Figure 11–8. The vas deferens is preserved during nephroureterectomy: **A.** The distal ureter is clipped securely and divided. **B.** The distal ureter is then transposed anterior to the vas deferens, and the ureterovesical junction is rolled anteriorly for exposure.

nula. The procedure begins with dissection of the distal ureter. An incision is made medial to the ipsilateral medial umbilical ligament. The ipsilateral medial umbilical ligament and the superior vesical artery are each secured with two pairs of 9-mm clips and divided. In the male, the vas deferens is preserved. To preserve the vas deferens, it may be necessary to remove the ureteral catheter and divide the lower ureter between a pair of 9-mm clips; the distal ureteral stump can then be brought in front of the vas deferens so the ureterovesical junction can be rolled anteriorly (Figure 11–8). In the female, the round ligament can be secured with two pairs of clips and incised, thereby precluding any preliminary division of the ureter.

A 4-in. piece of umbilical tape is placed around the middle of the ureter as was previously described in the technique for nephrectomy. The ureter is then dissected cephalad to the level of the ureteropelvic junction. The rest of the nephrectomy procedure is as previously described, except that the ureter is not divided until later in the procedure.

If the child is of sufficient size, the flexible cystoscope or flexible ureteroscope can be introduced per urethra, and the rest of the procedure for securing a cuff of bladder can be performed under cystoscopic visualization to be certain that no damage occurs to the contralateral ureteral orifice and to ensure that the entire length of ureter is safely secured within the jaws of the stapler.

The Endo-GIA tissue stapler is introduced through the suprapubic 12-mm port. The ureteral occlusion balloon catheter and guidewire are removed. The jaws of the Endo-GIA stapler are opened and are carefully slid around the ureterovesical junction (Figure 11–9A). Upward traction on the ureter can be exerted with an atraumatic 5-mm forceps passed through the lower MCL port. The bladder immediately below the Endo-GIA stapler can be stabilized and pushed somewhat medially using a 5-mm grasper passed through the lower AAL port. This will help to feed the bladder into the Endo-GIA stapler and ensure that the bladder cuff is taken just below the ureterovesical junction, thereby ensuring the completeness of the ureterectomy. When the jaws of the Endo-GIA stapler are closed, the tissue to be incised must lie proximal to the "cut" mark on both jaws of the Endo-GIA stapler (Figure 11–9B). The trigger lock is released and the handles of the Endo-

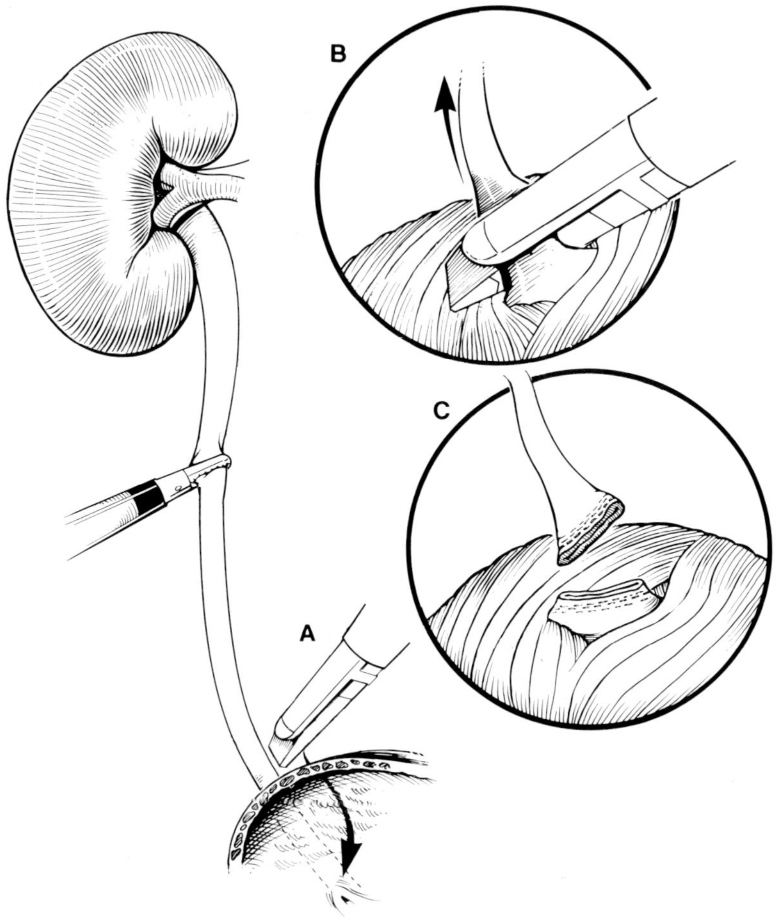

Figure 11–9. Ureterovesical ligation and division in a female child. The distal ureter has not been divided as described for a male patient (Figure 11–8). **A.** The ureter is pulled cephalad and anterior, thereby exposing the ureterovesical junction. **B.** The jaws of the Endo-GIA stapler are placed just below the ureterovesical junction and then closed around the cuff of bladder. The stapler is fired, the jaws are opened, and the stapler is removed from the surgical field. **C.** The cuff of bladder is closed with three rows of titanium staples.

TABLE 11–3. EXPERIENCE WITH LAPAROSCOPIC NEPHRECTOMY IN CHILDREN AT WASHINGTON UNIVERSITY AND BOSTON CHILDREN'S HOSPITAL

Patient	Age	Sex	Underlying Disease	Side	Operative Time	Estimated Blood Loss	Kidney Weight or Length
M.P.	17 y	F	Nonfunctioning, chronically infected kidney	R	290 min	150 mL	88 g
L.W.	16 y	F	Nonfunctioning, chronically infected kidney	R	265 min	100 mL	275 g
N.B.	8 m	M	Multicystic dysplastic kidney	R	55 min	Minimal	5 cm
J.H.	12 m	M	UPJ obstruction; nonfunctioning, chronically infected kidney	L	230 min	<25 mL	3 cm
P.T.	14 m	M	Multicystic dysplastic kidney	R	155 min	Minimal	6 cm

POD, postoperative day. UPJ, ureteropelvic junction.

GIA stapler are firmly apposed, thereby firing the six 3-cm-long rows of staples into the bladder and simultaneously cutting the cuff of bladder between the third and fourth rows of staples. The jaws of the Endo-GIA stapler are then opened and the stapler is removed from the site of the bladder cuff (Figure 11–9C). The bladder can then be filled via the Foley urethral catheter or cystoscope to rule out extravasation. The jaws of the Endo-GIA stapler are then closed and the stapler is withdrawn from the abdomen. The intraabdominal pressure is lowered to 5 mm Hg, and the bladder area and upper abdomen are thoroughly inspected for hemostasis.

The patient is returned to a supine position. The nephroureterectomy specimen can now be entrapped in a surgical sack as previously described. The specimen can be morcellated and removed via the suprapubic 12-mm port site. This part of the procedure is again completed under endoscopic control.

On completion of the procedure, the intraperitoneal pressure is again lowered to 5 mm Hg to search for any undetected venous bleeding. Lastly, all the ports are removed under optical control and the incisions closed as previously discussed.

COMPLICATIONS

Complications may occur intraoperatively (hypotension, gas embolus, hypertension, dysrhythmias, hypercarbia, hypoxemia, pneumothorax, vascular injury, or perforation of a viscus) or postoperatively (fever, peritonitis, azotemia, hernia, delayed hemorrhage). Complications of diagnostic laparoscopy are detailed in Chapter 2. As this is an extensive laparoscopic procedure, intestinal injury may occur but not be recognized at the time of the procedure. Perforation of a hollow viscus can be handled laparoscopically using intracorporeal suturing and knot-tying techniques; however, if there is any doubt as to the adequacy of the laparoscopic repair, then a formal laparotomy should be performed with appropriate tissue approximation. For a major vascular injury, open laparotomy and repair by a vascular surgeon are recommended.

Postoperatively, the development of increasing abdominal pain may be the first sign of a bowel perforation and associated peritonitis. Likewise, the development of postoperative fever should alert the surgeon to the possibility of a "missed" bowel perforation. It is noteworthy that a bowel perforation caused by a monopolar electrocautery injury may not develop for 5 days from the time of the procedure.

POSTOPERATIVE CARE

Oral intake is usually initiated 6 hours after the operation. Oral analgesics should suffice for pain control. On occasion the child may experience severe diaphragmatic and shoulder pain immediately following the laparoscopic procedure, usually as a result of diaphragmatic irritation from carbon dioxide. This discomfort can be controlled with parenteral narcotic analgesics and usually abates within 6 to 10 hours of the procedure.

THE WASHINGTON UNIVERSITY AND BOSTON CHILDREN'S HOSPITAL EXPERIENCES

We have performed laparoscopic nephrectomy in two adolescents (16 and 17 years) and three infants (8, 12, and 14 months).[31,32] The indications were a nonfunctioning chronically infected kidney (two cases), multicystic dysplastic kidney (two cases), and ureteropelvic junction obstruction and nonfunctioning kidney (one case) (Table 11–3). The average operative time was 109 minutes, and the mean postoperative hospital stay was 1.8 days. Our two adolescent patients returned to their usual activities after 1 week. No intraoperative or postoperative complications have developed. Similar results have recently been reported by Ehrlich and associates.[33] To date, we have completed

Pathologic Diagnosis Normal	Oral Intake	Amount of Analgesics Used	Postoperative Hospital Stay	Return to Activities
Nephrosclerosis	POD 1[b]	22 mg morphine IV	2 d	7 d
Nephrosclerosis, chronic inflammation	POD 1	10 mg morphine IV	3 d	7 d
Multicystic dysplastic kidney	After 12 h	None	<1 d	24 h
Dysplastic kidney	POD 1	1.6 mg morphine IV	2 d	Within 1 wk
Multicystic dysplastic kidney	POD 1	1 mg morphine IV	1 d	Within 1 wk

one laparoscopic nephroureterectomy in a 5-year-old girl; we are aware of two other cases being completed (S. Das; personal communication, 1992).

SUMMARY

The development of laparoscopic nephrectomy and laparoscopic nephroureterectomy is only one part of the overall surgical trend that has strongly emerged during the past decade under the general heading of "minimally invasive surgery." Although these less invasive procedures can be of great benefit to the patient, two critical areas need to be continuously addressed by the surgeon. First, there is a significant learning curve associated with these newer laparoscopic procedures; as such, it is essential for each surgeon to have proper training and clinical experience with these newer techniques to become facile in their performance. Second, these newer procedures, although initially exciting, must be carefully scrutinized and compared against their known open surgical counterparts. Only in this manner will the surgical community be able to judge whether a given "new" procedure is, indeed, an advance.

REFERENCES

1. Gans SL, Berci G. Peritoneoscopy in infants and children. *J Pediatr Surg.* 1973;8:399.
2. Cortesi N, Ferrari P, Zambarda E, et al. Diagnosis of bilateral abdominal cryptorchidism by laparoscopy. *Endoscopy.* 1976;8:33.
3. Silber SJ, Cohen R. Laparoscopy for cryptorchidism. *J Urol.* 1980;124:928.
4. Hamidinia A, Nold S, Amankwah KS. Localization and treatment of nonpalpable testes. *Surg Gynecol Obstet.* 1984;159:439.
5. Manson AL, Terhune D, Jordan G, et al. Preoperative laparoscopic localization of the nonpalpable testis. *J Urol.* 1985;134:919.
6. Scott JES. Laparoscopy as an aid in the diagnosis and management of impalpable testes. *J Pediatr Surg.* 1986;17:14.
7. Wright JE. Impalpable testes: A review of 100 boys. *J Pediatr Surg.* 1986;21:151.
8. Scott JES. Laparoscopy as an aid in the diagnosis and management of impalpable testes. *J Pediatr Surg.* 1986;17:14.
9. Weiss RM, Seashore JH. Laparoscopy in the management of the nonpalpable testis. *J Urol.* 1987;138:382.
10. Guiney EJ, Corbally M, Malone PS. Laparoscopy and the management of the impalpable testis. *Br J Urol.* 1988;63:313.
11. Bloom DA, Ayers JWT, McGuire EJ. The role of laparoscopy in management of nonpalpable testes. *J Urologie.* 1988;94:465.
12. Doig CM. Use of laparoscopy in children with impalpable testes. *Int J Androl.* 1989;12:420.
13. Naslund MJ, Gearhart JP, Jeffs RD. Laparoscopy: Its selected use in patients with unilateral nonpalpable testis after human chorionic gonadotropin stimulation. *J Urol.* 1989;142:108.
14. Donovan JF, Winfield HN. Laparoscopic varix ligation. *J Urol.* 1991;145:325A.
15. Donovan JF, Winfield HN. Laparoscopic varix ligation. *J Urol.* 1992;147:77.
16. Mehan DJ, Hagod PG, Worischeck JH, et al. Laparoscopic varicocelectomy: Preliminary report of a new technique, Part I. *J Urol.* 1991;145:242A.
17. Hagod PG, Mehan DJ, Worischeck JH, et al. Laparoscopic varicocelectomy: Preliminary report of a new technique. *J Urol.* 1992;147:73.
18. Schuessler WW, Vancaillie TG, Reich H, et al. Transperitoneal endosurgical lymphadenectomy in patients with localized prostate cancer. *J Urol.* 1991;145:988.
19. Winfield HN, See WA, Donovan JF, et al. A new cancer staging technique: Laparoscopic pelvic node dissection. *J Urol.* 1991;145:215A.
20. Winfield HW, Kavoussi LR. Laparoscopic lymphadenectomy. *Curr Surg Techn Urol.* 1991;4:2.
21. Kavoussi LR, Clayman RV. Organ entrapment system for removing nodal tissue during laparoscopic lymphadenectomy. *J Urol.* 1992;147:879.
22. Clayman RV, Kavoussi LR, Soper NJ, et al. Laparoscopic nephrectomy (letter) *N Engl J Med.* 1991;324:1370.
23. Clayman RV, Kavoussi LR, Soper NJ, et al. Laparoscopic nephrectomy: Initial case report. *J Urol.* 1991;146:278.
24. Clayman RV, Kavoussi LR, McDougall EM, et al. Laparoscopic nephrectomy: A review of 16 cases. *Surg Laparosc Endosc.* 1992;2:29.

25. Kerbl K, Figenshau RS, Clayman RV, et al. Retroperitoneal laparoscopic nephrectomy: Laboratory and clinical experience. *J Endourol.* 1993;7:23.
26. Clayman RV, Kavoussi LR, Long SR, et al. Laparoscopic nephrectomy: Initial report of pelviscopic organ ablation in the pig. *J Endourol.* 1990;4:247.
27. Figenshau RS, Albala DM, Clayman RV, et al. Laparoscopic nephroureterectomy: Initial laboratory experience. *Minimally Invasive Ther.* 1991;1:93.
28. McDougall EM, Clayman RV, Chandhoke PS, et al. Laparoscopic partial nephrectomy in the pig model. *J Urol.* 1993;149:1633.
29. Winfield HN, Donovan JF, Godet AS, Clayman RV. Human laparoscopic partial nephrectomy—Case report. *J Endourol.* 1992;6:59.
30. Clayman RV, McDougall EM, Chandhoke PS, et al. Laparoscopic ureteral reimplantation: Laboratory studies. *J Endourol.* 1992;6:S144.
31. Peters CA, Kavoussi LR, Retik AB. Laparoscopic nephrectomy in the infant. *J Urol.* 1993;149:189A.
32. Koyle MA, Woo HH, Kavoussi LR. Laparoscopic nephrectomy in the first year of life. *J Pediatr Surg.* in press.
33. Ehrlich RM, Gershman A, Fuchs G. Laparoscopic nephrectomy in a child: Expanding horizons for laparoscopy in pediatric urology. *J Endourol.* 1992;6:463.

CHAPTER 12

Thoracoscopy

BRADLEY M. RODGERS

The technique of thoracoscopy was first described by Jacobaeus, a Swedish Internist, in 1912.[1] He described the use of a cystoscope to visualize and lyse the adhesions in the pleural space in patients with pulmonary tuberculosis who were being subjected to collapse therapy. The technique proved to be very useful in this patient population and was used extensively in Europe and in the United States until effective antituberculous drug therapy became available in the 1950s. Jacobaeus later described the use of these instruments for biopsy of pleural lesions in a small number of patients, but this aspect of the technique did not gain widespread interest until the past decade when interest in endoscopic surgery stimulated the development of better instrumentation.[2] Although some children and adolescents were included in the large numbers of "closed intrapleural pneumonolysis" procedures performed for tuberculosis, there were no reviews evaluating the use of this technique in this particular patient population. Klimkovich et al were probably the first to describe the use of diagnostic thoracoscopy specifically in children.[3] In 1971, they reported on 43 children (aged 1 month to 14 years) in whom thoracoscopy had been performed for diagnosis. The clinical details of these patients are sketchy, and it is not clear whether complications were encountered or how helpful was the procedure. The modern era of thoracoscopy in children was introduced in 1976 with our description of pulmonary biopsy in 9 patients (aged 17 months to 15 years) with undiagnosed intrathoracic disease.[4] There were no significant complications in these patients and the diagnostic accuracy was 100%. Since that publication, several other reports have outlined the spectrum of utility of this procedure in the pediatric population.[5–8]

A review of reports in which thoracoscopic procedures performed in children can be identified clearly reveals significant differences in the indications for the procedure in children compared with those encountered in series of adult patients (Figures 12–1 and 12–2). The most common indication for thoracoscopy in the pediatric population has been for biopsy or resection of mediastinal and hilar masses. In the adult population, however, the most common indication for the procedure remains the diagnosis and treatment of idiopathic pleural effusions. The other common indications for thoracoscopy in children include biopsy of diffuse and localized pulmonary infiltrates, debridement and irrigation of pleural empyema, and bleb resection and pleurodesis for spontaneous pneumothorax. Many new and innovative uses of thoracoscopy have been discussed in the adult literature, but have yet to be reported as useful in children. Potentially, the most useful of these newer procedures for children appear to be creation of a pericardial window for pericardial effusion, esophagomyotomy for achalasia, and evaluation of the extent of injury in blunt and penetrating chest trauma.[9–11]

TECHNIQUE

The precise technique and instrumentation for thoracoscopy vary considerably depending on the size of the patient and the indication for the procedure. In general, a wider range of instrumentation is necessary for pediatric thoracoscopy than for similar procedures in the adult, and experience with all of these instruments is essential before undertaking this procedure. Moreover, none of these procedures should be performed by individuals who are not skilled in performing similar procedures by open thoracotomy. Thoracoscopy should be considered a true operative procedure. These cases should be performed in the operating room, where equipment and personnel are available to handle any potential complication.

Visualization of the intrathoracic pathology by thoracoscopy depends on the ability to establish an adequate pneumothorax to provide room for observation. Establishing and maintaining this pneumothorax

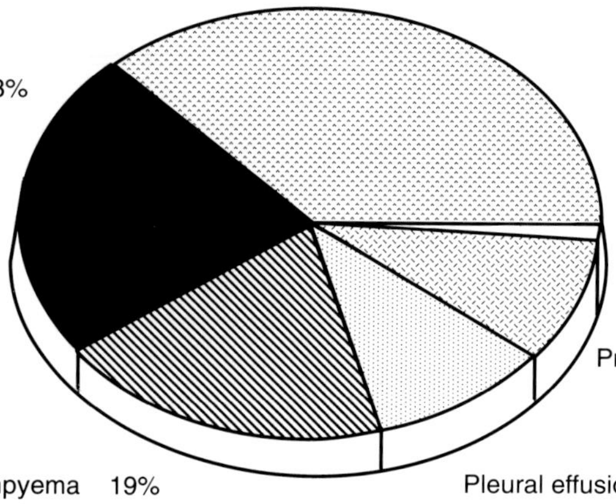

Figure 12–1. Indications for thoracoscopy in children since 1982 at the University of Virginia Health Sciences Center.

may be more difficult in children than in adults, and careful analysis of preoperative imaging studies becomes critically important in planning these operations in children. At a minimum, frontal and lateral chest roentgenograms should be obtained to localize the areas to be approached. In many cases, transthoracic ultrasound, chest computed tomography (CT) or magnetic resonance imaging (MRI) studies will further define the anatomic relationships involved. We have found transthoracic ultrasonography to be especially useful in patients with pleural effusions or empyemas to define the extent of the pleural fluid and to locate the largest locule. The positioning of the patient on the operating table is also more crucial for thoracoscopy than for open procedures and must be carefully considered prior to beginning the operation.

There are several important general considerations in performing these procedures in small patients, irrespective of the specific indication (Table 12–1). A complete thoracotomy tray should be available, although not necessarily unwrapped, in the operating room during the thoracoscopy. Adequate intravenous access must be obtained prior to starting the procedure. Although bleeding has not been a significant complication in our series, it has been described in adult patients and, at least theoretically, could be a major concern in children. The chest should be prepped and draped widely so as to allow for progression to an open thoracotomy if this should become necessary. Special care must be exercised to maintain

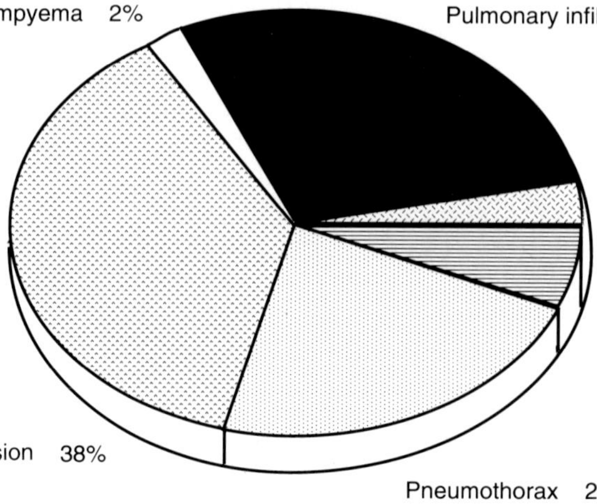

Figure 12–2. Compared with indications for children, indications for thoracoscopy differ in adults seen since 1982 at the University of Virginia Health Sciences Center (see Figure 12–1).

TABLE 12–1. GENERAL CONSIDERATIONS FOR THORACOSCOPY IN CHILDREN

Adequate intravenous access
Widely prepped and draped field
Maintenance of body temperature
Attention to careful padding in lateral decubitus position
Complete thoracotomy tray available in operating room

the patient's body temperature in the operating room, using overhead heaters and heating mattresses as appropriate. The patients should be carefully padded when placed in the lateral decubitus position to prevent injury to the skin.

The decision regarding the type of anesthesia to be employed for thoracoscopy depends to a great extent on the age of the patient and the anticipated procedure (see Chapter 18). Adequate anesthesia of the parietal pleura can be achieved with a multiple-rib intercostal nerve block, and some degree of analgesia from the pain of stimulation of the visceral pleura can be obtained with suitable intravenous sedation. For simpler procedures involving minimal manipulation within the pleural space, such as lung biopsy, regional anesthetic techniques with supplemental sedation may be sufficient.[7] The pain of more extensive and prolonged manipulation of the visceral pleura, however, as might be experienced by retraction of the lung for exposure of a mediastinal mass or for application of the Endo-GIA stapler (U.S. Surgical Corporation, Norwalk, CT), is more difficult to eliminate with sedation, and the use of general anesthesia is preferred in this setting. Even when general anesthesia is employed, it is useful to add a multiple-rib intercostal nerve block to anesthetize the area of trocar insertion, as this often allows a lighter level of anesthesia to be maintained during the procedure. For procedures involving extensive and lengthy exposure of mediastinal structures, unilateral ventilation has proven to be extremely helpful. This allows for complete collapse of the ipsilateral lung and facilitates wide exposure of the mediastinum. Unilateral ventilation, however, is not well tolerated by infants and children under the age of 2 years, presumably because of their limited functional residual capacity. Many of these patients become hypoxic even with a fraction of inspired oxygen of 1.00. A suitable ipsilateral pneumothorax can usually be maintained if the patient is allowed to breathe spontaneously and if excessive positive-pressure ventilation is avoided.

Surgeons performing thoracoscopy in children must have a broad range of instrumentation available. Three different sizes of telescopes and cannulas may be used, depending on the size of the individual patient. For patients under 2 years of age the 3.75-mm cannula and 0-degree telescope are used. The 5.0-mmcannula and telescope combination may be used for patients between the ages of 2 and 8 years. For older patients, the 10-mm cannula and telescope provide the best lighting and visibility. It should rarely be necessary to employ intrapleural gas insufflation to achieve an adequate pneumothorax in children; therefore, the valve assemblies found in the laparoscopic cannulas are not necessary. Several manufacturers now make an unvalved cannula for use in thoracoscopy and these are quite convenient for pediatric use (Figure 12–3). The 0-degree telescope optics should be sufficient for most intrathoracic work, although some authors have described using the 30-degree optics for visualizing the superior pulmonary hilum and the region of the inferior pulmonary ligament in adults. Working instruments must be able to pass through both the 3.75-mm cannula and the 5-mm cannula, although the 5-mm port will be used for the majority of these cases. The instruments should be properly insulated so that the cautery may be connected to them. Reusable instruments maintained on the thoracoscopy tray at the University of Virginia are listed in Table 12–2. Several instruments have been particularly useful for pediatric procedures. Fine-pointed, curved dissecting forceps (5 and 10 mm) are useful for retracting the parietal pleura and bluntly dissecting mediastinal lymph nodes. The disposable endoscopic scissors (5 mm) and hook cautery device (5 mm) are helpful for opening the mediastinal pleura and for coagulating small vessels. An endoscopic Allis clamp (5 mm) may be used to gently retract the lung, and larger (10-mm) Babcock and Duval clamps are available for grasping

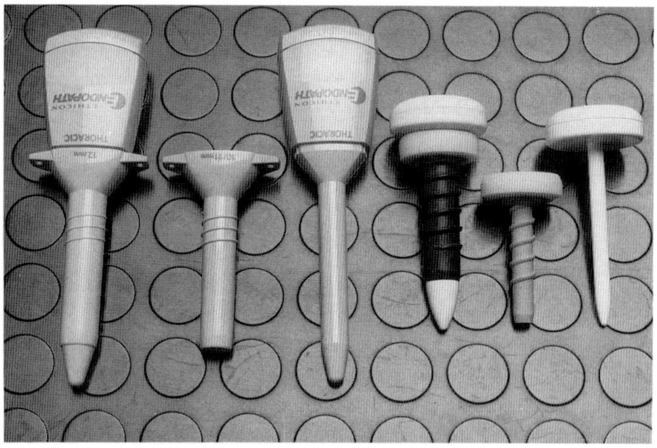

Figure 12–3. Thoracoscopic cannulas differ from laparoscopic ports. For example, the trocar does not have a sharp stylette with a retractable sleeve. In addition, one-way valves are not needed in the cannulas to prevent escape of carbon dioxide, as a pneumothorax is created naturally with the open cannula. On the *left* are thoracic cannulas made by Ethicon, Inc, and on the *right* are Thoracoports manufactured by U.S. Surgical Corporation.

TABLE 12–2. INSTRUMENTS CONSTITUTING THE THORACOSCOPIC TRAY AT THE UNIVERSITY OF VIRGINIA

2	metal cannulas (5 mm)
2	metal cannulas (3.5 mm)
3	cup biopsy forceps (insulated) (3.5 and 5 mm)
1	ratcheted grasping forceps (insulated) (5 mm)
2	dissecting forceps (insulated) (5 mm)
1	Allis tissue forceps (insulated) (5 mm)
2	Babcock tissue forceps (insulated) (5 and 10 mm)
1	stone forceps (10 mm)
1	hook scissors (insulated) (5 mm)
1	microscissors (insulated) (5 mm)
1	endoscopic needle
1	blunt probe (3.5 mm)
1	talc insufflator assembly
1	endoloop sleeve

the lung itself. Several types of fan lung retractors are available (5 and 10 mm), none of which are entirely satisfactory. The endoscopic clip applier, which passes through a 10-mm cannula, may be used for dividing larger intrathoracic vessels. The Endo-GIA stapling instrument, which passes through a 12-mm port, is useful for performing wedge biopsies and resecting bullae from the lung. This instrument places a 3-cm row of staples, and cartridges are available for vascular and tissue use. The instrument is cumbersome to use in smaller children, however, as 5 cm of the distal instrument must be within the chest to open the anvil. Therefore, it is important that this instrument be passed through a cannula placed as far caudally in the chest as possible to allow maximum intrathoracic manipulation.

At the conclusion of the operation the accessory cannulas are removed under direct visualization from within the chest to be certain that there is no bleeding through the cannula tracts. A suitably sized chest tube is inserted through one of these tracts and guided into appropriate position with the telescope. The posterior cannula site is used for placement of a small epidural catheter, which is used for postoperative pain relief. This catheter is manipulated into the posterior pleural gutter with the end of the thoracoscopy telescope. The telescope and its cannulas are removed last, observing this site for bleeding. This site and the other tracts are closed in layers using absorbable suture, and the chest tube and pleural catheter are secured to the skin with monofilament nylon. The chest tube is connected to 10 cm of underwater suction. A postoperative chest roentgenogram is obtained to ensure complete expansion of the ipsilateral lung and complete evacuation of fluid within that hemithorax. Daily chest roentgenograms are obtained while the chest tube is in place. The tube is placed to underwater seal without suction for 24 hours once it has stopped draining air and fluid and is then removed. Intrapleural analgesia is achieved postoperatively with 0.25% bupivacaine with epinephrine (0.75 mL/kg every 4 to 6 hours). As the positions of the ends of the pleural catheter and chest tube are separate, it is not necessary to clamp the chest tube when administering intrapleural bupivacaine. This catheter is usually removed at the time of removal of the chest tube, although occasionally it is left in place for a longer period. In cases in which the visceral pleura is not violated, the chest tube is usually removed on the day following surgery, and the patient may be discharged as soon as a chest roentgenogram confirms full expansion of the lung.

INDICATIONS

Mediastinal Masses

Thoracoscopy is most commonly performed in pediatric patients for the diagnosis or treatment of mediastinal masses. The involvement of anterior hilar and superior mediastinal lymph nodes with lymphomas, and chronic inflammation in children makes this technique particularly suited for diagnostic biopsies. With development of newer instrumentation, hilar and peritracheal cysts, such as bronchogenic cysts, may be completely dissected and removed with thoracoscopic techniques.[6,12] The utility of thoracoscopy in the management of posterior mediastinal masses remains to be fully explored. The majority of these lesions in children represent neurogenic tumors, and it is uncertain whether an adequate cancer resection can be performed for these lesions with this technique. On the other hand, posterior hilar lesions and posterior mediastinal lymphadenopathy can be readily visualized by thoracoscopy and a reliable diagnosis can be obtained.

Nowhere in pediatric thoracoscopy is precise preoperative imaging more important than in the approach to mediastinal lesions. Unlike an open thoracotomy, the exposure of the mediastinal lesions by thoracoscopy is dependent on the proper angulation of the telescope and operating instruments. In addition to standard frontal and lateral chest roentgenograms, chest CT or MRI scans provide critical anatomic information and define the relationships of the pathology to surrounding structures (Figure 12–4). These relationships dictate the proper position of the patient and the cannula sites for these procedures. In approaching anterior mediastinal masses, it is useful to tilt the patient 30 degrees posterior to a full lateral decubitus position (Figure 12–5). Likewise, for posterior mediastinal masses, rotating anteriorly 30 degrees provides a wider exposure. The discomfort from the manipulation required to expose most mediastinal lesions is difficult to ablate with regional anesthetic tech-

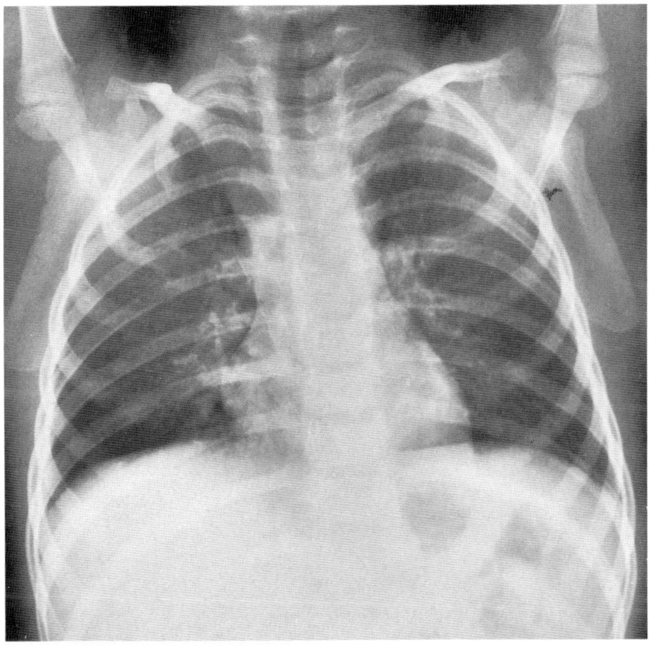

A

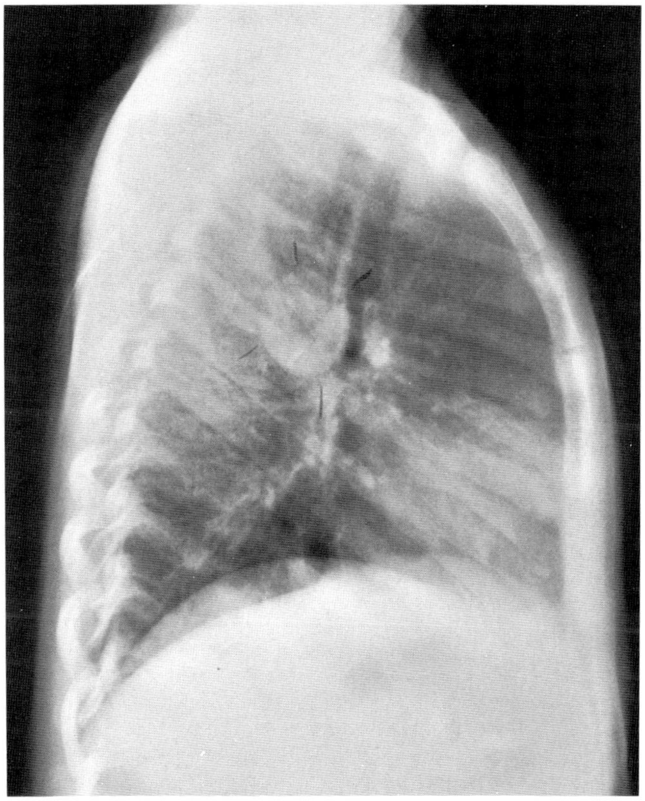

B

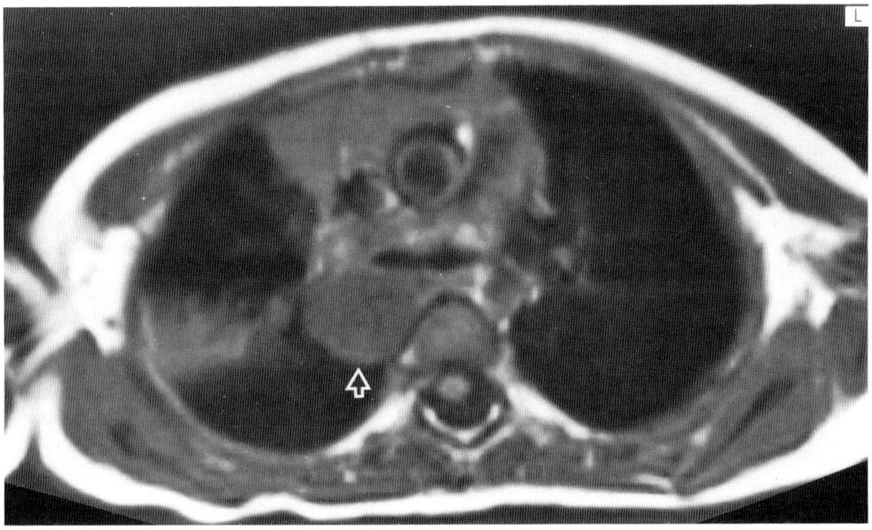

C

Figure 12–4. Frontal **(A)** and lateral **(B)** radiographs of a 3-year-old child with cough and fever show a well-circumscribed paratracheal lesion. **(C)** The MRI scan demonstrates that the lesion (*arrow*) has a uniform density and is located posterolateral to the trachea and carina. Atelectasis in the right middle lobe is also seen. This child underwent complete thoracoscopic resection of a bronchogenic cyst.

niques. Therefore, for the majority of mediastinal procedures, general anesthesia is preferred. The use of unilateral ventilation in older children allows the ipsilateral lung to be completely collapsed and maximizes both anterior and posterior exposure. With total collapse of the ipsilateral lung, the operating table can be rolled into an exaggerated position to use gravity to further expose the lesion to be approached. Successful dissection of mediastinal masses requires adequate visualization of the lesion and surrounding structures and therefore requires that the tip of the telescope be maintained at a modest distance from the lesion for maximum visibility. The initial telescope and cannula should be inserted slightly posterior to the midaxillary line for the approach to anterior mediastinal and hilar lesions (Figure 12–6) and slightly anterior to the midaxillary line for the approach to posterior lesions (Figure 12–7). Entry through the sixth intercostal space allows both cephalad and caudad visibility. The subcutaneous tract for cannula insertion should be made

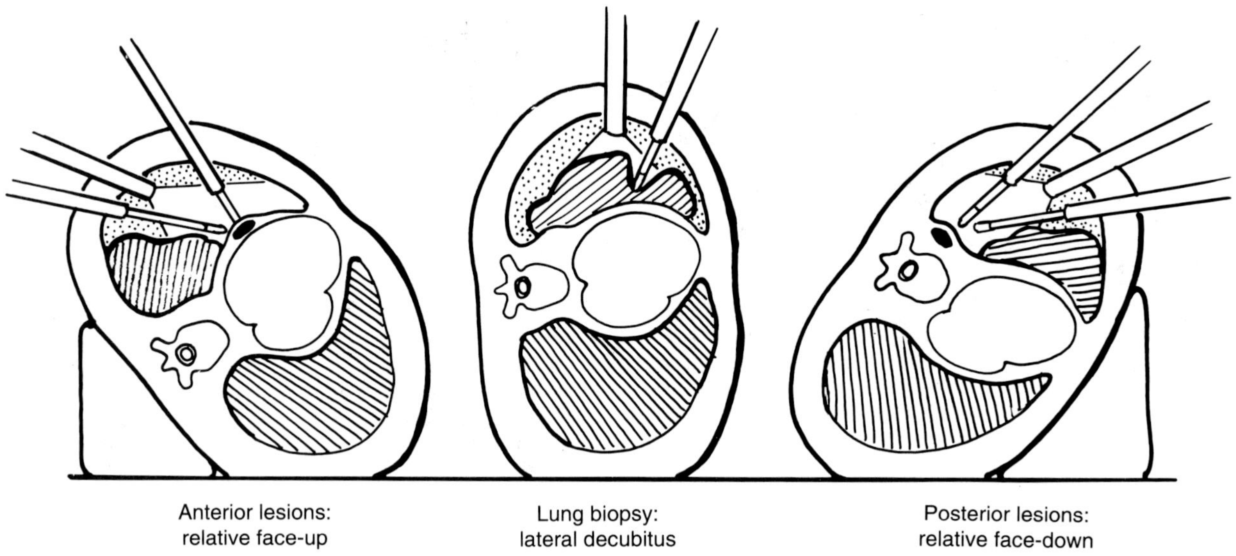

Figure 12–5. Patient positioning for the thoracoscopic approach to mediastinal and pulmonary lesions in children is important. The relative positions of the three cannulas are also illustrated for these lesions.

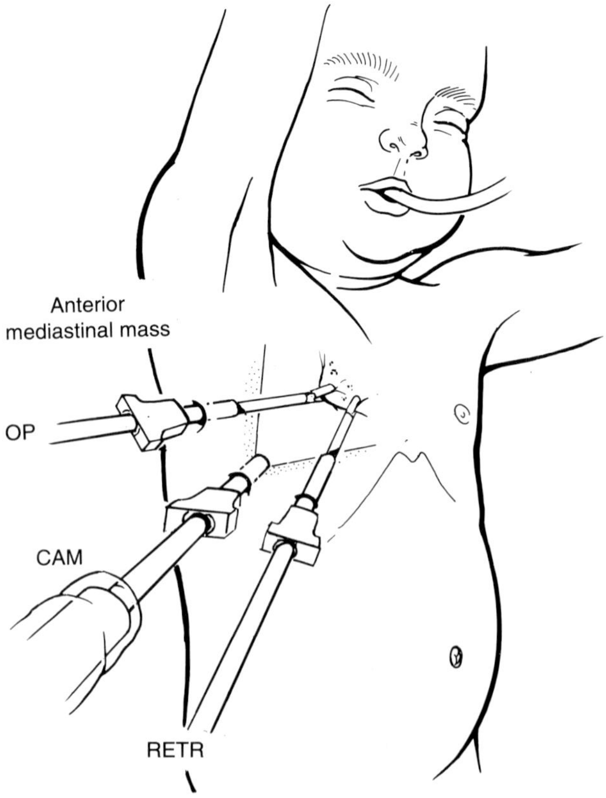

Figure 12–6. Placement of the instruments and camera for approach to anterior mediastinal lesions in children.

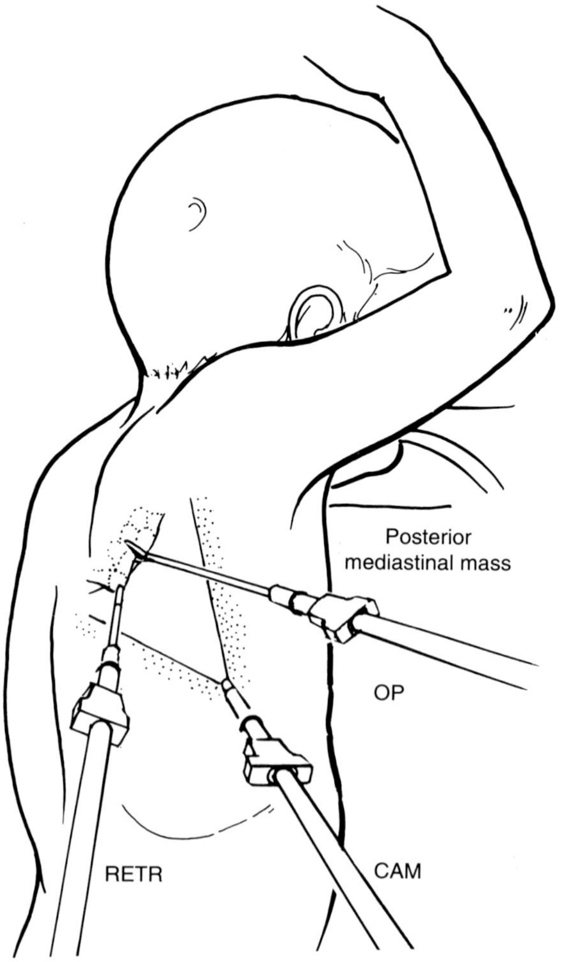

Figure 12–7. Placement of the instruments and camera for approach to posterior mediastinal lesions in children.

directly through the chest wall, rather than tunnelling as for placement of a chest tube. This allows cephalad and caudad rotation of the telescope and maximizes visibility.

Initial entry into the pleural space should be made with a fine-pointed hemostat. As the intercostal tract is dilated with this instrument, a pneumothorax is established, which minimizes the potential for injury to lung parenchyma with introduction of the sharp-pointed trocar. After the initial cannula and telescope are inserted, the lesion is identified and the positions of the accessory ports are planned. At this time an examination of the entire hemithorax should be performed to identify normal anatomic structures and to evaluate for possible unsuspected areas of involvement. Generally, the dissecting and operating instruments should be placed in the same axis as the telescope; the retraction instruments can be inserted in a different orientation. In the approach to the usual anterior mediastinal lesion, the dissecting port should be placed in the fourth or fifth intercostal space posteriorly and the retraction cannula in the same interspace anteriorly. The mediastinal pleura over the lesion can be picked up with a fine-pointed dissecting forceps and opened with either the endoscopic scissors or the hook cautery. Dissection about the mediastinal lesion is performed with a curved dissector and the spatula or hook cautery tip. It is not necessary to completely resect the enlarged lymph nodes when biopsying mediastinal adenopathy. They may be partially dissected from the surrounding structures and then biopsied generously with the cup biopsy forceps. If a complete dissection of the lesion is anticipated, additional ports may be necessary to retract and place the tissues being divided under tension. Prior to biopsy of any mediastinal lesion, consideration must be given to the possibility of it being a vascular structure. If there is any question in the surgeon's mind, a long aspirating needle can be passed through one of the cannulas and the contents of the lesion aspirated. This technique can also be employed to achieve cytologic preparations for suspected malignancies. After resection or biopsy of the lesion is completed, the area is irrigated and final hemostasis achieved with the cautery. A single chest tube is placed through the anterior cannula site. As the visceral pleura has not been violated in the majority of these procedures, a small (12-French) tube can be employed. This tube is positioned under direct visualization using a grasping forceps from the posterior trocar. A small epidural catheter is passed through the posterior port and positioned in the posterior vertebral gutter with the telescope. An immediate postoperative upright chest roentgenogram is obtained to ensure complete evacuation of the air from the operated hemithorax. If this appears satisfactory, the chest tube is placed to underwater seal and removed the following morning. The intrapleural analgesia catheter is usually removed at the same time as the chest tube, but may be left in place longer if the patient is experiencing discomfort.

One of the major advantages of thoracoscopy in approaching mediastinal masses, as well as in all of the indications to be discussed, is evident in the postoperative recovery time. Most of the patients with mediastinal masses are ready for discharge from the hospital the morning following the surgical procedure, and some surgeons have discussed discharging these patients on the same day if the visceral pleura has not been violated.[6] Postoperative discomfort is minimal and patients may resume all of their normal activities immediately following discharge. As there is no thoracotomy incision to heal, chemotherapy and irradiation therapy, if appropriate, may be instituted immediately following thoracoscopic biopsy. As with all endoscopic procedures there is a learning period in which the surgeon becomes facile in manipulating the various instruments required for these dissections. Once this facility is acquired, however, these procedures usually can be performed as quickly as comparable open thoracotomy procedures. An additional advantage of thoracoscopy is that proper planning of the cannula sites for thoracoscopy allows complete evaluation of the contents of the affected hemithorax without spreading the ribs. We reported a 31% incidence of discovery of unsuspected areas of pathology while approaching mediastinal neoplasms by thoracoscopy.[13]

The major disadvantage of thoracoscopy in evaluating mediastinal masses is that it is sometimes difficult to biopsy or resect more deeply located lymphadenopathy in the mediastinum. In an attempt to minimize this problem several biopsies through the same area of a given lymph node may be obtained to retrieve deeper tissue. Needle aspiration of the mediastinal structures may also minimize the false-negative biopsy rate. The overall diagnostic accuracy of thoracoscopy in approaching mediastinal lesions in children is reported as 85 to 100%.[6,12] Therefore, a negative biopsy result still requires careful follow-up of the patient and consideration for a more extensive open procedure in certain clinical situations.

Diffuse and Localized Pulmonary Infiltrates

The initial experience with thoracoscopy in children was acquired through pulmonary biopsy in patients with diffuse pulmonary infiltrates.[4,14] Most of these children were immunocompromised, either for treatment of neoplasms or following organ transplantation. With more aggressive use of broad spectrum antibiotics and bronchoalveolar lavage, the need for pulmonary biopsy has been reduced, although there still are patients in whom thoracoscopy and biopsy can be quite helpful (Figure 12–8). Similarly, thoracoscopy has proven to be helpful in the diagnosis of undiagnosed localized pulmonary infiltrates not responding to initial therapy. In these patients, frontal and lateral chest roentgenograms usually suffice for preoperative imaging, as the lesions are usually easily located with this study. In immunocompromised patients, who may be thrombocytopenic, preoperative platelet transfusions to raise the total platelet count to $50{,}000/mL^3$ are appropriate.

For most pulmonary biopsy procedures thoracoscopy can be performed satisfactorily under either general or regional anesthesia. If the procedure is anticipated to be short, regional anesthetic techniques work quite satisfactorily. There is some discomfort to the patient on obtaining the parenchymal biopsy itself, although this can usually be minimized with intravenous sedation. Procedures anticipated to be more lengthy are best performed under general anesthesia. If the indication for the biopsy procedure is a localized pulmonary infiltrate it is best to have the patient breathing spontaneously with double-lung ventilation. One of the most reliable endoscopic markers of a localized pulmonary infiltrate is regional atelectasis, and this may be difficult to appreciate if the entire lung is collapsed, as with unilateral ventilation. Positioning of these patients also depends on the specific indication for thoracoscopy. In children with diffuse pulmonary infiltrates a full lateral decubitus position allows reasonable access to the anterior and posterior surfaces of the lung (see Figure 12–5). In patients with more localized processes, rotation from a full lateral position, either anteriorly or posteriorly, may allow better access to the lesion. The initial telescopic cannula is placed in the fifth or sixth intercostal space in the posterior axillary line (Figure 12–9). The entire hemithorax is carefully evaluated, searching for unsuspected areas of involvement, and appropriate areas for biopsy are identified. A second port is placed anteriorly in the same interspace and any pleural fluid

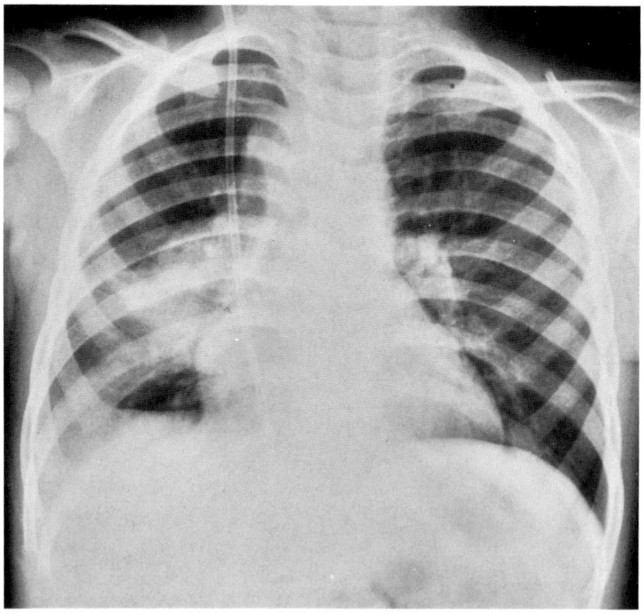

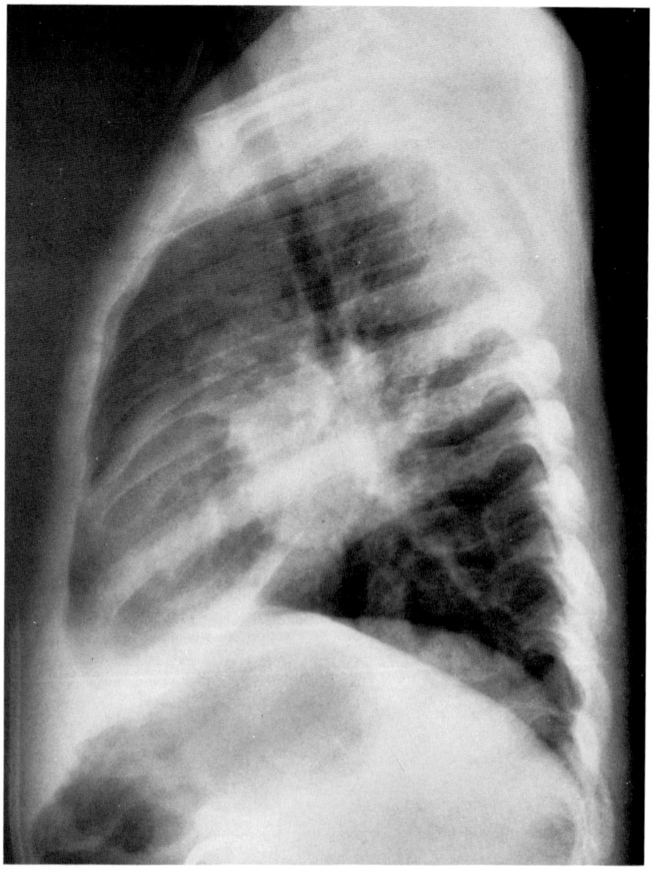

Figure 12–8. Frontal and lateral chest radiographs of a 2-year-old child with fever and a persistent pulmonary infiltrate revealed enlargement of hilar lymph nodes, particularly on the right. Thoracoscopic lung and hilar lymph node biopsies revealed pulmonary tuberculosis.

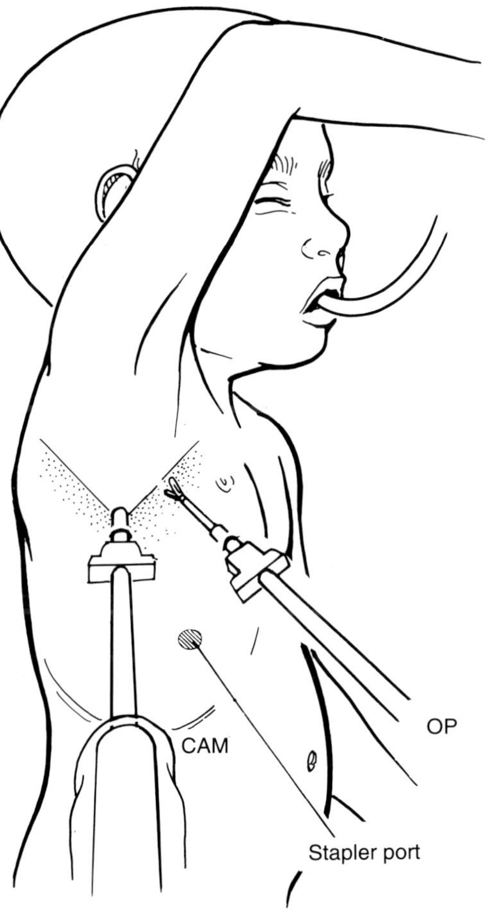

Figure 12–9. Placement of the camera and biopsy forceps for biopsy of diffuse parenchymal infiltrates. The location of the optional port for the endoscopic stapler is also shown.

present is suctioned into a collection trap. The insulated cup biopsy forceps may be used to grasp a small piece of lung (5–6 mm) as a biopsy specimen in patients with diffuse or localized infiltrates (Figure 12–10). The resulting parenchymal defect can be cauterized with these instruments, although this is often not necessary. In patients with diffuse processes, multiple biopsies should be obtained, including tissue from each pulmonary lobe. In patients with more localized processes, multiple biopsies should be performed in the same area to obtain deep as well as superficial specimens. In these patients it is often useful to obtain biopsies of more normal-appearing pulmonary parenchyma adjacent to the areas of inflammation to reconstruct the full pathologic picture. For all of these patients, specimens should be sent for pathologic evaluation as well as culture to maximize the diagnostic yield. Following biopsy, the area is irrigated and final hemostasis is achieved with the electrocautery. An appropriately sized chest tube is placed through the accessory instrument cannula site. A percutaneous epidural catheter may be placed posteriorly for postoperative intrapleural analgesia. Postoperatively, an upright portable chest roentgenograph is obtained to confirm complete evacuation of air and fluid from the operated hemithorax. The chest tube is left to 10 cm of underwater suction until all bubbling and drainage cease. It is then placed to underwater seal without suction for 12 to 24 hours prior to removal. Many patients with diffuse infiltrates have poorly compliant lungs and the chest tube should be left in place for an additional 24 to 48

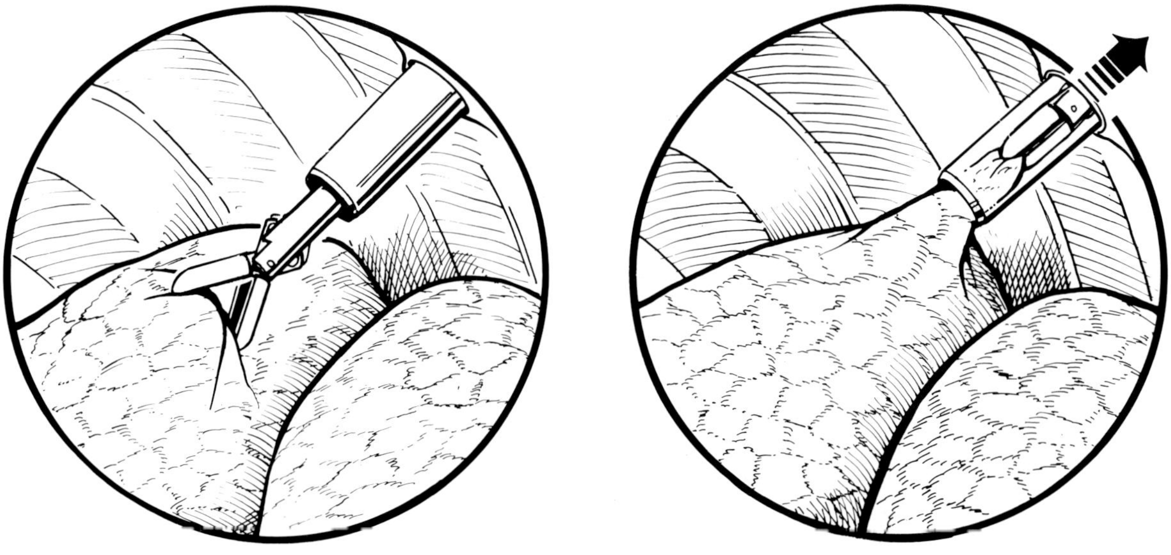

Figure 12–10. Pulmonary parenchymal biopsy can be obtained using an insulated cup biopsy forceps in young children with diffuse or localized pulmonary infiltrates.

hours to avoid recurrent pneumothorax after tube removal.

The diagnostic accuracy of pulmonary biopsy in children has consistently been greater than 95%.[5,6,14] In many cases, the results of these biopsies have significantly altered the therapy for these young patients. Thoracoscopy has the advantage of wide visualization of all of the visceral pleural surfaces, as compared with a limited open lung biopsy. This enhanced visibility allows for biopsy of all pulmonary lobes as well as evaluation for unsuspected areas of involvement. The major disadvantage of thoracoscopy is the potential for development of a bronchopleural fistula. Some of these children require high-pressure ventilator management prior to their biopsy and persistent air leak may complicate their management. The use of the Endo-GIA stapling device to obtain pulmonary biopsies may minimize the potential for air leak. This instrument is cumbersome to use in children weighing less than about 15 kg because of the length of the shaft that must be in the chest to open the anvil. In older children, however, wedge resection or tangential resection of a small piece of lung with this instrument provides excellent pneumostasis. Nonetheless, children who require very high inspiratory ventilator pressures are still probably best served with a limited thoracotomy and biopsy using staples and sutures for pneumostasis. Despite the fact that many immunocompromised patients are thrombocytopenic at the time of their biopsy, significant clinical bleeding does not seem to be a problem following thoracoscopy and biopsy, and blood transfusion has been necessary in less than 1% of the cases reported.[5,6,14]

Empyema

The goal of all forms of therapy for empyema is the complete evacuation of all purulent material from the pleural space, allowing full expansion of the underlying pulmonary parenchyma. In many patients with empyema, a tube thoracostomy will suffice for drainage. If the disease process is allowed to progress, however, into the fibrinopurulent stage of empyema, the pleural fluid begins to develop multiple loculations. It is in the management of children at this stage of the disease that thoracoscopy has been most beneficial (Figure 12–11). By use of the thoracoscope and dissecting forceps, the locules within the pleural space can be individually disrupted and the entire pleural space can be irrigated and manually debrided. Kern and Rodgers reported the use of this technique in nine children (aged 2 to 16 years) with loculated fibrinopurulent empyema with success in completely debriding the pleural space in each case.[15] One of these patients had an unsuspected leukemic infiltrate of the lower lobe diagnosed by thoracoscopic biopsy. This patient died of complications of the malignancy several months following thoracoscopy. All of the other patients fully recovered from their disease and all had normal chest roentgenograms months later. From this report, it appears that use of thoracoscopy in the early stages of empyema should eliminate the need for the more extensive open procedures described in the literature.

The technique for thoracoscopy in patients with empyema involves preoperative localization of the largest locule of pleural fluid by transthoracic ultrasound. This area is marked on the patient's chest wall by the radiologist. The choice of anesthesia in these patients is dictated by the complexity of the case. Extensive manipulation of the visceral and parietal pleura is uncomfortable for patients, and this pain may be difficult to alleviate with intravenous sedation. These patients are best treated with general anesthesia with unilateral ventilation. On the other hand, patients with relatively few, thin-walled locules may be debrided satisfactorily under regional anesthesia with intravenous sedation. Patients are usually placed in a full lateral position, but this may be modified depending on the location of the pleural fluid. The initial cannula and telescope are inserted directly into the previously identified major locule and the purulent material is evacuated from this cavity. Cultures and gram stains of this fluid and intracavitary debris are obtained. Adjacent pleural adhesions can usually be dissected down using the end of the 0-degree telescope. This enlarges the visible pleural space and allows a secondary working port for dissecting instruments and cautery to be inserted reasonably close to the initial cannula. The spatula cautery makes a particularly useful instrument with which to dissect pleural adhesions. All of the locules are disrupted, including those along the diaphragmatic surface of the lung. The pleural cavity is then irrigated forcibly with saline and larger collections of fibrinous material are mechanically debrided with the biopsy forceps. A large-bore chest tube is placed in the posterior thoracic gutter under visual control. Most of these patients have such severe pleural inflammation that the absorption of intrapleural analgesia agents is too irregular for this therapy to be used safely. Postoperatively these patients are followed with daily chest roentgenograms. If it appears that there is residual pleural fluid present, urokinase (500,000 U in 30 mL of normal saline) may be instilled through the chest tube and left in the hemithorax for 45 to 60 minutes. The chest tube is removed when the patient is afebrile and there is no evidence of continued fluid drainage.

Thoracoscopy in the clinical setting of empyema has the advantage over open procedures of allowing

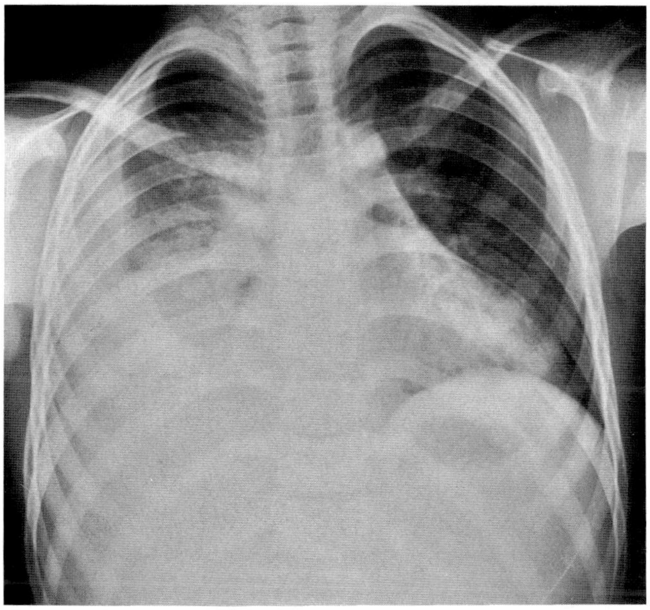

A

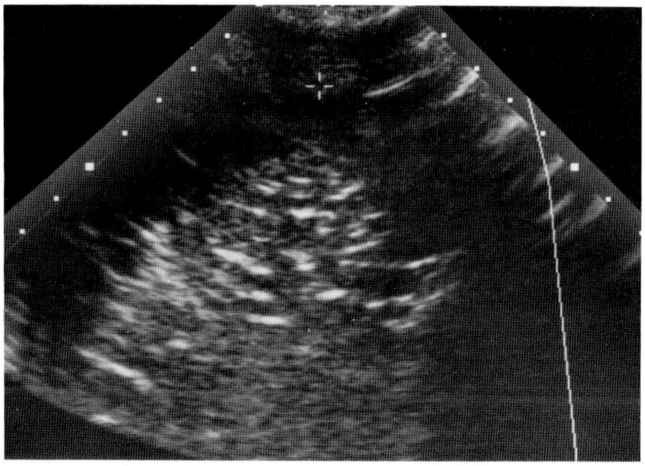

B

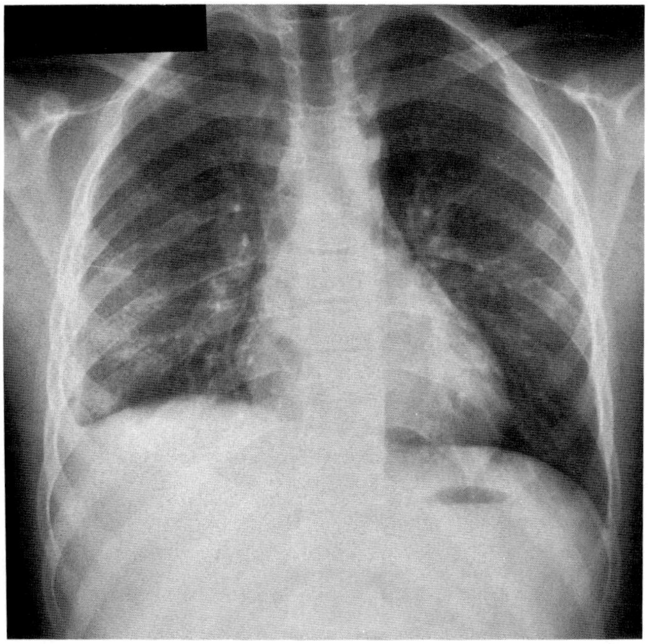

C

Figure 12–11. **A.** Frontal radiograph of an 8-year-old child with persistent fever and tachypnea following 10 days of antibiotics shows a persistent right pleural effusion with parenchymal entrapment. **B.** Transpleural ultrasound demonstrates multiple thick-walled locules of fluid within the pleural space. **C.** The frontal radiograph 1 month following thoracoscopic debridement of the right pleural cavity.

visualization of the entire pleural space through relatively limited access. The patient's respiratory mechanics appear to be better maintained postoperatively in the absence of a thoracotomy incision and patient morbidity is reduced. The simplicity of pleural debridement with thoracoscopy encourages an earlier approach to the fibrinopurulent stage of empyema and eliminates the potential for these patients to progress to the stage of fibrothorax.

Thoracoscopy should be considered in any child in whom more conservative measures have failed to clear the purulent fluid from the pleural space within

7 to 10 days. Even earlier intervention should be considered if the patient remains febrile and has evidence of loculated pleural fluid by transthoracic ultrasound.

Pneumothorax

Spontaneous pneumothorax is not an uncommon problem in the adolescent patient. In these patients the onset of symptoms is usually abrupt and the symptoms consist mainly of chest pain and mild dyspnea. The child with cystic fibrosis who develops a spontaneous pneumothorax, however, presents very differently. These patients are usually markedly symptomatic with respiratory distress and chest pain. The development of a tension pneumothorax is a significant cause of mortality in patients with cystic fibrosis. The treatment of a spontaneous pneumothorax depends on the etiology of the process and the circumstances of the individual patient. Patients with cystic fibrosis should be treated aggressively with the first episode of pneumothorax, whereas many physicians will await a second occurrence in otherwise healthy adolescents who have reasonable access to medical care. Thoracoscopy has provided an alternative method of managing these patients quite similar to that which would traditionally be performed with open thoracotomy. Preoperative imaging of these patients usually requires no more than frontal and lateral chest roentgenograms. These studies occasionally suggest the presence of pulmonary parenchymal cysts or blebs, but it is not necessary to perform more sophisticated studies to identify these lesions in children. If the patient is not in respiratory distress, the surgeon can proceed directly to thoracoscopy, prior to tube thoracostomy. In patients with cystic fibrosis, however, a tube thoracostomy should be performed prior to proceeding with thoracoscopic treatment, to control respiratory embarrassment.

The choice of anesthetic technique in patients with spontaneous pneumothorax is determined by the procedure planned. Induction of a talc pleurodesis can be achieved rapidly and without patient discomfort, and this procedure may be performed under regional anesthesia. Mechanical pleural abrasion, however, is more painful to the patient and is best performed under general anesthesia with unilateral ventilation. Many children with cystic fibrosis will not tolerate unilateral ventilation and the procedure can be performed with double-lung ventilation. In this case, the patient should be allowed to breathe spontaneously to avoid the necessity for positive-pressure ventilation.

These patients are best placed in the lateral decubitus position and the telescope and cannula are inserted in the posterior axillary line in the sixth intercostal space. This gives a complete view of the visceral pleural surface and allows identification of pleural blebs if present. If blebs are encountered, they may be managed either by ligation with an endoloop ligature (Ethicon, Inc, Cincinnati, OH) or by use of the Endo-GIA stapler (Figure 12–12). This stapling device must be passed through a 12-mm port and, because of the length of the anvil of the device, the introducing cannula must be inserted low in the hemithorax. This should be done under direct visualization with the telescope. If no blebs are visualized, the surgeon can proceed directly to creation of a pleural symphysis. This can be done either by mechanical abrasion of the parietal pleura or by talc insufflation. Talc insufflation appears to provide the surest protection against recurrent pneumothorax, and we continue to favor this technique for adolescents with repeated pneumothoraces.[16] Although our early experience with talc in children with cystic fibrosis suggested that it was extremely effective in eliminating recurrent pneumothoraces, the density of the pleural symphysis created by talc insufflation may complicate subsequent pulmonary transplantation.[17] For this reason we have abandoned its use in these patients. A thorough pleural abrasion can be accomplished thoracoscopically by using a small piece of polypropylene mesh (C.R. Bard, Inc) fastened to the end of a dissecting forceps. This can be passed through a 10-mm working cannula placed in the anterior axillary line in the sixth intercostal space. The position of the telescope and abrading forceps can be alternated to allow abrasion of both anterior and posterior pleural surfaces. Nearly the entire parietal pleural surface can be manually abraded with this technique with a satisfactory pleural symphysis.

The advantages of thoracoscopy over open thoracotomy in treating these patients with pneumothorax appears to be primarily in the avoidance of a thoracotomy incision and its attendant morbidity. The techniques appear to be comparable in their effectiveness in eliminating recurrent pneumothoraces and both techniques have a very low incidence of complications.[16] The ease with which a pleural symphysis may be created by thoracoscopy may encourage earlier definitive therapy in some of these children.

Other Indications

The most common indication for thoracoscopy in adult patients is for evaluation of idiopathic pleural effusions (see Figure 12–2). Although pleural effusions are uncommon in children, thoracoscopy may be helpful in certain circumstances. We have used thoracoscopy to assist in the management of four children with pleural effusions. Two of these patients had developed a chylothorax following complex cardiac surgery. Both

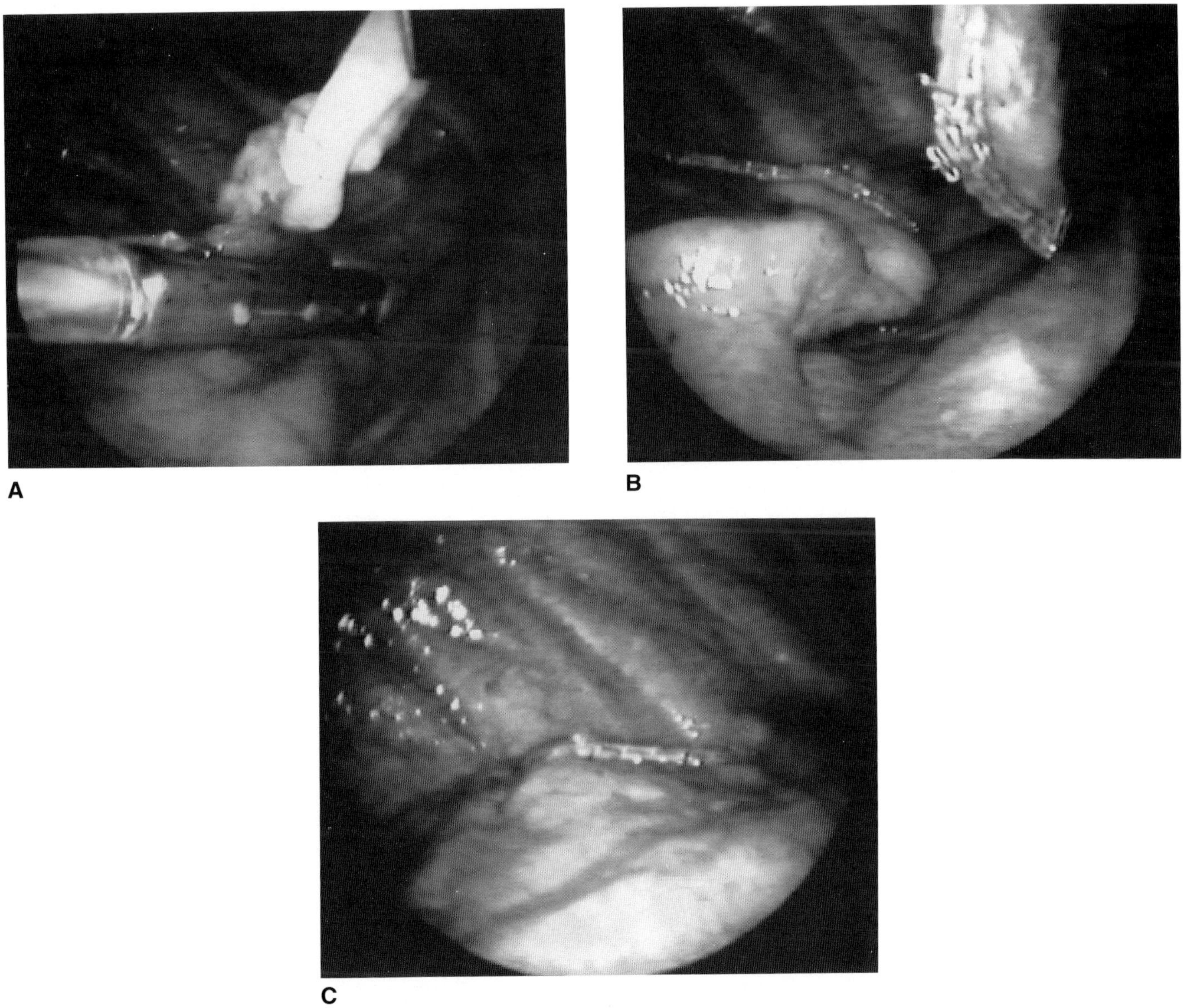

Figure 12–12. **A.** The Endo-GIA stapler has been inserted across the parenchymal bleb. **B.** The transection has been completed and the specimen is ready for removal. **C.** Reevaluation of the staple line demonstrates that it is intact without bleeding or air leak.

were considered candidates for a pleuroperitoneal shunt, but had evidence of loculated fluid by transthoracic ultrasound. Thoracoscopy was employed to disrupt the individual locules at the time of placement of the shunt and was successful in both instances. A third patient developed a unilateral pleural effusion following treatment for Wilms' tumor. Thoracentesis was nondiagnostic, and this patient was diagnosed by thoracoscopy as having metastatic Wilms' tumor on the pleural surface. The fourth patient developed a sterile pleural effusion several months following an episode of pneumonitis. This effusion was successfully evacuated and cultures were obtained by thoracoscopy.

The ability to clearly visualize the entire hemithorax with thoracoscopy has led to the development of several other innovative uses of the technique in adults. Several authors have now described partial pericardiectomy for chronic pericardial effusions in adults.[18,19] This technique has not been described in children, but technically could be performed in suitable patients. We have used the technique of thoracoscopy in one child, under regional anesthesia, to confirm congenital absence of the pericardium. Several authors have now described performing esophageal surgery by thoracoscopy in adult patients. Pellegrini et al reported performing esophagomyotomy in

15 adult patients with achalasia.[11] Shimi et al reported on three patients in whom a long esophagomyotomy was successfully performed for "nutcracker esophagus."[20] Three patients have also been reported in whom leiomyomas of the esophagus have been successfully resected by thoracoscopy.[21] None of these procedures has yet been described in pediatric patients, but they should be applicable in carefully selected situations.

CONTRAINDICATIONS

The only absolute contraindication to thoracoscopy appears to be the inability to create a sufficient pneumothorax to allow adequate visibility within the hemithorax (Table 12–3). In adult patients this would most commonly be caused by the presence of a complete and dense pleural symphysis. This would be an unusual circumstance in children and no patients have been described in the pediatric literature in whom thoracoscopy was abandoned for this problem. Janssen and Boutin described a technique of "extended thoracoscopy" used in adult patients, with limited dissection of the local pleural adhesions in the region of the initial thoracoscopy cannula.[22] They have performed this procedure under regional anesthesia in 20 patients with an 84% diagnostic accuracy. An adequate pneumothorax may be difficult to achieve and maintain in very small infants. We therefore have abandoned the use of this procedure in children less than 6 months of age, although Lobe and co-workers have successfully resected a bronchogenic cyst in a 4-month-old infant.[6] A relative contraindication to performing thoracoscopy includes the use of high-pressure ventilation, which limits the ability to create a satisfactory pneumothorax. A systemic coagulopathy that cannot be corrected with the use of blood products also constitutes a relative contraindication to thoracoscopy. Patients with thrombocytopenia can usually successfully undergo thoracoscopy with platelet transfusions. Prior to performing thoracoscopy for biopsy of pulmonary lesions, one must be reasonably convinced that the lesion may be visualized from the surface of the lung.

TABLE 12–3. CONTRAINDICATIONS TO THORACOSCOPY

- ABSOLUTE
  - Inability to create a sufficient pneumothorax
- RELATIVE
  - Small infant (<6 months)
  - Need for high-pressure ventilation
  - Systemic coagulopathy that cannot be corrected
  - Isolated lesions deep within parenchyma

Difficulties have been encountered in adult patients with metastatic or primary lung tumors in whom the lesion could not be visualized by thoracoscopy and open procedures had to be performed.

COMPLICATIONS

The relatively small number of papers describing thoracoscopy in children limits a discussion of the complications in these patients. Nonetheless, reviews of complications encountered in large numbers of thoracoscopy procedures in adults have documented an acceptably low complication rate for this procedure. Mortality attributed to the thoracoscopy procedure itself has rarely been reported. We have had experience with a single patient who underwent lung biopsy for a diffuse interstitial process following chemotherapy for a systemic malignancy. This patient was in severe respiratory failure and was maintained on a ventilator. She developed a bronchopleural fistula following thoracoscopic lung biopsy, which certainly complicated her respiratory management. She died of respiratory insufficiency 72 hours following surgery. This patient is the only mortality within 30 days of thoracoscopy in our series of 175 children. Viskum and Enk reviewed complications encountered in over 500 adult patients undergoing thoracoscopy.[23] One percent of these patients required transfusion for operative blood loss, but none required exploratory thoracotomy to control hemorrhage. We have had a single child who required transfusion after pulmonary biopsy by thoracoscopy. This patient was immunocompromised following a renal transplant and had a preoperative hematocrit of 15 vol%. The estimated operative blood loss was 200 mL, and this volume was replaced during the operative procedure. Otherwise, none of our patients has required transfusions because of blood loss from thoracoscopy and we have not had to convert to an open procedure for control of bleeding. Cardiac arrhythmias were encountered in less than 0.5% and air embolism in less than 0.2% of Viskum and Enk's patients. Infection, either at the cannula site or intrapleurally, was encountered in less than 2% of these adult patients. We have not experienced arrhythmias, air embolism, or infection in any of the pediatric patients in whom we have performed thoracoscopy. We have had one patient, a 9-month-old boy with a posterior mediastinal mass, in whom adequate exposure of the lesion could not be maintained by thoracoscopy and the procedure was converted to an open excisional biopsy. Exposure in the remainder of our patients has been adequate to achieve biopsy specimens in all cases.

SUMMARY

Experience with thoracoscopy in children over the past two decades has clearly shown this technique to be of benefit to pediatric surgeons in the management of carefully selected patients. Thoracoscopy is well tolerated by pediatric patients and provides the surgeon with an extensive view of the contents of the hemithorax. The postoperative morbidity appears significantly less than after open thoracotomy with the division of the intercostal muscles and rib retraction. Thoracoscopic biopsy of pulmonary and mediastinal lesions can be performed rapidly and safely and has been shown to have a diagnostic yield of 85 to 100%. The technique has also proven useful in treating pleural empyemas and pleural effusions in children. The complications of this technique in children have been infrequent, and the operative mortality for all indications is less than 1%. The extent of the role of thoracoscopy in children will depend on the development of new endoscopic instruments and the imagination of the individual surgeon. One could speculate that development of suitable endoscopic vascular clamps may lead to thoracoscopic lobectomies or resection of pulmonary sequestrations. Further experience with endoscopic suturing techniques could allow such procedures as division of H-type tracheoesophageal fistulas or repair of traumatic diaphragmatic hernias by thoracoscopy. Whatever the future applications of thoracoscopy will be, this procedure already has a well-demonstrated utility in the management of children with chest disease, and pediatric surgeons will have to become facile with these procedures to properly serve their patient population.

REFERENCES

1. Jacobaeus HC. Über die moglichkeit die zystoskopie bei untersuchung seroser hohlungen anzuwenden. *Munch Med Wochenschr.* 1910;40:2090.
2. Jacobaeus HC. The practical importance of thoracoscopy in surgery of the chest. *Surg Gynecol Obstet.* 1922;34:289.
3. Klimkovich IG, Geldt VG, Okulou AB, Ovchinnikov AA, Polyakova ON, Pikaleva EE. Thoracoscopy in children. *Khirurgikila.* 1971;47:19.
4. Rodgers BM, Talbert JL. Thoracoscopy for diagnosis of intrathoracic lesions in children. *J Pediatr Surg.* 1976;11:703.
5. Janik JS, Nagaraj HS, Groff DB. Thoracoscopic evaluation of intrathoracic lesions in children. *J Thorac Cardiovasc Surg.* 1982;83:408.
6. Rogers DA, Philippe PG, Lobe TE, et al. Thoracoscopy in children: An initial experience with an evolving technique. *J Laparoendosc Surg.* 1992;2:7.
7. Rodgers BM. Thoracoscopy in children. *Poumon-Coeur.* 1981;37:301.
8. Ryckman FC, Rodgers BM. Thoracoscopy for intrathoracic neoplasia in children. *J Pediatr Surg.* 1982;17:521.
9. Kern JA, Tribble CG, Spotnitz WD, Rodgers BM, Daniel TM. Thoracoscopy: A potential role in the subacute management of patients with thoraco-abdominal trauma. *Chest.* 1992;104.
10. Mack MJ, Aronoff RJ, Acuff TE, Douthit MB, Bowman RT, Ryan WH. Present role of thoracoscopy in the diagnosis and treatment of diseases of the chest. *Ann Thorac Surg.* 1992;54:403.
11. Pellegrini C, Wetter LA, Patti M, et al. Thoracoscopic esophagomyotomy. *Ann Surg.* 1992;216:291.
12. Kern JA, Daniel TM, Tribble CG, Silen ML, Rodgers BM. Thoracoscopic diagnosis and treatment of mediastinal masses. *Ann Thorac Surg.* In press.
13. Rodgers BM, Ryckman FC, Moazam F, Talbert JL. Thoracoscopy for intrathoracic tumors. *Ann Thorac Surg.* 1981;31:414.
14. Rodgers BM, Moazam F, Talbert JL. Thoracoscopy: Early diagnosis of interstitial pneumonitis in the immunologically suppressed child. *Chest.* 1979;75:126.
15. Kern JA, Rodgers BM. Thoracoscopy in the management of empyema in children. *J Pediatr Surg.* In press.
16. Daniel TM, Tribble CG, Rodgers BM. Thoracoscopy and talc poudrage for pneumothoraces and effusions. *Ann Thorac Surg.* 1990;50:186.
17. Tribble CG, Selden RF, Rodgers BM. Talc poudrage in the treatment of spontaneous pneumothoraces in patients with cystic fibrosis. *Ann Surg.* 1986;204:677.
18. Lewis RJ, Caccavale RJ, Sisler GE, MacKenzie JW. One hundred consecutive patients undergoing video-assisted thoracic operations. *Ann Thorac Surg.* 1992;54:421.
19. Wakabayashi A. Expanded applications of diagnostic and therapeutic thoracoscopy. *J Thorac Cardiovasc Surg.* 1991;102:721.
20. Shimi SM, Nathanson LK, Cuschieri A. Thoracoscopic long oesophageal myotomy for nutcracker oesophagus: Initial experience of a new surgical approach. *Br J Surg.* 1992;79:533.
21. Bardini R, Segalin A, Ruol AL, Pavanello M, Peracchia A. Videothoracoscopic enucleation of esophageal leiomyoma. *Ann Thorac Surg.* 1992;54:576.
22. Janssen JP, Boutin C. Extended thoracoscopy: A biopsy method to be used in case of pleural adhesions. *Eur Respir J.* 1992;5:763.
23. Viskum K, Enk B. Complications of thoracoscopy. *Poumon-Coeur.* 1981;37:25.

CHAPTER 13

Rigid Esophagoscopy

ARTHUR J. ROSS III • JAMES A. O'NEILL, JR

Kussmaul is credited with the technical description and performance of the first esophagoscopy in 1870. Interestingly, he performed the examination on a professional sword swallower who acted as his "volunteer" for the study! Early attempts at upper gastrointestinal (GI) tract endoscopy by Kussmaul and others used rigid, hollow metallic tubes with a reflected lamp light. The relatively straight course of the esophagus was amenable to such examination and the mouth, pharynx, esophagus, and stomach could be visualized with rigid equipment. The field of upper GI endoscopy then blossomed with the development of flexible esophagogastroscopes only a decade after Kussmaul's pioneering studies. Endoscopy as both an art and a science peaked in what some have termed the *Philadelphia School of Bronchoesophagology* under the direction of Chevalier Jackson. Jackson raised bronchoesophagology to a specialty and his clinic attracted worldwide attention. Jackson's teachings also produced most of the early leaders in the field including Tucker, Jackson, and Holinger.

Conceptually, the current practice of hollow (or rigid) -tube esophagoscopy remains the same as that initially practiced by Kussmaul. Advances in technology in terms of visualization and illumination have represented the most significant advances within the field. In 1968, the introduction of the Hopkins rod-lens optical system for use with rigid open-tube esophagoscopy added a new dimension to endoscopy and this advance in optical technology allowed significantly more investigation and manipulation of the upper GI system than was previously possible.[1]

ROLE OF RIGID ESOPHAGOSCOPY IN THE ERA OF FLEXIBLE INSTRUMENTATION

New generations of flexible fiberoptic esophagogastroscopes provide excellent visualization and are significantly miniaturized. Although many procedures formerly undertaken with the rigid esophagoscope (variceal sclerotherapy, evaluation of esophagitis, evaluation of upper GI bleeding) are now performed with flexible instrumentation, definite indications remain for the use of rigid esophagoscopic examination and evaluation, such as management of esophageal foreign bodies and strictures.

In this era of increasing specialization, the "complete" esophagologist should have facility with both rigid and flexible instruments. There are very clear advantages and disadvantages to each approach, and one trained to use both flexible and rigid instruments is far better equipped to make the optimal choice for means of evaluation and treatment of the patient.

CLINICAL PRESENTATION

Foreign Bodies

The most common indication for rigid esophagoscopy is removal of foreign bodies from the pharynx and esophagus. The esophagus is a relatively passive organ with weak peristalsis, so it has a tendency to retain foreign bodies.

Retention of foreign bodies is largely a problem affecting the pediatric population. As small children are naturally inclined to place objects into their mouths, it is easily understood why foreign body ingestion and aspiration are so common. Ingestions significantly outnumber aspirations. The 1992 statistics from the National Safety Council demonstrate that suffocation from foreign body ingestion and aspiration is the third leading cause of accidental death in children younger than 1 year of age and the fourth leading cause in children aged 1 to 4 years. Moreover, these statistics do not reflect the additional morbidity and mortality related to subsequent complications.[2]

The majority of foreign bodies ingested pass uneventfully; however, retained foreign bodies within the esophagus are still common problems in all pediatric surgical clinics. Once a foreign body arrests in the esophagus its removal is important as soon as the diagnosis is made, because edema and erosion of the foreign body into the esophageal wall make manipulation and removal more difficult.

When an esophageal foreign body creates symptoms acutely, immediate medical help is usually sought. In many instances, though, symptoms are lacking and the presence of the foreign body may go unnoticed for a long time. Most ingestions are unwitnessed so an accurate history may not be obtainable. Furthermore, the diagnosis may be delayed because of an asymptomatic period between the time of ingestion and the development of significant signs and symptoms. In children who do not have a clear, acute, documentable history of foreign body ingestion, the diagnosis should be suspected if the child presents with dysphagia, weight loss, fever, or airway symptoms, especially if there is any prior history of gagging, choking, drooling, or unexplained coughing or vomiting episodes (Table 13–1). Most esophageal foreign bodies become impacted at a point just distal to the cricopharyngeal musculature (Figure 13–1). As this site is in close proximity to the larynx and trachea, it is easy to understand why airway symptoms are common. Foreign bodies may also lodge at the site of physiologic narrowing in the midesophagus, related to aortic and/or left mainstem bronchus compression, and at the gastroesophageal junction.

In the otherwise normal child, coins are the most commonly encountered pediatric esophageal foreign body (Figure 13–2). A penny will be the likely coin removed, as pennies are the most common coin left on floors for infants to swallow. Pins, especially safety pins used in diapers, were frequently encountered in the past. In recent years, plastic foreign bodies have become a common injuring agent and most of these are not radiopaque.[3] Also, there has been an increase in the number of small acid-containing disk batteries ingested during the 1980s.[4] In children with esophageal narrowing or motility disturbances of either a structural or functional nature, such as following repair of esophageal atresia, there is a great propensity to retain food material.

If a patient is suspected of having an esophageal foreign body, anteroposterior (AP) and lateral roentgenograms of the neck and chest are obtained; if the object is radiopaque, the diagnosis is clear (Figure 13–3). With negative radiographs but strong clinical suspicion or negative radiographs with suspicious ancillary findings (paraesophageal inflammation or hyperinflation of the hypopharynx and proximal esophagus), a contrast esophagram should be performed to search for a persistent filling defect around a radiolucent foreign body. If the child's symptoms are severe with airway compromise or drooling and evidence of esophageal obstruction, one should proceed immediately to rigid esophagoscopy.

Esophageal foreign bodies can cause severe complications. Foreign bodies may present with dysphagia or respiratory distress acutely. Chronically, a foreign body may erode into and even through the wall of the esophagus, causing vascular problems (aorto-esophageal fistula, innominate esophageal fistula, ca-

TABLE 13–1. SYMPTOMS OF ESOPHAGEAL FOREIGN BODIES

Dysphagia
Unexplained weight loss
Unexplained airway symptoms
Drooling, choking, gagging, or coughing
Vomiting
Unexplained fever

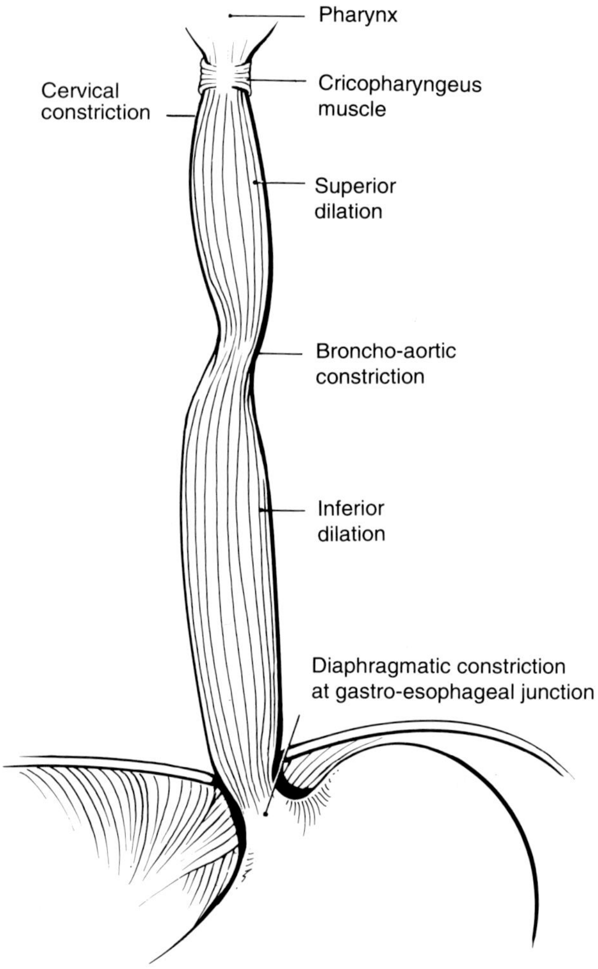

Figure 13–1. Normal anatomic sites of narrowing in the esophagus. Most esophageal foreign bodies become impacted at the site of anatomic cervical constriction, which is just distal to the cricopharyngeal musculature.

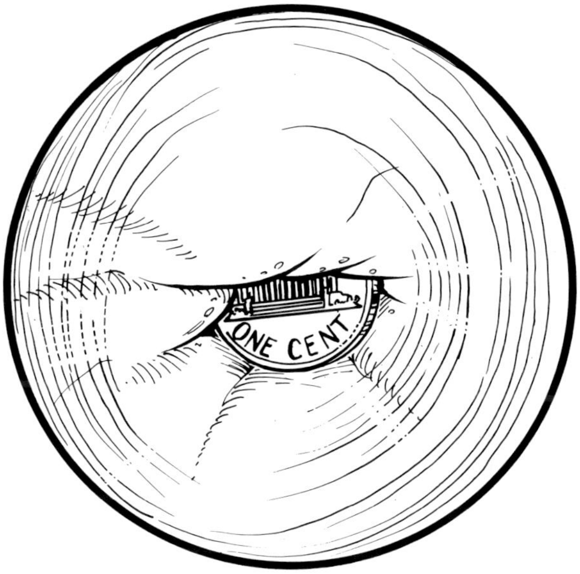

Figure 13–2. A penny is the most common coin extracted from the esophagus.

rotid rupture), suppurative problems (mediastinitis with or without abscess, paraesophageal abscess, retropharyngeal abscess, thyroid abscess), or other problems (esophagitis, pericarditis, esophageal stricture, vocal cord paralysis).[5] Therefore, once a foreign body has lodged within the esophagus, it should be removed as soon as the diagnosis is made to avoid esophageal perforation.

Anatomic Abnormalities of the Esophagus

Children may present with anatomic abnormalities of the esophagus including stricture, congenital stenosis, cartilaginous rings within the esophageal wall, leiomyomas, and cystic duplications. Such children have dysphagia as their most common presenting symptom. Strictures are most commonly seen in children who have previously undergone repair of esophageal atresia or in those with chronic esophagitis. Symptoms of dysphagia are progressive in such children. Children with congenital stenosis and cartilaginous rings within the esophageal wall as well as leiomyomas, corrosive injury, and cystic duplications often have symptoms of dysphagia that can be dated to infancy but usually do not tend to present as precipitously as those with acquired strictures. In all patients who present with dysphagia, the initial workup includes AP and lat-

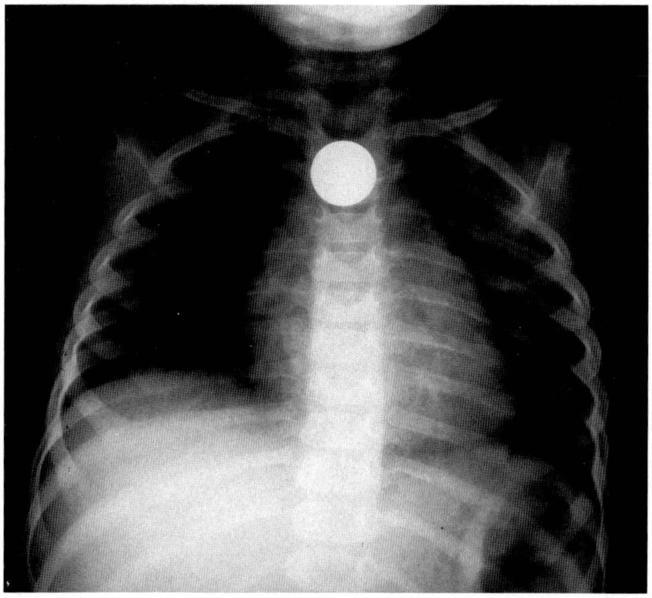

Figure 13–3. Typical chest radiograph showing a swallowed coin lodged in the cervical esophagus.

eral cervical and thoracic radiographs followed by a contrast esophagogram. These abnormalities are best managed by esophagoscopy. Although the initial examination and treatment may well be carried out with a flexible esophagoscope, most would prefer to manage an esophageal stricture with a rigid scope.

TREATMENT OPTIONS

Most foreign bodies can be removed using either a rigid or flexible esophagoscope; however, use of a rigid scope with a Hopkins rod-lens telescope gives the best magnification and visualization for grasping foreign bodies. Although currently available flexible esophagoscopes do provide adequate visualization, only small foreign bodies can be extracted with this technique. Coins and solid objects with discrete edges may be removed with a flexible scope, but soft foreign bodies such as meat, vegetable matter, and objects without discrete edges are difficult to manage with flexible equipment.

Although the flexible esophagoscope allows both aspiration and biopsy, the size of the operating channel used for children tends to limit the amount of tissue that can be obtained. Similarly, the retrieval of foreign bodies using this instrument is hampered by the size of the forceps and the channel through which the foreign body is removed. With flexible systems, sharp foreign bodies cannot be drawn up into the esophagoscope as can usually be done with a rigid scope so as to protect the esophageal mucosa from the foreign body as it is withdrawn. The Hopkins–Storz system is optimal for management of esophageal foreign bodies and their optical forceps are ideal in that they pass through the esophagoscope. The telescope is coupled to the grasping element, with the position of the tip controllable within the rigid scope sheath (Figure 13–4). Furthermore, there are far more options available in the form of small forceps, graspers, basket snares, and balloons which are able to be passed through the instrument channel of the rigid scope sheath while it is positioned in the esophagus. Food impactions are managed more expeditiously using the rigid esophagoscope as the larger forceps and lumen of the rigid esophagoscope permit more efficient removal of food material.

Another option available for the removal of a smooth esophageal foreign body is the use of a contrast-filled Foley balloon catheter under fluoroscopic control.[6,7] Foreign bodies that are neither sharp nor embedded within the mucosa from long-term presence may be removed with this technique. The balloon extraction technique should not be used in patients with preexisting esophageal abnormalities. Although it is commonly employed in many centers, including ours, a large number of otolaryngologists condemn the use of this technique. They feel that even with an appropriately prepared and positioned pa-

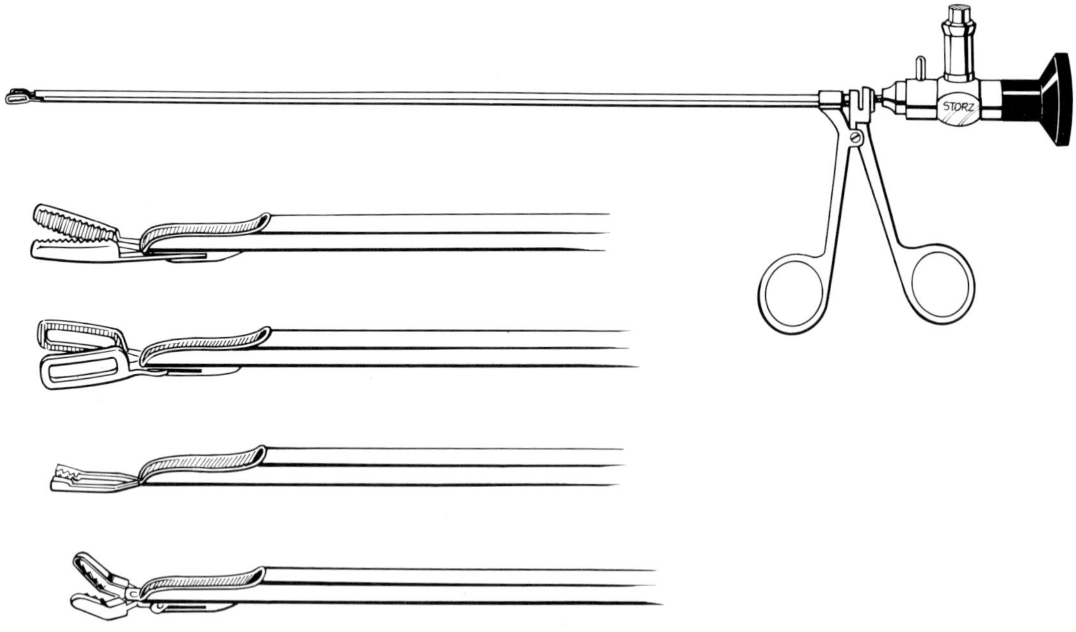

Figure 13–4. A variety of forceps are available for use with the Storz esophagoscopes, allowing the examiner to individualize his or her choice of equipment as dictated by the specific needs for management of the foreign body. Note that some tips are better for grasping hard foreign bodies, whereas others are better for grasping soft foreign bodies. The forceps' tips are also able to rotate.

tient, there is not adequate assurance as to the protection and safety of the child's airway, although there is little evidence for the validity of this concern.

Evaluation of a child with dysphagia may be undertaken with either the rigid or flexible esophagoscope. There are several alternative techniques for dilation of an esophageal stricture using the rigid esophagoscope, whereas one's ability is limited with the flexible esophagoscope. The broad blunt-tipped flexible esophagoscope does not pass through strictures easily. Esophageal dilation with the flexible scope is best managed using the Rigiflex balloon (Microvasive, Watertown, MA). We prefer to manage esophageal strictures with the rigid esophagoscope because it is possible, even with small tight strictures, to manipulate a small rigid esophagoscope through the stricture under direct vision. Should the stricture be so tight that the rigid scope cannot be safely passed, a guidewire, ureteral catheter, or balloon or rigid dilator can be passed down the instrument channel of the esophagoscope and through the stricture.

Other causes of dysphagia such as esophagitis, leiomyoma, duplication, congenital stricture, and cartilaginous rings may be diagnosed by either technique. Evaluation of the child who has had a caustic ingestion may be performed with either the rigid or the flexible system and is best approached according to the experience and comfort of the examining physician; however, it is preferable if the examining physician is adept with both techniques.

TECHNIQUE

Equipment

In performing rigid esophagoscopy in children we employ the Hopkins–Storz lens system of esophagoscopes, which are available in lengths of 20 and 30 cm. These esophagoscopes vary in outer diameter from 4.8 to 8.2 mm. Although the smaller esophagoscopes were designed for use in newborn infants, we have found that the size 4 scope (length 30 cm, outer diameter 6.7 mm) can be used in all but the smallest of newborns. In larger children we usually begin with at least the size 5 (length 30 cm, outer diameter 7.7 mm). Optical forceps are easily employed through these esophagoscopes, and a variety of forceps tips are available for use in the management of several different types of foreign bodies (see Figure 13–4). The esophagoscopes have an air inflation channel and suction capabilities. Flexible suction catheters as large as 7 French can be passed through the instrument channel, as can Fogarty balloon catheters and a variety of additional types of forceps. For larger children and patients with difficult impactions, we have occasionally used larger Storz esophagoscopes of the Roberts–Jesberg type with Hopkins optical forceps. In addition, these operating esophagoscopes have both distal and proximal illumination capability and good magnification sources, so that excellent optics is still present even when the procedure must be performed without the telescope. Finally, in larger children, we have found that the Forbes-type esophageal speculum allows good visualization of the hypopharynx down to the cricopharyngeus, which will permit removal of a foreign body with laryngeal forceps under direct vision.

Method

Rigid esophagoscopy requires the use of a general anesthetic. The patient is positioned supine on the operating table with a rolled towel placed underneath the shoulders, allowing extension of the neck. This permits freedom of motion of the head so that introduction and manipulation of the esophagoscope can be safely performed (Figure 13–5). It is not necessary to have an assistant hold the head extending over the end of the operating table.

The endoscopist opens the mouth with the left hand, and both the patient's mandible and maxilla are supported by this hand or by a laryngoscope, so that when the esophagoscope is grasped proximally by the right hand (as one might grasp a pencil) it can be introduced under direct vision into the posterior pharynx. The esophagoscope is initially held in an almost vertical position as it is inserted into the right side of the mouth. The patient's tongue is displaced to the left as the esophagoscope is advanced. As the esophagoscope is advanced it is slowly brought down to a near-horizontal orientation, allowing it to travel in a straight direction through the mouth and hypopharynx into the esophagus itself. The lip of the beveled portion of the esophagoscope should be oriented anteriorly, and as the esophagoscope passes through the mouth into the hypopharynx, the left hand continues to support the mandible and maxilla while permitting the left thumb and index finger to hold the distal esophagoscope in a pinching-type maneuver (see Figure 13–5). When this procedure is appropriately performed, the endoscopist is permitted precise two-handed control of the esophagoscope while completely protecting both the upper and lower lips and teeth.

It cannot be overemphasized that complete visualization of the esophageal lumen must be maintained throughout passage of the esophagoscope through the mouth and hypopharynx into the esophagus. We have found that precise exposure of the esophageal lumen is achieved by using the anterior lip of the esophago-

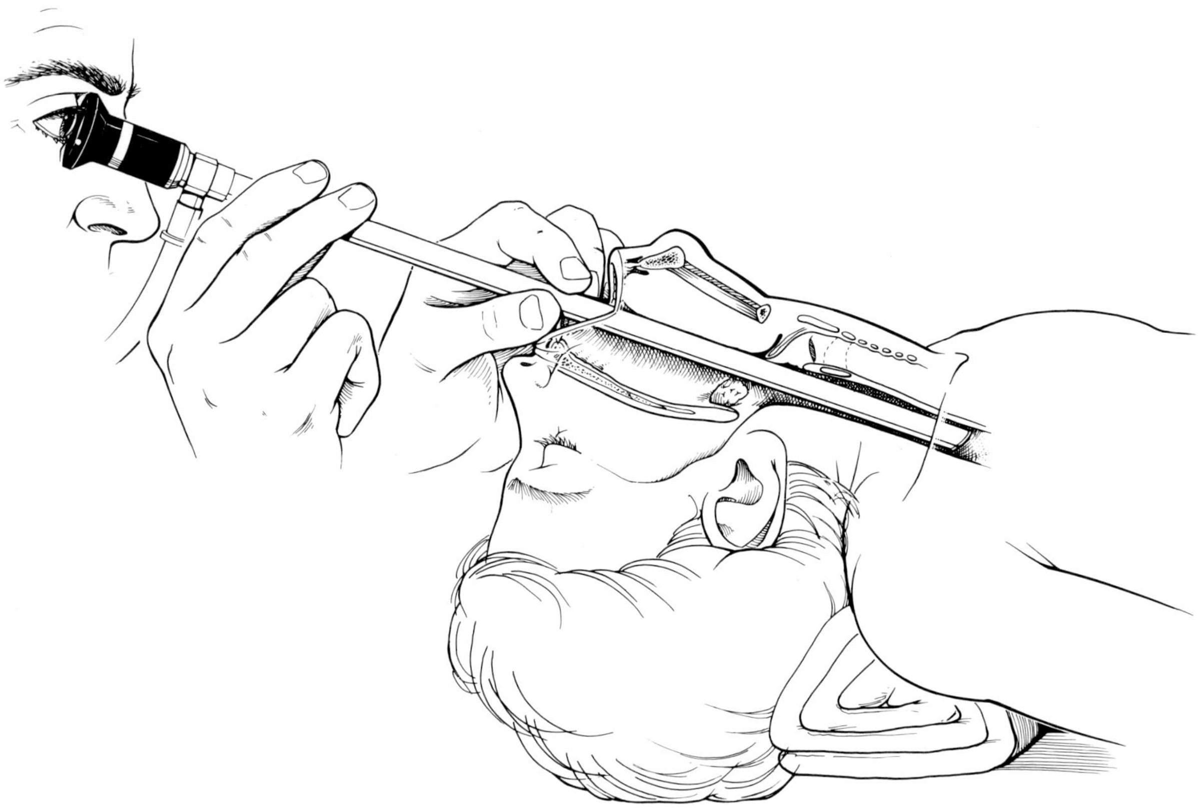

Figure 13–5. A child is appropriately positioned for rigid esophagoscopy. The large rolled towel placed underneath the child's shoulder allows the neck to be extended. Note that the endoscopist's left hand supports the mandible and maxilla while protecting the lips and teeth. Also note that precise two-handed control of the esophagoscope is maintained, to minimize the risk of perforation during introduction of the esophagoscope through the cricopharyngeal musculature.

scope to elevate the larynx and open the cricopharyngeal muscle. As many patients undergoing esophagoscopy are intubated, this feat may easily be accomplished by advancing the scope behind the endotracheal tube, allowing exposure of the cricopharyngeal muscle and esophageal lumen. We often use a laryngoscope to elevate the larynx, allowing passage of the esophagoscope just behind the arytenoids into the esophageal lumen. Regardless of the technique employed, it is critical not to advance the esophagoscope until the lumen is clearly visualized. Moreover, passage through the cricopharyngeal musculature requires precise visualization because it is at this site that perforation is most likely to occur (Figure 13–6). It is also important to understand the child's laryngeal and hypopharyngeal anatomy because the small size and contraction of the cricopharyngeal muscle frequently make passage of the scope difficult. Adequate identification of the pyriform sinuses aids in avoiding hypopharyngeal perforation (Figure 13–7). It is also useful, on occasion, to pass a soft suction catheter into the upper esophagus to make identification of the lumen easier. The catheter may be introduced into the esophageal lumen through the esophagoscope itself, with the esophagoscope then passed over it, or the catheter may be passed separately with the esophagoscope placed beside, keeping it in direct vision. An esophagoscope must never be advanced unless the lumen is clearly visualized ahead.

With respect to foreign bodies, the use of appropriate instrumentation is emphasized. Soft objects such as food impactions are removed either piecemeal or by the passage of a distal balloon catheter that, on inflation of the balloon, can move the impaction up into the esophagoscope. Perhaps the most challenging foreign bodies are those with sharp points or edges. In designing the appropriate removal of these types of foreign bodies it is well to heed one of Chevalier Jackson's great teaching rules: "Advancing points perforate; trailing points do not."[8] Thus, in managing pins, it is best to try to bring them out of the esophagus with their sharp point trailing rather than advancing. When faced with an open safety pin within the esophagus with the pin pointing upward, the operator is best

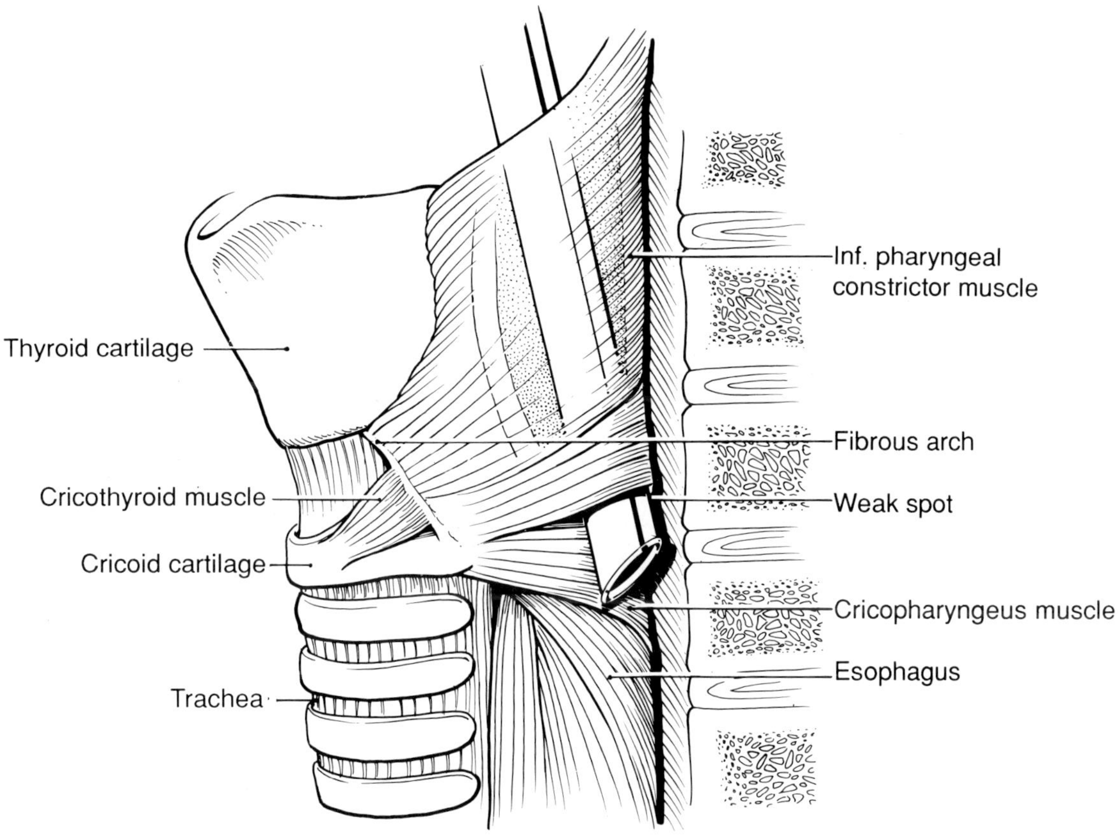

Figure 13–6. The relative weak spot of the esophagus at the level of the cricopharyngeal musculature. Pressure exerted on this weak spot causes perforation, emphasizing the need for the esophagoscope to be passed with complete visualization of the esophageal lumen at all times.

advised to grasp the spring loop with a forceps and advance the entire pin into the stomach where it can be rotated and extracted with the open point pointing downward. It is always reasonable to try and manipulate large or sharp objects into the protecting sheath of a rigid open-tube esophagoscope.

In managing esophageal strictures one can try to gently insinuate the rigid esophagoscope through the stricture in a rotary fashion. If successful, the stricture can be dilated progressively with standard dilators. If the stricture is too tight to permit safe passage of the esophagoscope, several options are available. Small dilators can be passed via the esophagoscope through the stricture under direct visualization to initiate the dilation procedure. A Rigiflex balloon system may also be passed alongside the esophagoscope under direct vision to perform the initial dilation. Filiform catheters and followers may similarly be used. Another useful technique is passage of a deflated Fogarty balloon catheter via the instrument channel through the stricture, followed by inflation of the balloon and dilation of the stricture. Should all such efforts fail, a final option is passage of a ureteral catheter through the instrument channel of the esophagoscope and past the

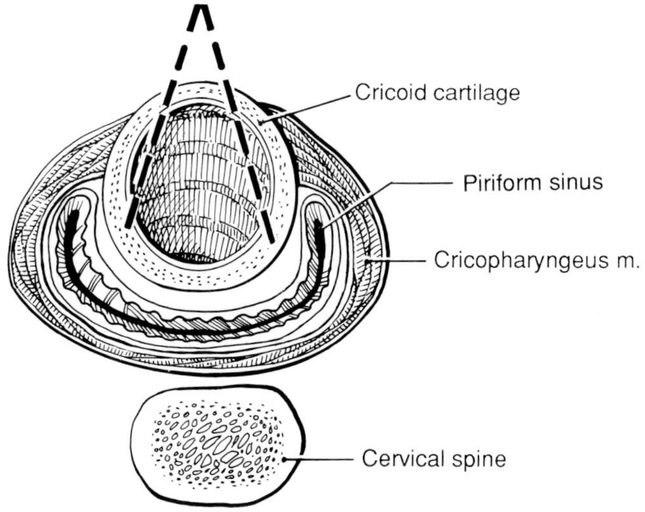

Figure 13–7. This diagram demonstrates how the relationship between the cricoid cartilage and cricopharyngeal muscle allows the esophageal opening to be closed in a pinchcock-type fashion. To safely introduce the esophagoscope and minimize risk of perforation, the endoscopist must feel comfortable in identifying the pyriform sinus. Passage of a luminal finder such as a soft suction catheter can also be helpful in ensuring the safety of the examination.

stricture into the stomach, where it may be retrieved via gastrotomy. A string may then be tied to the ureteral catheter and looped through the nose and gastrostomy site so that guided dilation can be performed later. It is also helpful to inject strictures with triamcinolone acetonide 40 mg/mL to soften the scar using a sclerotherapy needle passed through the instrument channel.

COMPLICATIONS

Complications occur in less than 2% of patients. Perforation is the most common complication of rigid esophagoscopy and generally occurs in one of two locations. The most frequent site of perforation is in the cervical esophagus at the level of the cricopharyngeal muscle. Although less frequent, perforation can also occur just above the gastroesophageal junction, where the esophagus deviates slightly laterally. It may happen during the time of stricture dilation, especially if the dilation is either forceful or undertaken without complete luminal visualization. In addition, manipulation of the esophagoscope during the removal of a difficult foreign body could cause perforation, as could a biopsy if taken too deeply; however, complications related to the removal of foreign bodies are usually related to the foreign body itself. Late presentation with esophageal erosion by the foreign body predisposes to perforation.

In addition to perforation, other complications such as pneumothorax, pneumomediastinum, mediastinitis, croup, pneumonia, airway obstruction, dysphagia, and loss of teeth can occur following esophagoscopy. In the past, posterior pharyngeal perforation was an occasional complication when rigid esophagoscopy was performed on a child who was not fully sedated, but the current use of flexible scopes in unanesthetized children has proven to be quite safe in this regard. Therefore, we believe that all children undergoing rigid esophagoscopy should have general anesthesia.

POSTOPERATIVE CARE

Following completion of the esophagoscopy, careful assessment of their breath and heart sounds should be performed. Signs of perforation would include diminished breath sounds with pneumothorax or Hamman's mediastinal crunch sound indicative of mediastinal air. If either is noted, an immediate chest radiograph is performed before leaving the operating room. Otherwise, a chest film is obtained on the majority of patients approximately 1 hour following the procedure in the recovery room. In the absence of any immediate signs of complication, the patient is not permitted to eat, is maintained on intravenous fluids for 4 to 8 hours, and is observed for signs of esophageal perforation, which may include fever, chest or back pain, as well as evidence of cervical emphysema or crepitus. Routine leukocyte counts are not obtained unless symptoms are present. Should clinical suspicion of a perforation be aroused, chest and neck radiographs are obtained. If any question still remains, a water soluble contrast esophagogram is performed. If no symptoms are evident after 4 to 8 hours, the child is permitted to consume clear liquids until the following day when the diet may be liberalized. In children in whom strictures have been dilated, we have administered sucralfate (Carafate) slurpees (1 g sucralfate mixed in 20 mL of ice water) three times daily for a month to reduce the incidence of stricture reformation.

Although all children who have undergone rigid esophagoscopy must be watched closely for signs and symptoms of perforation, the incidence of this complication is minimal with proper technique. In the authors' combined experience of several hundred cases of rigid esophagoscopy, no esophageal perforations or other major complications have occurred.

REFERENCES

1. Berci G. History of endoscopy. In Berci G, ed. *Endoscopy.* New York: Appleton-Century-Crofts; 1976.
2. *Accident Facts, 1992.* Itasca, IL: National Safety Council; 1992.
3. Manning S, Stool SE. Foreign body detection: Don't overlook plastic. *J Resp Dis.* 1987;8:33.
4. Moves MD, Corithers JS, Birck HG. Esophageal burns secondary to disc battery ingestion. *Ann Otol Rhinol Laryngol.* 1984;93:364.
5. Burton DM, Stith JA. Extralumenal esophageal coin erosion in children. Case report and review. *Int J Pediatr Otorhinol.* 1992;23:187.
6. Bigler FC. The use of a Foley catheter for removal of blunt foreign bodies from the esophagus. *J Thorac Cardiovasc Surg.* 1966;51:754.
7. O'Neill JA Jr, Holcomb GW Jr, Neblett WW. Management of tracheobronchial and esophageal foreign bodies in childhood. *J Pediatr Surg.* 1983;18:475.
8. Jackson C, Jackson CL. *Diseases of the Air and Food Passages of Foreign Body Origin.* Philadelphia: WB Saunders; 1936.

CHAPTER 14

Percutaneous Endoscopic Gastrostomy

GEORGE W. HOLCOMB III • MICHAEL W.L. GAUDERER

Gastrostomy is becoming one of the most common procedures performed by pediatric surgeons. Historically, the Stamm gastrostomy has been the most widely used technique. Another open procedure is the Janeway gastrostomy, in which a permanent stoma is created, tubularizing a portion of the gastric wall. With the revolution in minimally invasive surgery, laparoscopic gastrostomy is an additional option promising several advantages over the open technique (see Chapter 9). Percutaneous endoscopic gastrostomy (PEG), initially developed for children, was reported in 1980.[1] Since then, its popularity has increased and PEG has become the procedure of choice for those surgeons who are skilled in gastroscopy.

INDICATIONS

The most common indication for gastrostomy is the inability of the child to swallow effectively.[2] Other indications include feeding supplementation, continuous enteral feedings, and administration of long-term nonpalatable medications or feedings. Expanded applications of this principle include endoscopic gastrostomy for bile administration, for esophageal stenting, for management of gastric volvulus, for control of bleeding from a Stamm gastrostomy, for gastric decompression, and for temporary correction of stomal prolapse. Central nervous system (CNS) disease is the most common reason for a child's inability to swallow. Included in this myriad of diagnoses are anoxic brain injury, oropharyngeal and laryngotracheal malformations, cleft lip and palate, trauma, chromosomal and metabolic abnormalities, and other unclassified neurologic disorders.

Children requiring gastrostomy for feeding supplementation include those patients with severe failure to thrive, bronchopulmonary dysplasia, congenital heart disease or malignancies, esophageal dysmotility, biliary atresia, as well as those with acquired immunodeficiency syndrome (AIDS). Continuous enteral feedings may be required for children with short bowel syndrome, malabsorption, Crohn's disease, and intestinal pseudo-obstruction.

Percutaneous gastrostomy may also be indicated in patients who cannot tolerate medications or special diets. Included in this group would be patients with Alagille syndrome, chronic renal failure, and severe chronic constipation.

ANTIREFLUX PROCEDURE?

Gastroesophageal reflux (GER) is often present in patients requiring gastrostomies.[3–5] Therefore, it is important to evaluate these children for the presence of GER and to decide whether a gastrostomy should be performed alone or in conjunction with a fundoplication. This question remains controversial.[4–9]

Our basic assumption is that not all severely impaired and high-risk children need a fundoplication, which may expose them to a new set of complications and problems. It is not surprising that antireflux procedures performed in these candidates have a high complication rate.[10] These patients are often malnourished and may have increased abdominal pressure secondary to spasticity or seizures, musculoskeletal or other anatomic deformities, associated systemic diseases, ventriculoperitoneal shunts, and other problems. Their inability to swallow contributes to the aspiration of saliva and complicates their pulmonary care. For these reasons, any laparotomy is a major procedure and may provoke undesirable early or late complications.

A careful preoperative evaluation for these patients is required. This usually includes an upper gastrointestinal barium study, esophageal manometry, and 24-hour esophageal pH studies. Moreover, some children require gastric emptying studies. Our personal experience has been that only those patients with severe reflux (defined as the inability to tolerate nasogastric feedings for a period of 4 to 6 weeks) will need an antireflux procedure and Stamm gastrostomy rather than just a PEG.

Studies aimed at defining the degree of preoperative GER do not necessarily correlate with the incidence of post-PEG reflux.[11] In addition, some children who have had occasional bouts of emesis in the first few months following PEG have gradually improved, particularly after adjustments have been made in the feeding regimen. This finding reinforces the concept that correction of malnutrition may improve foregut function. Moreover, as all PEG candidates have been evaluated in a standardized fashion, there has been a good correlation between preoperative nasogastric tube feeding tolerance and absence of post-PEG GER. Post-PEG fundoplication or conversion to feeding jejunostomy has been required only in the group consisting of neurologically impaired children.[12] Therefore, gastrostomy and fundoplication are recommended only in children who are unable to tolerate tube feedings because of reflux. As PEG is a simple procedure and does not interfere with possible future fundoplication, it is placed initially in children without symptomatic reflux. With careful follow-up, an antireflux procedure can be performed later if necessary.

TECHNIQUE

Percutaneous endoscopic gastrostomy in infants and young children is performed in the operating room. In older children and in those able to tolerate endoscopy without compromise of the upper airway, local anesthesia and sedation may be employed. In younger children, however, general endotracheal anesthesia is preferred, primarily because of anticipated difficulties with airway management. The patient receives one dose of a broad-spectrum antibiotic intravenously prior to the procedure.

Equipment

Prior to 1988, a dePezzer mushroom catheter with a diameter of 12 to 20 French, depending on the patient's size, was employed. In the past 4 years, a 15-French silicone rubber PEG catheter developed for children has been used routinely (Gauderer PEG, Bard Interventional Products, Tewksbury, MA) (Figure

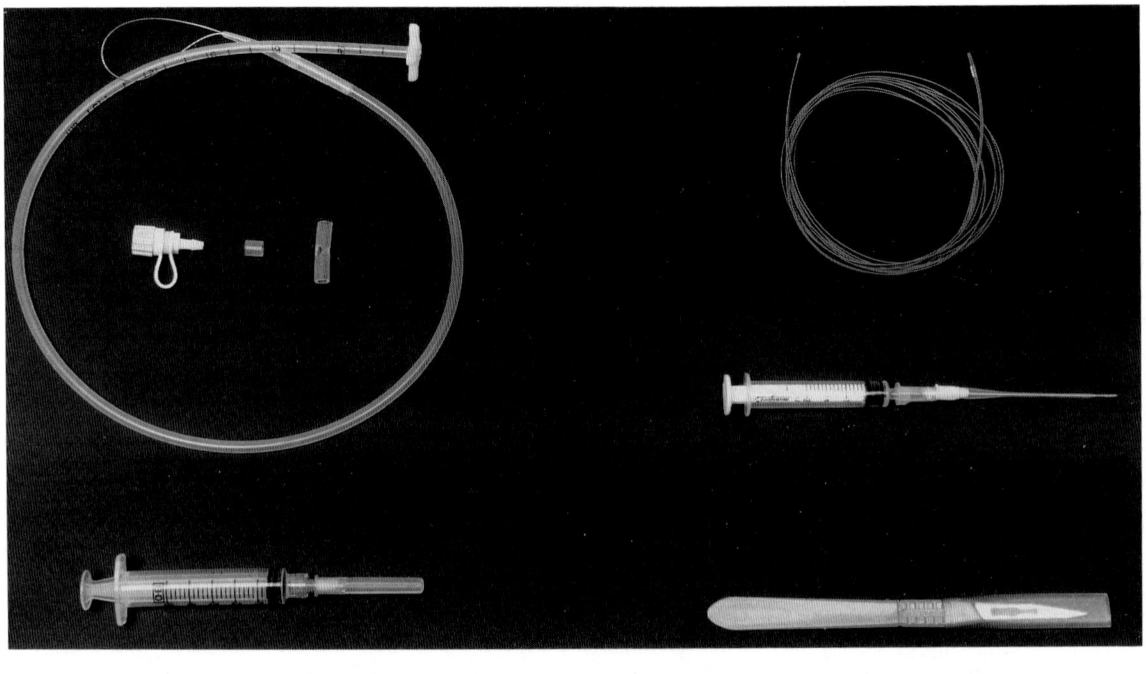

Figure 14–1. Basic components of the pediatric percutaneous endoscopic gastrostomy tray: 15-French silicone rubber catheter with flexible internal retaining crossbar, tapered catheter end and wire loop, and shaft markings; external retaining bolster and ring; external cap; flexible stainless-steel traction wire; 16-gauge cannula; syringe and scalpel. (*Courtesy of Bard Interventional Products, Tewksbury, MA.*)

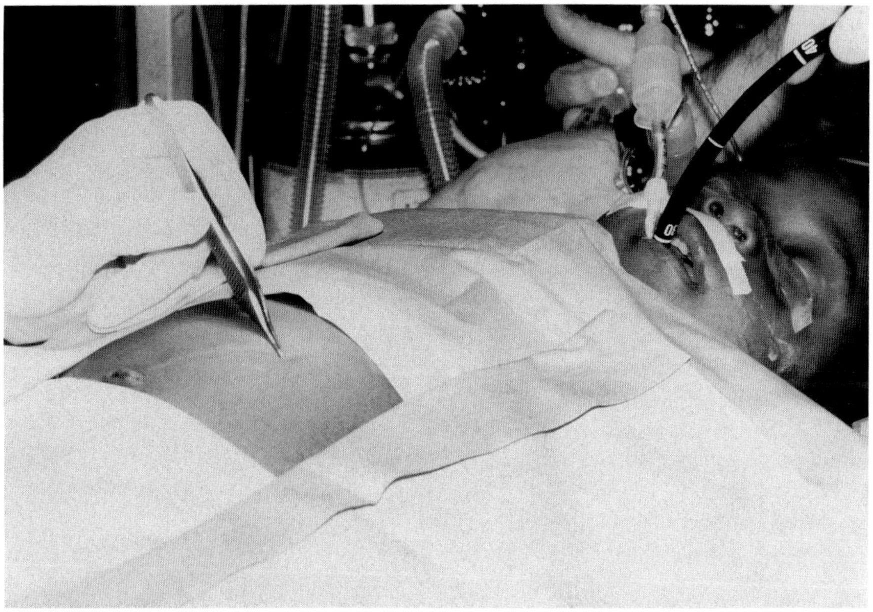

Figure 14–2. Four-year-old 10-kg child with chronic granulomatous disease requiring long-term continuous enteral feedings. The endoscope has been inserted in the stomach. Pressure is being exerted over the point of maximal transillumination.

14–1). This tube has a tapered tip with a loop of fine, flexible stainless-steel wire. Special markings on the shaft allow the surgeon to determine the length of the remaining tube segment during the pulling process. The cross-shaped gastric retainer is nondetachable, but the wings of this retainer collapse to allow passage through the esophagus and subsequent catheter removal.

Procedure

For the procedure, two operators are required. The child is positioned in the supine position and, following anesthesia, the abdomen is widely prepared and draped in a sterile fashion. The site for exteriorization of the gastrostomy tube is tentatively marked over the midportion of the left upper rectus abdominis muscle. Usually, this site corresponds to the junction of the lower two thirds and upper one third of a line drawn between the umbilicus and the midportion of the left inferior costal margin. The eventual exit site must, however, correspond to the point of maximum transillumination (Figure 14–2).

The fiberoptic or videogastroscope is introduced through the child's mouth and advanced into the stomach. Esophagogastroduodenoscopy is rapidly performed. Gastric insufflation pushes the liver, spleen, and colon away from the gastrostomy site and brings the anterior gastric wall into contact with the abdominal wall. The tip of the gastroscope is flexed toward the anterior gastric wall. Both the gastric contour and position of the gastroscope can be better discerned when the operating room lights are dimmed. As the child's stomach is small, the gastroscope should be moved gently and in limited increments during endoscopy.

Having identified the illuminated stomach, the surgeon exerts digital pressure over the proposed gastrostomy site where the transillumination is brightest. With finger manipulation, the anterior abdominal wall is pushed inward, producing an indentation in the anterior gastric wall (Figure 14–3). It is imperative that the endoscopist clearly identify this "mound." If absolute confirmation is not possible, the finger is moved to adjacent sites until the clearest identification is achieved.

A polypectomy snare is then advanced through the channel of the endoscope and a small transverse skin incision is made at the site of the gastrostomy. A curved hemostat is introduced into the incision and

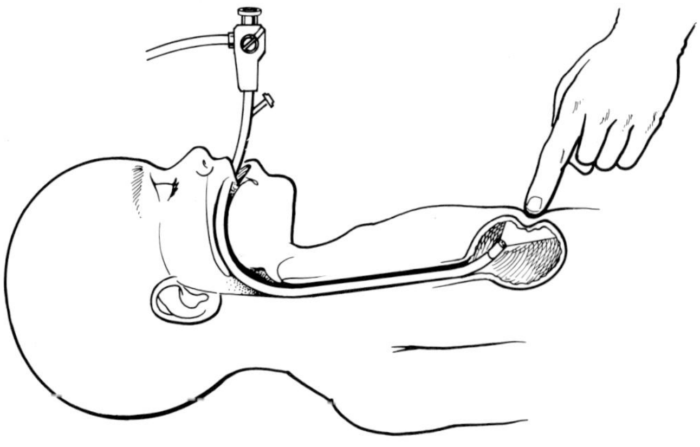

Figure 14–3. Following gastroscopy, the surgeon firmly indents the anterior abdominal wall and produces a "mound," which is visualized by the endoscopist.

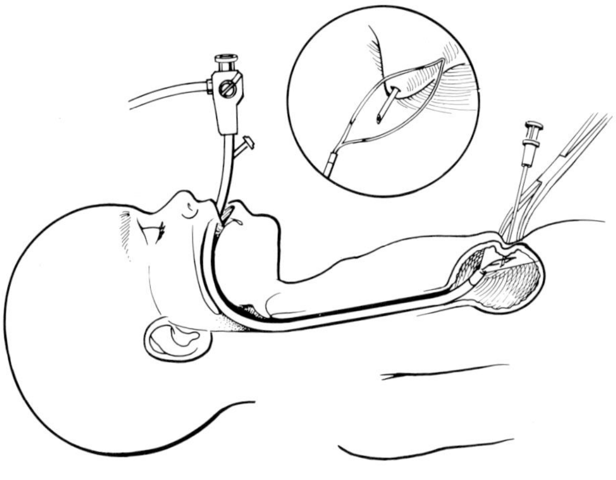

Figure 14–4. The endoscopist continues to visualize this site and a 5-mm incision is made externally by the surgeon. The incision is then spread using a hemostat, and an Intramedicut cannula is inserted through the abdominal wall and into the stomach at this site. The endoscopist places a snare around the cannula and the needle is withdrawn from the cannula.

pressure is again applied to reproduce the gastric in-Zdentation. As the surgeon maintains pressure on the hemostat, the endoscopist manipulates the open polypectomy snare around this intragastric mound. The surgeon then introduces the 16-gauge needle and cannula through the center of the incision between the prongs of the hemostat, piercing the muscular layer, peritoneum, and gastric wall with a quick motion to avoid separating the stomach from the abdominal wall (Figure 14–4). The endoscopist positions the snare loosely around the cannula and the needle is removed by the surgeon, leaving the plastic sheath in place. A looped wire is inserted through the cannula by the surgeon, and the wire is ensnared by the endoscopist (Figure 14–5). Alternatively, the wire can be grasped with a biopsy forceps introduced through the side channel of the endoscope. After the wire is secured, it is exteriorized through the mouth together with the endoscope. This establishes the guide for the PEG catheter. Gastric insufflation is maintained throughout the procedure to avoid separating the stomach from the abdominal wall.

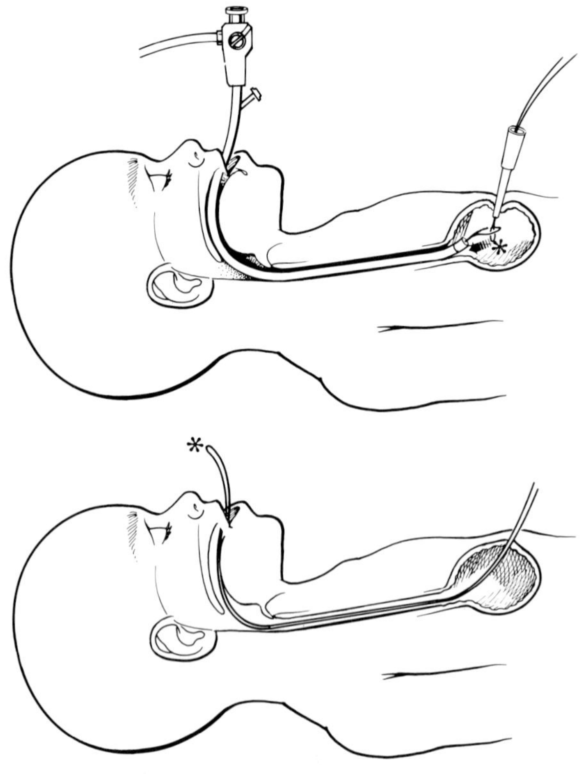

Figure 14–5. The wire is threaded through the cannula and is snared by the endoscopist. The wire and endoscope are then removed. The gastrostomy tube is then secured to the wire, which has exited from the mouth.

The PEG catheter is attached to the oral end of the guiding loop. The two wires are interlooped which eliminates the need for a knot. A water soluble lubricant is applied to the catheter and traction is placed on the transabdominal portion of the loop. The catheter is pulled through the patient's mouth, esophagus, and upper stomach and across the gastric and abdominal walls (Figure 14–6). This described catheter is long and, when the tapered end exits through the abdominal wall, the other end is still outside the patient's mouth (Figure 14–7). As the catheter has markings, the surgeon can estimate the location of the retaining inner crossbar. Markings corresponding to the appropriate thickness of the abdominal wall can be added to unmarked catheters.

The endoscope is repositioned in the stomach and the position of the crossbar is documented. Tension is

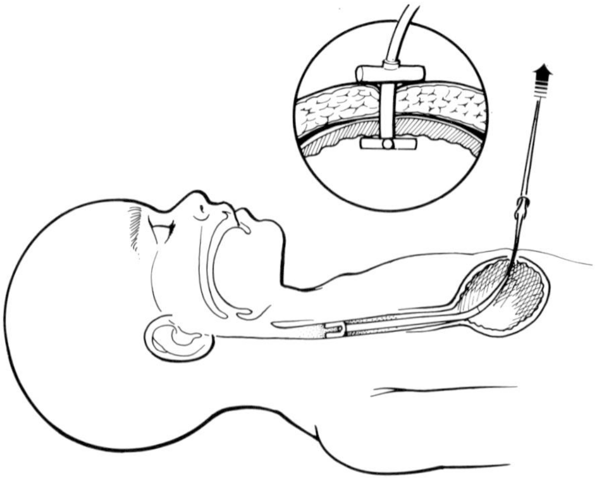

Figure 14–6. After the wire is tied to the gastrostomy tube, the wire and tube are then pulled in an antegrade direction down the esophagus and stomach and out the anterior abdominal wall. The gastrostomy tube is pulled firmly against the anterior abdominal wall; the crossbar on the tube prevents its external migration.

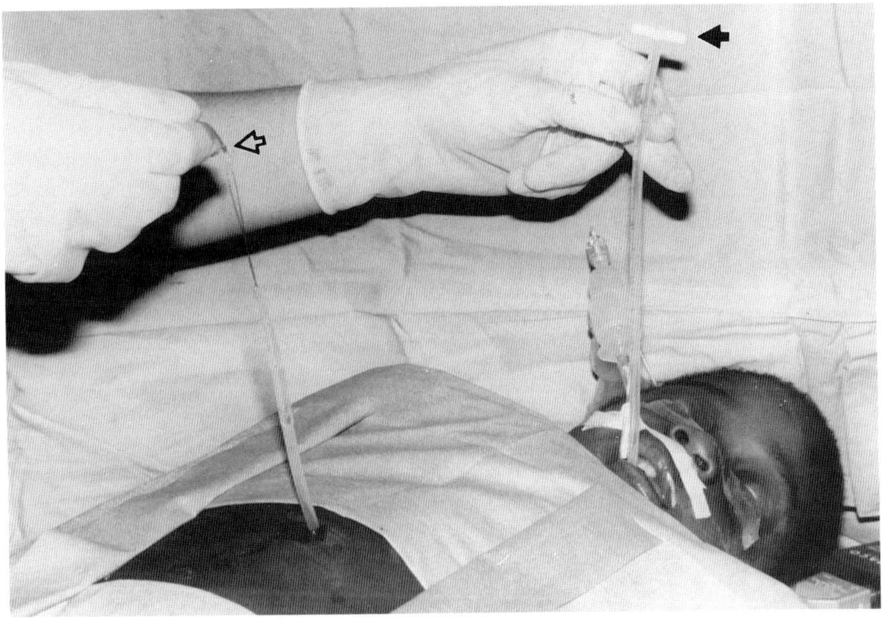

Figure 14–7. The catheter has been pulled through the patient's mouth and esophagus and across gastric and abdominal walls. Note the interlooped wires (*open arrow*) and the internal retaining crossbar (*solid arrow*). Two of the four prongs were cut off to facilitate subsequent removal.

applied to the catheter outside until it is judged that the gastric and abdominal walls are in loose contact. The inner crossbar should move freely and not be embedded in the gastric mucosa. The external retaining crossbar and the immobilizing ring are then applied with the help of the hemostat. It is important not to indent the skin with application of the external retaining crossbar.

Following removal of the endoscope, the catheter is cut to the desired length and an adapter is attached. The catheter is then attached to an opened container, providing gravity drainage (Figure 14–8). A small dressing is applied to the exit site. Anchoring sutures are no longer employed but the catheter is immobilized with tape for several days.

POSTOPERATIVE CARE

A careful abdominal examination is performed postoperatively to ensure that peritonitis has not developed. Feedings are started 12 to 24 hours postoperatively and small volumes of dilute formula are given. These can be advanced to full volume and concentration over 1 to 2 days. Patients are discharged without dressings, but special attention is required to ensure that the external crossbar has a little "play." A postoperative visit is arranged at 1 to 2 weeks, when the skin–catheter interface is inspected for the formation of granulation tissue. Silver nitrate is applied to reduce the granulation tissue and, if necessary, excised.

When no longer needed, removal of the catheter is accomplished in the office with simple traction. The fistulous tract is covered with a dry dressing and will usually close within a few days. On the other hand,

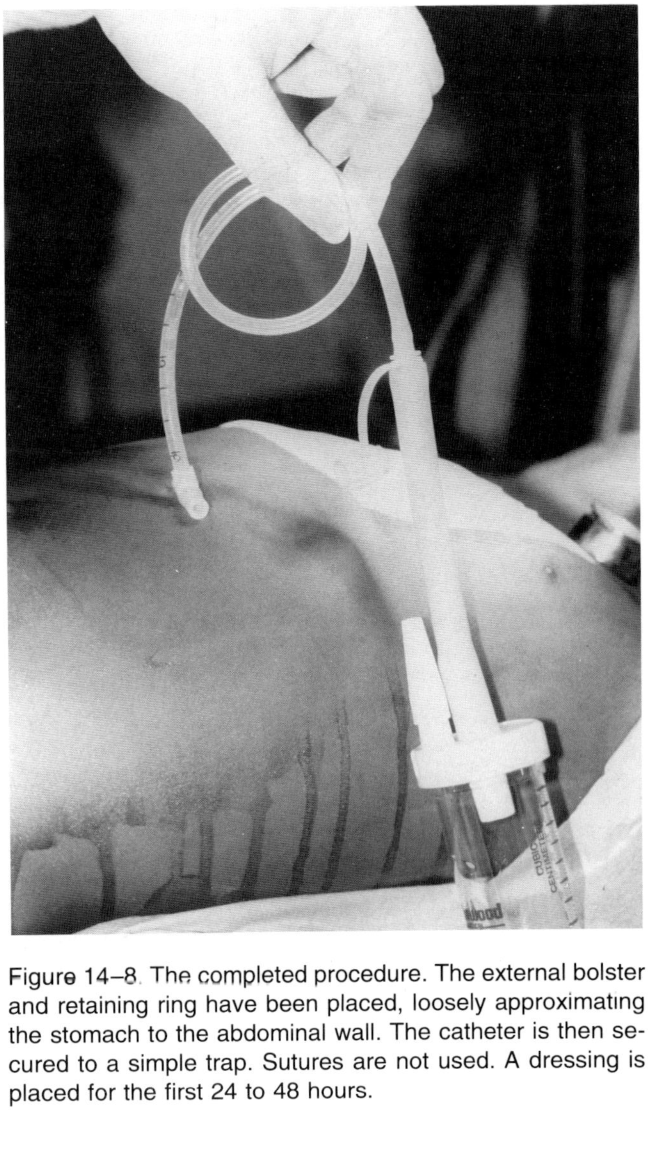

Figure 14–8. The completed procedure. The external bolster and retaining ring have been placed, loosely approximating the stomach to the abdominal wall. The catheter is then secured to a simple trap. Sutures are not used. A dressing is placed for the first 24 to 48 hours.

chronic fibrosed tracts may need excision and closure. When desired, removal of the catheter and insertion of a gastrostomy button are usually not accomplished until at least 3 to 6 months after the procedure to ensure that adequate adhesion has developed between the stomach and the abdominal wall.

COMMENTS

The operating room is the preferred location for the procedure. The attendance of a surgical and anesthetic teams affords maximum patient safety. Moreover, should complications or an open gastrostomy be required, these can be managed best in this location.

The gastrostomy site should be carefully chosen prior to an incision. The midline should be avoided as it is thin and could predispose to leaks. Epigastric vessels can often be seen during transillumination and should be avoided. Gastrostomies situated too close to the costal margin have a tendency to leak because of increased catheter motion secondary to breathing. In addition, chondritis may develop.

It is important to control the amount of air instilled into the stomach. Gastric underinflation will not push the colon caudally and will make it more vulnerable to puncture. Gastric hyperinflation may rotate the colon anteriorly, again making it more vulnerable. Prolonged upper endoscopy prior to needle placement should also be avoided, as air-filled small bowel loops may push the colon and stomach cephalad.[13] Unequivocal transillumination and digital pressure on the central portion of the stomach are the two most important safeguards for preventing complications with this procedure. Failure to demonstrate either should lead the surgeon to seriously consider an open procedure.

The inner and outer crossbars should not be tight as either one may result in pressure necrosis with embedment of the catheter, which leads to external migration and difficulty with feeding, pain, and leakage problems. Moreover, even though the catheter is no longer sutured to the skin, accidental catheter removal has not occurred. The use of the external crossbar and immobilizing ring reinforced with tape has been adequate to secure the catheter.

THE CASE WESTERN RESERVE EXPERIENCE

From 1979 to 1992, 335 PEGs were performed in 330 patients at Rainbow Babies' and Children's Hospital, Cleveland, Ohio. One child required the procedure three times, and three children had two procedures each.

Two hundred and twenty-eight (68.7%) children underwent gastrostomy for inability to swallow. Within this group there were 27 different diagnoses, mainly CNS lesions. Feeding supplementation was the indication in 78 patients (23.5%). Seventeen patients (5.1%) required continuous enteral feedings. In the remaining 7, PEG was used for the administration of long-term nonpalatable medications and/or diet.

The patients ranged in age from 1 month to 24 years. One hundred and thirty-two patients (39.7%) were less than 1 year of age and 47 were less than 1 month. Twenty percent weighed less than 5 kg and four weighed 2.5 kg. Forty-six (13.8%) children had previously undergone an abdominal operation, 35 (10.5%) underwent a concomitant procedure, and 2 had a mild coagulopathy. Twelve patients (3.6%) had severe cardiac lesions and one had esophageal varices. All procedures were performed in the operating room and general anesthesia was employed in 215 PEG placements (63.7%).

COMPLICATIONS

Five children developed gastrocolic fistulas diagnosed between 4 and 21 months following the procedure. Analysis of these cases revealed problems with gastric insufflation in three (underinflation in two and overinflation in one). In the other two patients, transillumination and digital indentation were not clearly evident from the outset. One child had severe scoliosis and one, who had previously undergone repair of a diaphragmatic hernia, had intestinal malrotation. The gastrocolic fistula closed following catheter removal in three patients, but operative correction was needed in the other two.

Partial gastric separation occurred 1 month post-PEG in a 9-month-old child with cyanotic congenital heart disease. The small leak was identified and corrected using a limited celiotomy. One late partial gastric separation occurred 3 years post-PEG in a 3½-year-old with short bowel syndrome during insertion of a "button." The small leak was promptly identified and corrected using a limited celiotomy. No major complications have occurred in the last 6 years.

In the past few years, two important trends have been observed in our institution: a decrease in the complication rate and a decrease in the median age of patients referred for PEG. Because of satisfaction with the principle of the PEG, applications of the concept have been expanded to include percutaneous jejunostomy,[14] PEG for gastric decompression, and a nonendoscopic modification to correct severe gastrostomy leakage.[15]

A substantial body of literature has developed

since 1980 demonstrating the efficacy, simplicity, and safety of PEG; however, as with any other type of stoma placement, careful patient selection, attention to technical details, and a willingness to systematically follow these children are essential.

REFERENCES

1. Gauderer MWL, Ponsky JL, Izant RJ. Gastrostomy without laparotomy: A percutaneous endoscopic technique. *J Pediatr Surg.* 1980;15:872.
2. Gauderer MWL. An updated experience with percutaneous endoscopic gastrostomy in children. *Gastrointest Endosc Clin North Am.* 1992;2:195.
3. Abrahams P, Burkitt BFE. Hiatus hernia and gastroesophageal reflux in children and adolescents with cerebral palsy. *Aust Paediatr J.* 1970;6:41.
4. Holmes TW Jr. Chalasia, peptic esophagitis, and hiatal hernia: A common syndrome in patients with nervous system disease. *Chest.* 1971;60:441.
5. Wesley JR, Coran AG, Sarahan TM, et al. The need for evaluation of gastroesophageal reflux in brain-damaged children referred for feeding gastrostomy. *J Pediatr Surg.* 1981;16:866.
6. Jolley SG, Smith EI, Tunell WP. Protective antireflux operation with feeding gastrostomy, experience with children. *Ann Surg.* 1985;201:736.
7. Mollitt DL, Golladay ES, Seibert JJ: Symptomatic gastroesophageal reflux following gastrostomy in neurologically impaired patients. *Pediatrics.* 1985;75:1124.
8. Berezin S, Schwartz SM, Halata MS, et al. Gastroesophageal reflux secondary to gastrostomy tube placement. *Am J Dis Child.* 1986;140:699.
9. Jolley JG, Tunell WP, Hoelzer DJ, et al. Lower esophageal pressure changes with tube gastrostomy: A causative factor of gastroesophageal reflux in children? *J Pediatr Surg.* 1986;21:624.
10. Dedinsky GK, Vane DW, Black T, et al. Complications and reoperations after Nissen fundoplication in childhood. *Am J Surg.* 1987;153:177.
11. Grunow JE, Al-Hafidh AS, Tunell WP. Gastroesophageal reflux following percutaneous endoscopic gastrostomy in children. *J Pediatr Surg.* 1989;24:42.
12. Gauderer MWL. Percutaneous endoscopic gastrostomy: A 10 year experience with 220 children. *J Pediatr Surg.* 1991;26:288.
13. Stefan MM, Holcomb GW, Ross AJ III. Cologastric fistula as a complication of percutaneous endoscopic gastrostomy. *J Parenter Enter Nutr.* 1989;13:554.
14. Ponsky JL, Gauderer MWL, Stellato TA, et al. Percutaneous approaches to enteral alimentation. *Am J Surg.* 1985;149:102.
15. Gauderer MWL. A simple technique for correction of severe gastrostomy leakage. *Surg Gynecol Obstet.* 1987; 165:170.

CHAPTER 15

Bronchoscopy and Endobronchial Procedures

ROBERT E. WOOD • RICHARD G. AZIZKHAN

Bronchoscopy is being used increasingly for both diagnostic and therapeutic purposes in infants and children.[1–12] Until recently, pediatric bronchoscopy was performed exclusively with rigid instruments and was considered the domain of the surgeon. The introduction of flexible bronchoscopes in the early 1970s revolutionized the practice of adult pulmonary medicine, and most bronchoscopic procedures in adults today are performed by pulmonologists rather than by surgeons. In pediatrics, however, such a shift in technique and practice has been slower to evolve because of the delay in development of flexible instrumentation suitable for children.

THE UNIVERSITY OF NORTH CAROLINA EXPERIENCE

With specialists from different disciplines performing the same procedure, there exists potential for conflicts at several levels. Who will do the bronchoscopy? What technique will be used? At the University of North Carolina (UNC), we have developed a practice model for the management of pediatric bronchoscopy that we believe combines the best of both specialties. The majority of the diagnostic procedures are performed by pediatric pulmonologists using flexible instruments, and the majority of therapeutic procedures are performed by surgeons (pediatric surgery or pediatric otolaryngology) using rigid instruments. Whenever warranted, a combined procedure is done. The essential elements of this practice model include skilled specialists in both areas, suitable equipment and facilities, videoendoscopy capability, and effective cooperation and communication among the various physician specialists. The results of the diagnostic procedures are recorded on videotape and reviewed with the appropriate surgical specialist who is able to plan the best procedure (surgical or endoscopic) for therapeutic management. With this team approach, operating room time is used efficiently and there are fewer surprises. The major disadvantage, however, is that a few patients undergo two procedures rather than one.

Such a practice model assumes appropriately trained and skilled nonsurgical endoscopists, who are not available in all institutions. There has been a trend in recent years for medical specialists other than pulmonologists (ie, anesthesiologists, neonatal and pediatric intensivists) to perform bronchoscopy in certain settings. This is not necessarily inappropriate, but it is important that the performing physician be knowledgeable about the technique and also about the findings that may be observed. For example, a flexible bronchoscope is often used to facilitate the difficult intubation. Abnormalities of the airway are frequently encountered in this setting; the person performing the bronchoscopic intubation must be able to recognize and manage effectively these findings.

INSTRUMENTATION

Rigid Bronchoscopes

Rigid bronchoscopes range from 2.5 to 8.5 mm in diameter and from 20 to 50 cm in length. The most salient feature of the rigid bronchoscope is that it is sufficiently large to function as an endotracheal tube. The airways distal to the tip of the bronchoscope are illuminated either with a prism inserted partially into the lumen or by fiberoptics through the glass rod telescope.

The optical characteristics of rigid bronchoscopes are either superb or abysmal. The optical quality of the image with the glass rod telescope is spectacular and unequaled by any other bronchoscope; however, when the prism is used for optical quality, visualization through the bronchoscope can be difficult. This mode is often necessary with manipulation of instruments passed through the bronchoscope.

Although the lumen of the rigid bronchoscope is relatively large, the glass rod telescope occupies the majority of the lumen and special instruments are required for use in association with the telescope. These include the "optical forceps," a specially designed forceps that operates in conjunction with the telescope, and an "ultrathin" forceps, which can be passed alongside the telescope. Certain other tools can be passed through the bronchoscope in parallel with the telescope; these include suction catheters, balloon-tipped (Fogarty and Gruentzig) catheters, snares, and retrieval baskets.

The presence of the glass rod telescope results in a significant increase in resistance to ventilation through the bronchoscope.[13] Thus, the use of a rigid bronchoscope and telescope does not guarantee that ventilation will be easily accomplished. For example, the bronchoscope most commonly used in infants has a 3.5 mm internal diameter, whereas the diameter of the corresponding telescope is 2.5 mm. It is therefore essential that the patient's oxygenation and ventilation be carefully monitored during rigid bronchoscopy.

Flexible Bronchoscopes

Flexible bronchoscopes differ from rigid bronchoscopes in many ways, not the least of which is their pliability. In contrast to rigid scopes, they are solid instruments and the patient breathes around the flexible instrument rather than through it. For this reason, the diameter of the flexible bronchoscope must be relatively small.

The standard pediatric flexible bronchoscope is approximately 3.5 mm in outer diameter. Within this scope, a suction channel measures 1.2 mm in diameter. Flexible instruments used in adults range up to 6 mm in outside diameter with a suction channel as large as 2.7 mm; however, as the trachea of a newborn infant is only about 5 to 5.5 mm in diameter, such instruments are clearly not suitable for pediatric use. Smaller flexible bronchoscopes are available with the smallest being 2.2 mm in outside diameter.

The flexible bronchoscope is distinguished by its ability to flex its distal end as much as 180 degrees. Thus it can easily be guided into the upper lobes or other places that are difficult to visualize with rigid bronchoscopes. Flexible bronchoscopes are usually inserted through the nose rather than through the mouth and can be passed through endotracheal or tracheostomy tubes of appropriate size.

The image produced by a flexible bronchoscope is composed of several thousand "points" of color and light intensity; each "point" represents the light transmitted by a single glass fiber. The resolution of this image is inherently much lower than that obtained with the glass rod telescope. In practice, however, the image quality is quite good and the operator's eye rapidly compensates for the low resolution.

Flexible nasopharyngoscopes are often used to evaluate the upper airway in pediatric patients and have some utility.[14,15] Although less expensive than flexible bronchoscopes, these instruments have limitations. They are much shorter than bronchoscopes. Because they have no suction channel, it is not possible to suction secretions or to deposit topical anesthetic agents on the larynx. As a result, it may be difficult to examine the subglottic airway with such an instrument unless effective laryngeal anesthesia is achieved in another fashion.

Semidisposable image guides are marketed for utilization through endotracheal tubes and have been used to examine the lower airways of intubated patients.[16] These instruments have very limited utility, however, as they lack the ability for controlled angulation of the tip. This makes their use very difficult except through an endotracheal or tracheostomy tube. Moreover, it is difficult to examine the airways distal to the end of the tube. If the tip of the endotracheal tube is situated in one of the mainstem bronchi, it may be difficult to identify the anatomic site as the tip of the image guide cannot be manipulated.

The sizing of the bronchoscopes can be confusing.[13,17] The size designation for rigid bronchoscopes applies to the outer diameter of the largest instrument that can be passed through the bronchoscope, not to the outer diameter of the bronchoscope itself. On the other hand, the size designation for a flexible bronchoscope refers to the actual diameter of the bronchoscope. For example, a 3.5-mm flexible bronchoscope will easily pass through a 3.5-mm rigid bronchoscope.[1]

ANESTHESIA

Although it is possible to perform either rigid or flexible bronchoscopy with minimal or no anesthesia, the object is not to see how much the patient can tolerate. For a safe and effective procedure, it is important for the patient to be comfortable.[18,19] In practice, this means general anesthesia for children undergoing

TABLE 15–1. LOCATIONS WHERE FLEXIBLE BRONCHOSCOPY WAS PERFORMED AT UNIVERSITY OF NORTH CAROLINA

Bronchoscopy laboratory	62%
Pediatric intensive care unit	22%
Neonatal intensive care unit	7%
Operating rooms	7%
Other intensive care units	2%

rigid bronchoscopy. On the other hand, flexible bronchoscopy is most commonly performed with sedation and topical anesthesia. At our institution, we generally use a combination of an intravenously administered narcotic and a benzodiazepine, with topical lidocaine applied to the mucosa of the nose and larynx (and trachea or bronchi).

The passage of the bronchoscope and the associated anesthesia/sedation alters the patient's ability to breathe and may place him or her at risk for other complications as well. Therefore, it is essential that the patient be monitored appropriately throughout the procedure.[19] Procedures should be performed in a facility that has adequate monitoring and is appropriately staffed and equipped to deal with any and all contingencies. At UNC, we perform the majority of our flexible procedures in a bronchoscopy laboratory. The remainder are performed in the operating rooms or various intensive care units (Table 15–1). In appropriate circumstances, flexible bronchoscopy can be safely and effectively performed on outpatients. In fact, 27% of our procedures were performed on an outpatient basis; however, it must be recognized that pediatric patients have special needs and special risks and overnight hospitalization may be necessary. We often use a "23-hour admission," which most third parties recognize as an outpatient event although such patients are included as inpatients in our data.

COMPLICATIONS

The patient must be properly prepared and monitored before, during, and after the procedure. The bronchoscopist must be well trained, equipped, and prepared to recognize and deal with any complication that may arise (Table 15–2). In general, bronchoscopic complications can be classified into several groups.

Mechanical Complications

Although relatively unusual, mechanical complications are the most common problem encountered from bronchoscopy. These complications include mucosal trauma, hemoptysis or epistaxis, pneumothorax, subglottic edema, tracheal or bronchial perforation, and trauma to the vocal cords. All are more common with rigid instruments than with flexible ones because of the nature of the instruments and the type of patients selected for rigid bronchoscopy. For example, flexible bronchoscopes are rarely used for foreign body extraction, a situation in which mucosal tears or bronchial perforation may occur.

TABLE 15–2. COMPLICATIONS REPORTED FOR PEDIATRIC FLEXIBLE BRONCHOSCOPY

	Series						Total
	Wood[26]	C. G. Green[a]	Fitzpatrick et al[27]	Fan and Flynn[28]	Nussbaum[29]	Raine and Warner[30]	
Procedures	1095	262	129	104	96	50	1736
Complications	32	14	3	3	8	7	67
Major							11
Lung abscess	1						
Pneumothorax	2	1					
Laryngospasm	1						
Respiratory depression		2				2	
Pneumonia						2	
Minor							54
Bradycardia	13		1	2			
Laryngospasm	2					1	
Epistaxis	8	5		1	6		
Hemoptysis (<10 mL)			2				
Anesthetic complication	5						
Atelectasis		1					
Transient cyanosis		4				2	
Endobronchial bleeding		1					

[a] Unpublished data.

Physiologic Complications

Physiologic complications include hypoxia, hypercarbia, bradycardia or other cardiac arrhythmias, laryngospasm, and bronchospasm.[20] Hypoxia and hypercarbia may occur because a flexible instrument obstructs the airway or because ventilation and oxygenation are impaired with prolonged instrumentation through the rigid bronchoscope. Cardiac arrhythmias and laryngospasm may result from direct vagal stimulation, which is usually the result of inadequate topical anesthesia. As a consequence of inadequate sedation or topical anesthesia, coughing can result in mechanical trauma. Aspiration may result if the patient's stomach is not empty.

Bacteriologic Complications

Bacteriologic complications may occur when microorganisms are carried into the distal airways by the bronchoscope or when the child aspirates from laryngeal anesthesia. Great care must be taken to ensure that instruments are properly cleaned and sterilized between patients, as nosocomial infection from contaminated bronchoscopes has been reported.[21–23] Contamination of the instruments or ancillary equipment can also result in false diagnoses.[24]

Anesthetic Complications

Anesthetic complications may result from either too much or too little anesthesia. A patient who is inadequately sedated or anesthetized may move unexpectedly, producing mechanical trauma. Too much sedation can result in a depressed respiratory drive, resulting in hypoxia and hypercarbia. This is a particular risk of flexible bronchoscopy, as the patients usually are not intubated and must breathe spontaneously during the procedure. Rarely, a patient may have an adverse reaction to an anesthetic agent. Toxic reactions to topical anesthetic agents such as lidocaine may result in hypotension, seizures, or other adverse effects.

In general, the risk of complications appears lower with flexible bronchoscopes than with rigid bronchoscopes, but the experience in a given institution will depend greatly on the skill and training of the bronchoscopist and the selection of patients.

CHOICE BETWEEN RIGID AND FLEXIBLE BRONCHOSCOPES

The instrument chosen for a particular patient and a particular procedure depends on several factors including the personal preference and experience of the bronchoscopist, the indications for the procedure, and the characteristics and size of the patient. In general, flexible instruments appear to have significant advantages for many diagnostic procedures, whereas rigid instruments have advantages for most therapeutic procedures. Foreign body extractions in children should be undertaken with a flexible instrument only as an adjunct to rigid bronchoscopy or in very unusual clinical circumstances.[25]

INDICATIONS

In general, diagnostic bronchoscopy is indicated when it is the safest, most effective, and most appropriate method to obtain information needed for the care of the patient. If the same information can be obtained by another, less invasive or less risky technique, then bronchoscopy is not indicated.

Similarly, therapeutic bronchoscopy is indicated when it is the best way to accomplish the therapeutic goals. For example, a foreign body could be removed via a bronchotomy, but in most cases, bronchoscopy will suffice and is therefore the indicated procedure.

The advent of the flexible bronchoscope resulted in a considerable increase in indications for diagnostic bronchoscopy, as previously most indications were therapeutic in children. Flexible bronchoscopy allows evaluation of airway structure, airway dynamics, and airway contents. In addition, it provides access to secretions and washings from the lower airways. Over the past 9 years, flexible bronchoscopy has been performed on 2115 children less than 10 years of age at UNC (Tables 15–3 and 15–4).

TABLE 15–3. INDICATIONS FOR FLEXIBLE BRONCHOSCOPY AT UNIVERSITY OF NORTH CAROLINA (SEPTEMBER 1983–MAY 1992)

Airway obstruction	475
Stridor	379
Atelectasis	176
Tracheostomy evaluation	269
Pneumonia	
Persistent	132
Recurrent	70
Compromised host	43
Unspecified	21
Hemoptysis	49
Aid to intubation	88
Aid to extubation	61
Research	139
Cough	52
Persistent wheezing	109
Suspected foreign body	52
Total	2115

TABLE 15–4. AGE OF PATIENTS UNDERGOING FLEXIBLE BRONCHOSCOPY AT UNIVERSITY OF NORTH CAROLINA

<1 month	7.9%
<6 months	31.2%
<1 year	44.9%
<2 years	63.2%
<10 years	91.8%

The Upper Airway

The advantage of flexible instruments for examination of the pediatric airway is that they are usually passed transnasally. Thus, evaluation of the nasopharynx becomes part of the exam. It is not unusual to find significant pathology in this area that was not suspected. The upper airway can be examined with the patient's head in a neutral position without extending or flexing the neck. When evaluating a child with stridor, it is important not to place abnormal tension on the larynx or other airway structures. Stridor is always visible. If the child is making noise at the time of the examination, the vibrating structure should always be visualized. As a significant percentage of children with stridor have more than one airway lesion, the entire upper and lower airway should be examined unless contraindicated (ie, critical subglottic narrowing).[26,31]

The nasal airway can also be explored with rigid telescopes. The posterior nasopharynx can be viewed with a rear-viewing (120-degree) telescope, especially if the soft palate is elevated. The dynamics of the larynx (vocal cord movement, supraglottic structures) can easily be observed with a rigid instrument if the patient is breathing spontaneously and vocalizing.

The Lower Airway

The structure and dynamics of the lower airway can be observed with either a rigid or a flexible bronchoscope, and either can be used to obtain specimens (Figure 15–1). Flexible instruments can be passed much further into the airways than rigid bronchoscopes, although a glass rod telescope can be extended beyond the tip of the rigid bronchoscope if indicated.

In general, a rigid bronchoscope will allow direct visualization of segmental bronchi, but the standard pediatric flexible bronchoscope can be inserted several generations further. The 2.2-mm ultrathin bronchoscope can be passed to 12 to 16 generations, even in infants. The upper lobe bronchi are perhaps more readily visualized and more easily entered with a flexible than a rigid bronchoscope.

Often, it is important to evaluate airway dynamics in infants and children. Airway dynamics may be altered by anesthesia or sedation, depending on the type and level used. It is important to examine the airway with the patient spontaneously breathing as dynamic airway collapse can be missed easily during positive-pressure ventilation.[32,33] The bronchoscope itself can alter dynamics either by stenting the airway or by changing airway resistance and, therefore, the pressure relationships.

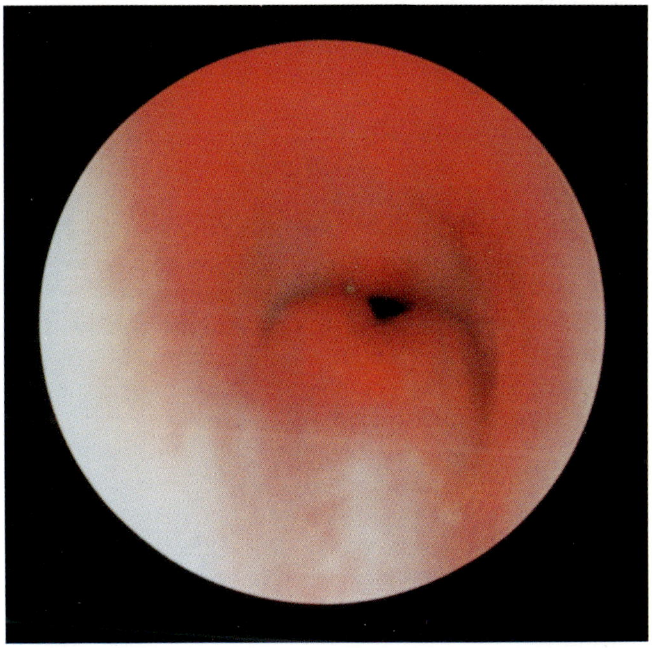

Figure 15–1. Rigid bronchoscopy in an infant with stridor reveals a subglottic hemangioma, which is almost completely occluding the tracheal lumen.

Bronchoscopes can be used to obtain specimens from the lower airways and lung parenchyma. Secretions can be directly aspirated or washings can be performed. Bronchial lavage is a useful technique to obtain a specimen that may be more representative than simple aspiration, as a larger area is sampled. In children, the difference between "bronchial lavage" and "bronchoalveolar lavage" may be semantic and there is no standardization of either technique.[34] Nevertheless, this technique is very useful in the diagnosis of infectious or inflammatory process and often obviates the need for open lung biopsy.

Transbronchial lung biopsy is commonly used in adults but rarely is used in children.[35] With the advent of pediatric lung transplantation, however, this procedure may be increasingly employed.[36] The smallest commercially available flexible bronchoscope that can be readily used for biopsy is 4.9 mm in diameter and is difficult to use in children younger than 3 to 4 years of age. Flexible forceps are used for mucosal biopsy, and brushings allow epithelial scraping for microbiologic or cytologic analysis.

APPLICATIONS

Extraction of Foreign Bodies

Foreign body extraction should be performed with the rigid bronchoscope. Several reports of foreign body extraction with flexible bronchoscopes have been published[37,38]; however, a limited array of instruments can be passed through the flexible instrument to grasp the foreign body and more of the airway is obstructed by the flexible bronchoscope compared with the rigid instrument. Nevertheless, in selected circumstances, the flexible bronchoscope can be very helpful. Specifically, when a foreign body is suspected but not proven, a flexible examination can diagnose or exclude a foreign body. In older children, examination of airways distal to the range of the rigid bronchoscope may reveal foreign bodies that would not be seen with the rigid technique. The flexible instruments have also proven useful in the follow-up examination of patients who have had a foreign body extracted.[25]

In the extraction of a bronchial foreign body, it is important to have as much information as possible before manipulating the object. For this purpose, the patient's history and radiographs should be fully evaluated (Figure 15–2). Identification of the object prior to bronchoscopy can help in planning the endoscopic approach and the instruments to be used. Many foreign bodies are surrounded by granulation tissue or secretions. Careful lavage and suctioning may help identify and make extraction easier. In selected cases, an argon laser has been used to remove granulation tissue surrounding a foreign body,[39] but this maneuver could result in damage to the bronchial walls. The optical forceps is often the most useful instrument to grasp the object, but a Fogarty catheter is also a useful instrument[40] (Figure 15–3). Care must be taken to avoid pushing the foreign body more distally or perforating the bronchus.

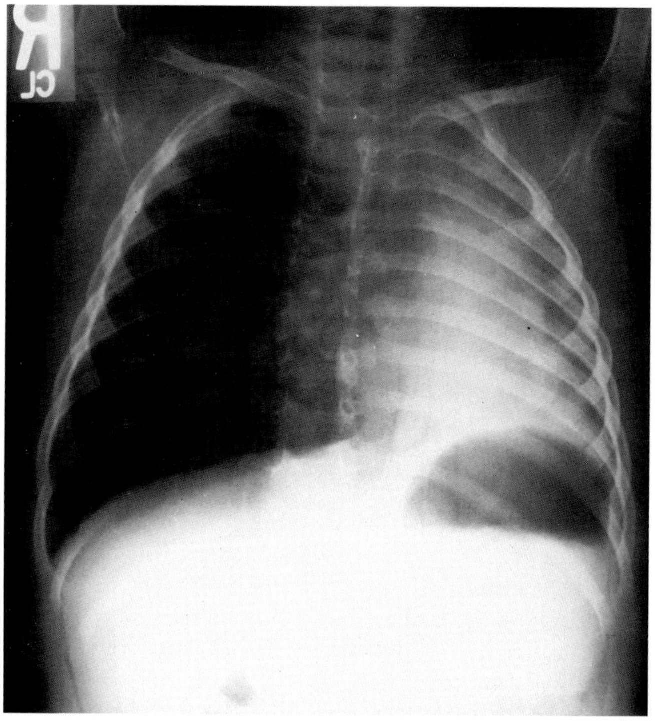

Figure 15–2. Chest radiograph in an infant with sudden coughing and wheezing indicates collapse of the left lung and mediastinal shift to the left. There is compensatory hyperinflation of the right lung. The foreign body is suspected to be in the left mainstem bronchus.

Removal of Tissue Masses

Removal of tissue masses from the airway is usually most easily accomplished with a rigid bronchoscope and forceps. Unless the patient is large enough to allow the use of an adult bronchoscope, forceps cannot be used through flexible instruments. In selected circumstances, however, a mass lesion can be ablated with an argon laser placed through a flexible bronchoscope.[41]

Diagnosis of Tracheal or Bronchial Stenosis

Tracheal or bronchial stenosis can usually be readily diagnosed with either rigid or flexible instruments (Figure 15–4). Examination of the airway distal to the stenosis helps identify the extent of the problem and additional anatomic anomalies. The ultrathin flexible bronchoscope is especially useful in this regard, as it can often be passed through the area of stenosis without producing mucosal edema. Alteratively, a localized small-volume bronchogram or high-resolution computed tomography scan can clarify the anatomy beyond the stenotic area.

Congenital tracheal stenosis has been treated with balloon dilation,[42] and we have treated several children with this modality. The ultrathin flexible bronchoscope is passed through the rigid bronchoscope to observe the positioning of the balloon catheter prior to inflation. In one case, we were able to pass the ultrathin flexible scope through the glottis and leave the entire lumen of the rigid scope available for the balloon catheter. Another useful application of the ultrathin flexible scope in patients with complete tracheal rings has been the intraoperative evaluation of the tracheal lumen as the graft is placed.[43]

Acquired bronchial or tracheal stenosis often results from suction trauma in infants and children with prolonged endotracheal intubation. This may or may not respond to simple dilation performed with the bronchoscope itself or with an instrument (such as an

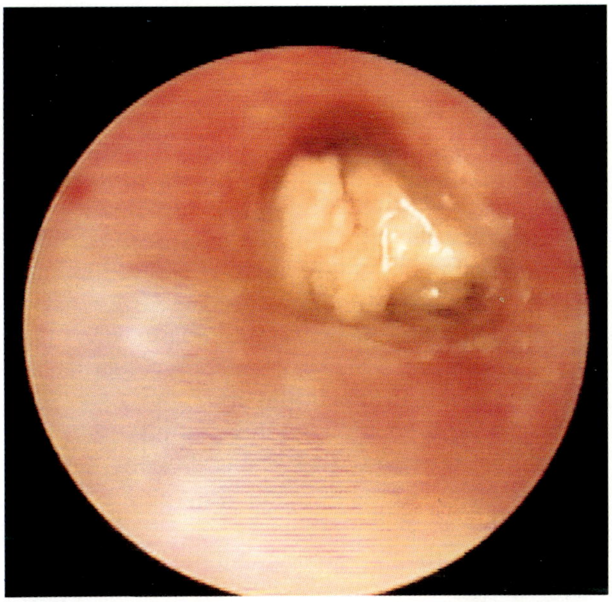

A

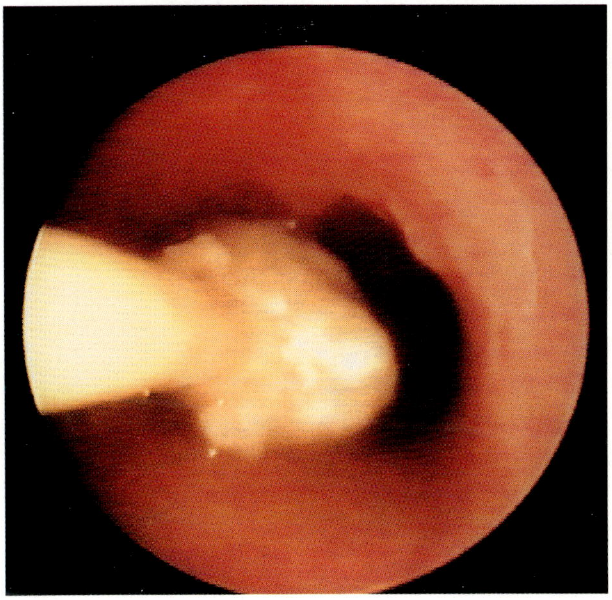

B

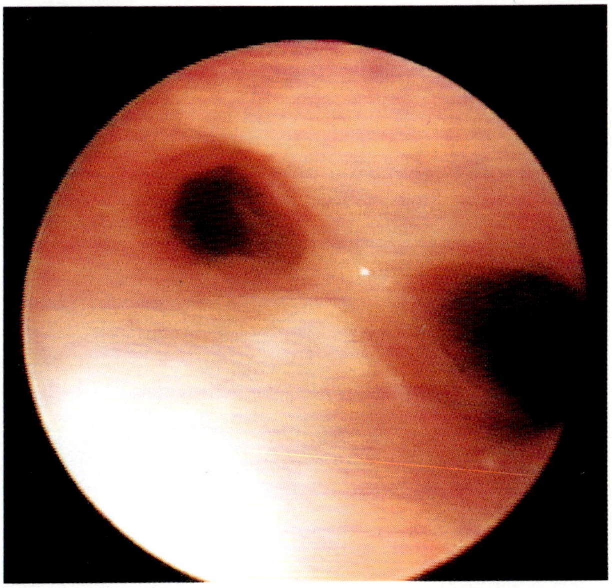

C

Figure 15–3. **A.** Rigid bronchoscopy for presumed foreign body reveals complete occlusion of the left mainstem bronchus with a piece of food material. **B.** The material is grasped with a bronchoscopic forceps and extracted. **C.** Repeat bronchoscopy reveals patency of both the right and left mainstem bronchi.

angioplasty balloon) passed through the rigid bronchoscope. We have had considerable experience with an argon laser in this setting.[41] A quartz laser fiber can be passed through either a rigid or a flexible bronchoscope; however, we have found control of the fiber much easier through the flexible scope. The fiber is passed through the suction channel and manipulated accurately. We have used the argon laser with a 300-μm fiber for this purpose. In contact with the lesion, a 2.5-W, 0.5-second laser emission produces a lesion about 0.5 mm in diameter and 1 mm deep. Thus, the ablation can be done precisely. The laser is fired with the beam roughly parallel to the bronchial wall to minimize the risk of penetration injury.

Laser application through flexible bronchoscopes mandates the use of general anesthesia. This causes difficulties with airway management, as the 3.5 mm flexible bronchoscope cannot be passed through an endotracheal tube smaller than 4.5 mm i.d. Patients cannot be adequately ventilated through an endotracheal tube smaller than 5.0 mm i.d., even with positive-pressure assistance. Most of the patients in whom we have used the argon laser have had tracheostomies. The flexible scope was passed through the glottis and directed down the trachea parallel to the tracheostomy tube. In infants without a tracheostomy, the baby was ventilated through a nasopharyngeal tube. There was sufficient space around the 3.5-mm flexible scope for adequate ventilation.[44]

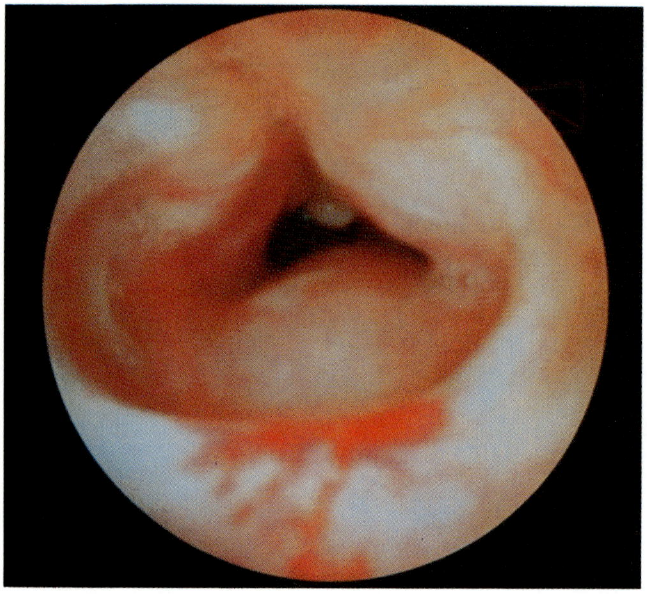

Figure 15–4. Bronchoscopy performed in this infant with prolonged endotracheal intubation reveals critical subglottic stenosis.

The argon laser has been well tolerated by our patients and no complications have been encountered. The use of low power (2.5 W, 0.5 second) avoids the potential problems of localized heat from steam arising from the vaporized tissue, so the effects are quite localized. We routinely treat the patients with steroids for 2 to 3 days and reexamine the airway in 2 weeks. Several treatment sessions are often needed to avoid ablation of large portions of airway at one time. This protocol avoids the residual scarring and stricture formation likely to occur with one prolonged laser application. The combination of laser excision and balloon dilation has been very effective in selected patients. We now have long-term endoscopic follow-up in several patients; all have done well.

Placement of Endobronchial Stents

Endoscopic placement of endobronchial stents for localized stenosis or severe tracheomalacia or bronchomalacia is now a relatively well-established technique in adult patients. There have been a few reports of the use of stents for nonmalignant disease in children.[33,45,46] The relatively small diameter of the pediatric airway is a serious impediment to this therapeutic option and long-term results have not been reported. Nevertheless, it is an attractive possibility for some children with severe tracheomalacia or bronchomalacia, especially if the disease process is localized.

Bronchoalveolar Lavage

Bronchoalveolar lavage (BAL) is an important diagnostic technique which is being increasingly used in children.[33,47] Bronchoalveolar lavage can be defined as the instillation of fluid into and aspiration from the airways in sufficient volume and in such a manner as to ensure that the effluent contains some alveolar fluid. It is a useful procedure to obtain a representative sample of airway surface liquid from the lower airways. BAL can be used for a variety of purposes, but clinically is most often used for microbiologic or cytologic diagnosis.

Bronchoalveolar lavage is easily performed with a flexible bronchoscope. The tip of the instrument is gently wedged into a distal airway, with the bronchial generation being determined by the relative size of the patient and the bronchoscope. Sterile saline is alternately instilled and aspirated. In adults, typical volumes are 50 to 100 mL per exchange. In children, there has been no standardization of technique and various bronchoscopists use different volumes ranging from 1 to 3 mL/kg to fixed volumes of 10 to 25 mL.

It is possible to perform BAL with a rigid bronchoscope, but this can be challenging. To ensure that the saline reaches the alveolar spaces and does not spill into wide areas of the lung, it is necessary to occlude the bronchus being lavaged. With a flexible bronchoscope, this is done by passing the bronchoscope distally until it wedges. This cannot be done with a rigid instrument; some form of catheter must be passed through the scope. Instillation of saline through the rigid bronchoscope followed by aspiration does not constitute BAL.

Because of their pliability, flexible bronchoscopes can be used to visualize otherwise inaccessible locations within the airways. An example is the examination of the lower airways in patients with endotracheal tubes. Although in many cases it would be feasible to extubate the patient and use a rigid bronchoscope, the flexible bronchoscope can be passed through the endotracheal or tracheostomy tube. This is now possible even in the smallest of intubated infants, as the 2.2-mm ultrathin flexible instrument will pass through a 2.5-mm-i.d. tube. In some situations, extubation and the use of a rigid bronchoscope are not viable options. We have successfully used the flexible bronchoscope to visualize the lower airways and direct the application of rigid instruments passed through a tracheostomy stoma in patients with an unstable cervical fracture or with extreme mandibular hypoplasia.[43]

Evaluation of Atelectasis

Atelectasis is a relatively common indication for bronchoscopy and may be due to a variety of lesions that obstruct the airways. Flexible bronchoscopes are very useful for diagnostic evaluation, which should include cytologic and microbiologic evaluation of washings from affected areas. In patients in whom discrete mucus plugs are found, the flexible bronchoscope can also be useful therapeutically. Despite the relatively small suction channel, surprisingly large mucus plugs can be removed.[26] Occasionally, lavage with mucolytic agents may be necessary, and rarely, a rigid instrument with forceps must be used. If the atelectasis is due to an impacted foreign body or a tissue mass, then rigid bronchoscopy will be needed.

Intubation

Bronchoscopic intubation is a very important application of flexible bronchoscopes.[26,32,48] Children with mandibular hypoplasia or ankylosis, oropharyngeal or cervical mass lesions, and other anatomic problems that make conventional intubation techniques difficult or impossible can usually be intubated successfully with this technique. In brief, a flexible bronchoscope is passed through the appropriate tube and then the bronchoscope is advanced into the trachea. The endotracheal tube is positioned in the trachea by sliding it over the bronchoscope and the position of the tip of the tube is verified visually (Figure 15–5). The standard 3.5-mm pediatric flexible bronchoscope can be used with endotracheal tubes between 4.5 and 6.5 mm i.d.; smaller tubes require the use of an ultrathin bronchoscope. Although this technique makes it possible to intubate in almost any circumstance, special maneuvers are occasionally necessary.[32] If the upper airway is obscured by tissue or secretions, it is helpful to pass oxygen (1–2 L/min) through the suction channel (analogous to insufflation of air through gastrointestinal endoscopes). Sometimes, gentle traction on the tongue will also help expose the glottis. The visual evaluation of the airway that is obtained in the process of bronchoscopic intubation is often very helpful in the subsequent management of the patient.

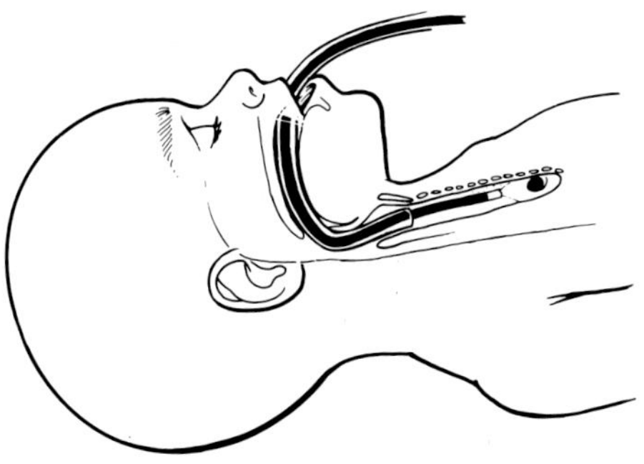

Figure 15–5. Difficult intubations can be facilitated with the use of bronchoscopy. The endotracheal tube is positioned over the bronchoscope and the bronchoscope is inserted into the trachea. The endotracheal tube is then slid over the bronchoscope into the trachea and its position confirmed.

Extubation

Endoscopic techniques can also be an aid to extubation in selected patients. When a child has failed extubation, direct examination of the airway can help define the problem. Our usual approach is to examine the lower airways through the endotracheal tube and then to examine the nasopharynx and larynx with a flexible bronchoscope that has been passed through a clean endotracheal tube of appropriate size. With the tip of the bronchoscope positioned just over the glottis, the existing endotracheal tube is withdrawn. If no abnormalities are noted after thorough examination, the bronchoscope is withdrawn. If problems arise, the bronchoscope is advanced into the trachea and the new endotracheal tube is passed over the bronchoscope. It should be noted that subglottic edema sufficient to prevent successful extubation may not become apparent for 5 to 10 minutes after extubation, so the airway should be examined thoughtfully.

Other Applications

Pediatric bronchoscopes, both rigid and flexible, can be used to great advantage in areas of the body other than the airways. Although there are significant disadvantages to using flexible bronchoscopes in the gastrointestinal tract, their application may be useful in selected circumstances. For example, we have used a flexible bronchoscope to pass a string through a tight esophageal stricture to facilitate dilation. The bronchoscope was inserted retrograde through a gastrostomy stoma and flexible biopsy forceps were passed through the stricture and out the nose.

Retrograde direct laryngoscopy is sometimes useful in the evaluation of children with laryngeal stenosis or other glottic or subglottic lesions. This may be accomplished with a glass rod telescope with provision for side viewing or a flexible bronchoscope (Figure 15–6). In either case, the bronchoscope is inserted through the tracheostomy stoma and directed upward. If the stoma is small, ventilation can be accomplished during the examination by passing oxygen into the distal trachea through a small catheter.

Computed tomography has in large part made

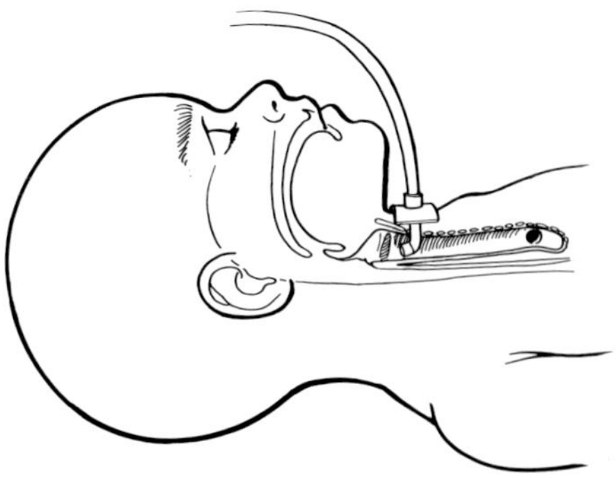

Figure 15–6. Retrograde endoscopy for evaluation of the subglottic and glottic structures can be performed through the tracheostomy stoma.

bronchography obsolete, but this is still indicated in selected patients. Bronchographic contrast material can be instilled through a catheter passed blindly into the trachea, but it is more convenient to use a flexible bronchoscope for this purpose. The tip of the bronchoscope can be wedged into the desired bronchus similar to BAL, and the contrast material injected through the suction channel. This technique has many advantages over the more conventional procedure. In some patients, visual examination of the airways will document a finding that makes the bronchogram unnecessary or even contraindicated. In addition, with this technique, the amount of contrast used is minimized and the airways are well filled. This results in a very high quality bronchogram.

REFERENCES

1. Green CG, Eisenberg J, Leong A, et al. Flexible endoscopy of the pediatric airway. *Am Rev Respir Dis.* 1992;145:233.
2. Hoeve LJ, Rombout J. Pediatric laryngobronchoscopy. 1332 procedures stored in a data base. *Int J Pediatr Otorhinolaryngol.* 1992;24:73.
3. Lindahl H, Rintala R, Malinen L, et al. Bronchoscopy during the first month of life. *J Pediatr Surg.* 1992;27:548.
4. Finer NN, Etches PC. Fiberoptic bronchoscopy in the neonate. *Pediatr Pulmonol.* 1989;7:116.
5. Holinger LD. Diagnostic endoscopy of the pediatric airway. *Laryngoscope.* 1989;99:346.
6. Puhakka H, Kero P, Valli P, et al. Pediatric bronchoscopy: A report of methodology and results. *Clin Pediatr Phila.* 1989;28:253.
7. Cohn RC, Kercsmar C, Dearborn D. Safety and efficacy of flexible endoscopy in children with bronchopulmonary dysplasia. *Am J Dis Child.* 1988;142:1225.
8. Hein J, Gulzow HU, Breuel K, et al. Bronchoskopie und bronchographie bei neugeborenen und sauglingen. *Z Erkrank Atmungsorgane.* 1988;171:117.
9. Myer CM III, Thompson RF. Flexible fiberoptic bronchoscopy in the neonatal intensive care unit. *Int J Pediatr Otorhinolaryngol.* 1988;15:143.
10. Wood RE, Postma D. Endoscopy of the airway in infants and children. *J Pediatr.* 1988;112:1.
11. DeBlic J, McKelvie P, Le-Bourgeois M, et al. Value of bronchoalveolar lavage in the management of severe acute pneumonia and interstitial pneumonitis in the immunocompromised child. *Thorax.* 1987;42:759.
12. Godfrey S, Springer C, Maayan C, et al. Is there a place for rigid bronchoscopy in the management of pediatric lung disease? *Pediatr Pulmonol.* 1987;3:179.
13. Lockhart CH, Elliot JL. Potential hazards of pediatric rigid bronchoscopy. *J Pediatr Surg.* 1984;19:239.
14. Silberman HD. The use of the flexible fiberoptic nasopharyngoscope in the pediatric upper airway. *Otol Clin N Am.* 1978;11:365.
15. Wang D, Clement P, Kaufman L, et al. Fiberoptic examination of the nasal cavity and nasopharynx in children. *Int J Pediatr Otorhinolaryngol.* 1992;24:35.
16. Visicath imaging probes. *Surg Endosc.* 1987;1:186.
17. Stankiewicz JA, Holinger LD. Endoscopic sizing: An attempt at uniformity. *Laryngoscope.* 1986;96:997.
18. Guidelines for the elective use of conscious sedation, deep sedation, and general anesthesia in pediatric patients. *Pediatrics.* 1985;76:317.
19. American Academy of Pediatrics Committee on Drugs. Guidelines for monitoring and management of pediatric patients during and after sedation for diagnostic and therapeutic procedures. *Pediatrics.* 1992;89:1110.
20. Schnapf BM. Oxygen desaturation during fiberoptic bronchoscopy in pediatric patients. *Chest.* 1991;99:591.
21. Wheeler PW, Lancaster D, Kaiser AB. Bronchopulmonary cross contamination and infection of suction valves of bronchoscopes. *J Infect Dis.* 1989;159:954.
22. Nelson KE, Larson PA, Schraufnagel DE, et al. Transmission of tuberculosis by flexible fiberbronchoscopes. *Am Rev Respir Dis.* 1983;127:97.
23. Wood RE, Gauderer MW. Flexible fiberoptic bronchoscopy in the management of tracheobronchial foreign bodies in children: The value of a combined approach with open tube bronchoscopy. *J Pediatr Surg.* 1984;19:693.
24. Pappas SA, Schaaff DM, Dicostanzo MB, et al. Contamination of flexible fiberoptic bronchoscopes. *Am Rev Respir Dis.* 1983;127:391.
25. Siegman-Igra Y, Inbar G, Campus A. An "outbreak" of pulmonary pseudoinfection by *Serratia marcescens. J Hosp Infect.* 1985;6:218.
26. Wood RE. Spelunking in the pediatric airways: Explorations with the flexible fiberoptic bronchoscope. *Pediatr Clin North Am.* 1984;31:785.
27. Fitzpatrick SB, Marsh B, Stokes DC, et al. Indications for flexible fiberoptic bronchoscopy in pediatric patients. *Am J Dis Child.* 1983;137:595.
28. Fan LL, Flynn JW. Laryngoscopy in neonates and infants: Experience with the fiberoptic bronchoscope. *Laryngoscope.* 1981;91:451.
29. Nussbaum E. Flexible fiberoptic bronchoscopy and laryngoscopy in children under 2 years of age: Diagnostic and therapeutic applications of a new pediatric flexible fiberoptic bronchoscope. *Crit Care Med.* 1982;10:770.

30. Raine J, Warner JO. Fiberoptic bronchoscopy without general anaesthetic. *Arch Dis Child.* 1991;66:481.
31. Gonzalez C, Reilly JS, Bluestone CD. Synchronous airway lesions in infancy. *Ann Otol Rhinol Laryngol.* 1987;96:77.
32. Wood RE. Pitfalls in the use of the flexible bronchoscope in pediatric patients. *Chest.* 1990;97:199.
33. Mair EA, Parsons DS. Pediatric tracheobronchomalacia and major airway collapse. *Ann Otol Rhinol Laryngol.* 1992;101:300.
34. Wood RE. Bronchoalveolar lavage in infants and children. In: Baughman RP, ed. *Bronchoalveolar Lavage.* St. Louis, MO: Mosby-Year Book; 1992.
35. Fitzpatrick SB, Stokes DC, Marsh B, et al. Transbronchial lung biopsy in pediatric and adolescent patients. *Am J Dis Child.* 1985;139:46.
36. Scott JP, Higenbottam TW, Smyth RL, et al. Transbronchial biopsies in children after heart–lung transplantation. *Pediatrics.* 1990;86:698.
37. Monden Y, Morimoto T, Taniki T, et al. Flexible bronchoscopy for foreign body in airway. *Tokushima J Exp Med.* 1989;36:35.
38. Cunanan OS. The flexible fiberoptic bronchoscope in foreign body removal: Experience in 300 cases. *Chest.* 1978;72(suppl):725.
39. Hayashi AH, Gillis DA, Bethune D, et al. Management of foreign-body bronchial obstruction using endoscopic laser. *J Pediatr Surg.* 1990;25:1174.
40. Kosloske AM. The Fogarty balloon technique for the removal of foreign bodies from the tracheobronchial tree. *Surg Gynecol Obstet.* 1982;155:72.
41. Azizkhan RG, Lacey SR, Wood RE. Acquired symptomatic bronchial stenosis in infants: Successful management using an argon laser. *J Pediatr Surg.* 1990; 25:19.
42. Bagwell CE, Talbert JL, Tepas JJ III. Balloon dilatation of long-segment tracheal stenosis. *J Pediatr Surg.* 1991;26:153.
43. Wood RE, Azizkhan RG, Lacey SR, et al. Surgical applications of ultrathin flexible bronchoscopes in infants. *Ann Otol Rhinol Laryngol.* 1991;100:116.
44. Bailey AG, Valley RD, Azizkhan RG, et al. Anaesthetic management of infants requiring endobronchial argon laser surgery. *Can J Anaesth.* 1992;39:590.
45. Loeff DS, Filler RM, Gorenstein A, et al. A new intratracheal stent for tracheobronchial reconstruction: Experimental and clinical studies. *J Pediatr Surg.* 1988;23: 1173.
46. Mair EA, Parsons DS, Lally KP. Treatment of severe bronchomalacia with expanding endobronchial stents. *Arch Otolaryngol Head Neck Surg.* 1990;116:1087.
47. Reynolds HY. State of the art: Bronchoalveolar lavage. *Am Rev Respir Dis.* 1987;135:250.
48. Rucker RW, Silva WJ, Worcester CC. Fiberoptic bronchoscopic nasotracheal intubation in children. *Chest.* 1979;76:56.

CHAPTER 16

Endourology

JOHN W. BROCK III

Endoscopic evaluation of the urinary tract has been a mainstay of urology practice for a number of years. Introduction of the modern cystoscope by Nitze more than 100 years ago heralded the onset of the modern era of endoscopic examination of the urinary tract. Since that time, remarkable refinements have been made not only in equipment but also in the indications for these procedures. Advances in equipment technology have also allowed improved investigation of the upper urinary system, including ureteroscopic and nephroscopic management for several diseases. A systemic approach to the endoscopic management of urologic problems in the pediatric patient is now possible because of technologic advances in this aspect of genitourinary surgery.

CYSTOSCOPY

As in adult urology, the early days of pediatric endoscopy were hindered by the lack of sophisticated equipment to evaluate the lower urinary system adequately; however, technologic improvements have permitted the development of better and smaller infant cystoscopes with sizes ranging down to 7 French. As cystoscopic equipment improved so did radiologic evaluation of the urinary tract. This advancement in noninvasive technology made obsolete many of the previous indications for cystoscopy in the child. Furthermore, cost containment has been a major impetus in medical practice and in the indications for anesthetic cystoscopy. Several authors have proposed a very narrow range of indications for cystourethroscopy based on a high anticipation of positive findings.

Endoscopic evaluation of the lower urinary system in the child is usually accomplished under general anesthesia. This necessity is a consideration when contemplating the procedure; however, the morbidity associated with general anesthesia in major centers has been minimal. In addition to the endoscopic evaluation, the anesthetized child presents an opportunity for careful examination of the genitalia, the lower abdominal area, and the rectum. Cystourethroscopy includes accurate calibration of the meatal size with normal meatal sizes well documented.[1] The opportunity to evaluate the pendulous, bulbar, and membranous urethra for stricture, polyps, and inflammatory lesions should not be overlooked. Entrance into the membranous and prostatic urethra provides the opportunity to evaluate for posterior urethral valves, abnormalities of the utricle, verumontanum, and the bladder neck. On entry into the bladder, the mucosa is carefully examined for its integrity, status of inflammation, and appearance. Furthermore, the amount of trabeculation and cellule formation is an indicator of possible urologic abnormalities. The trigone is well inspected including ureteral orifices and the position and appearance of the orifices are documented. This information is important in evaluating urinary symptoms, especially in patients with vesicoureteral reflux. Finally, the opportunity is taken to inspect urine draining from each kidney. From this examination further studies can be initiated as indicated, including retrograde pyelography or ureteroscopy. In girls the vagina should be examined for abnormalities and the presence of foreign bodies or ectopic ureteral orifices. Rectal examination is performed as the final portion of the examination under anesthesia.

Although the relative indications for cystoscopy in children are decreasing, they can be grouped into four main categories: hematuria, voiding dysfunction, urinary tract infection, and reflux.[2,3] As discussed later, however, absolute indications are rare. The indications for cystoscopy in the pediatric patient with hematuria are few. Gross hematuria with normal radiographs and lab studies in many cases will obviate the need for cystoscopy. Clinical judgment, however, may dictate a need in selective cases. On the other hand, gross hematuria and abnormal x-rays may require endoscopy for further pathologic delineation. The bloody urethral spotting of urethrorrhagia does warrant cystoscopy, especially in those children with symptoms persisting for more than 6 months.[4] Microscopic hematuria with greater than 10 red blood cells per high-power field (RBC/HPF), even with normal laboratory and radiographic studies, may be an indication for endoscopy; however, the documented inability of cystoscopy to provide data that would change treatment in patients with fewer than 10 RBC/HPF and negative radiographic and laboratory findings makes its usefulness limited in this situation. A second major indication for cystoscopy is voiding dysfunction, especially with abnormal radiographic studies. Urethral calibration and dilation have been of little benefit, and blind comparisons of dilation and urethrotomy with medication alone have shown no difference.

In children with cystitis cystica and urinary tract infection, cystoscopy may be helpful in determining the need for long-term antibiotics. This is rarely, if ever, indicated in normal children with initial or noncomplicated urinary tract infections.

Routine use of cystoscopy to evaluate ureteral orifices in management of vesicoureteral reflux has been the subject of great controversy (Figure 16–1). The International Reflux Study Group has compared use of this technique in both Europe and United States. Only the finding of a golf hole orifice was a significant prognostic indicator. Therefore, the routine use of cystoscopy to evaluate this group of patients is unwarranted.

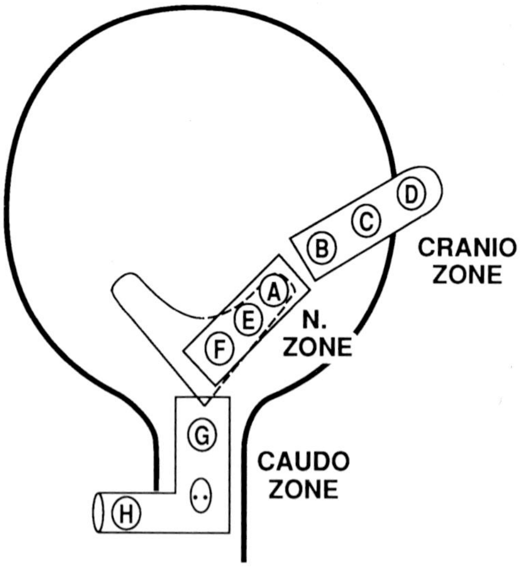

Figure 16–1. Normal and ectopic ureteral orifice positions. Such a classification allows communication between physicians regarding findings at cystoscopy.

Endoscopic Management of Lower Genitourinary Problems

Perhaps nowhere in pediatric urology are the refinements of instrumentation more apparent than in endoscopic management of lower urinary problems, especially in the neonate. The optical improvements have allowed several manufacturers to decrease the size of endoscopic equipment and provide working channels for treatment of urologic problems.

Availability of smaller sheaths with refined telescopes has enabled the pediatric urologist to treat posterior urethral valves primarily without the need for an antecedent vesicostomy or even supravesical diversion. It has been shown that primary valve ablation in the newborn provides decompression as well as vesicostomy and usually does not require secondary procedures.

Several techniques are used for ablation of posterior ureteral valves.[5] The usual procedure involves passage of a cystoscope per urethra with the knowledge that the size of a full-term infant's meatus is generally an instrument size 7 or 8 French. A Bugbee electrode (3-French) is passed down the working channel of the cystoscope for fulguration of the valves under direct vision. Children with larger urethras will accommodate a 10- to 11-French cystoscope and allow a wire electrode for valve destruction. Also, valves may be ablated by a perineal urethrostomy approach through a suprapubic cystostomy. The antegrade approach allows easy access to the valves with either a rigid or flexible scope, and valve ablation is accomplished with either Bugbee electrodes or contact laser probes.[6,7]

In the past, complications of neonatal valve ablation have been significant and have led the pediatric urologist away from primary valve ablation. The incidence of stricture has been as high as 25% with transurethral ablation and strictures have been reported following perineal urethrostomy. Urinary incontinence may be caused by damage to the external sphincter during ablation, although this problem is often multifactorial. The proper transurethral technique for valve destruction involves calibrating the urethra and performing a meatotomy if necessary. A zero-degree telescope provides the best graphic view of the valves. The valve may be engaged with a wire hook or loop (Figure 16–2). The 3-French Bugbee may also be used. Prior to ablation, it is imperative that the valves are visualized unequivocally. The non-current-bearing loop may be swept along either side of the verumontanum engaging the valves. Only after the valves are elevated away from the urethral wall is cutting current employed and the valve cusp incised

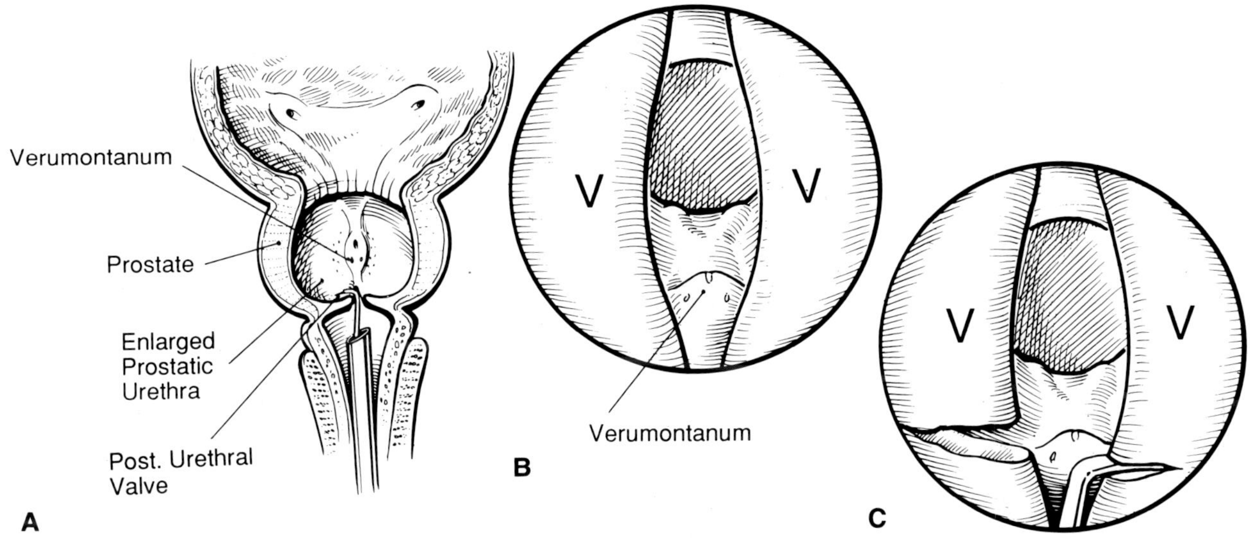

Figure 16–2. Ablation of posterior urethral valves can be performed endoscopically. The valves are located proximal to the verumontanum, and the prostatic urethra distal to the valves is dilated **(A)**. The valves are visualized endoscopically **(B)** and incised at the 5, 7, and 12 o'clock positions with a wire hook or loop **(C)**.

at the 5, 7, and 12 o'clock positions. The depth of the cut does not extend to the urethral wall.

Endoscopic management of urethral stricture disease remains an important technique.[8,9] Direct vision urethrotomy for discrete short strictures is the procedure of choice. Extensive stricture disease has been managed endoscopically with the knowledge that subsequent procedures or intermittent catheterization may be necessary to maintain an open urethra.[10,11]

In recent years, especially in Europe and Ireland, subureteric injection of substances has been used for management of vesicoureteral reflux.[12] The cystoscopic injection subureterally of polytetrafluoroethylene (Teflon) paste (STING procedure) has been shown to result in success in all types of vesicoureteral reflux, approaching that of surgical treatment. This technique involves injecting polytetrafluoroethylene paste under the ureteral orifice using a 1-mL syringe connected to a fine 4-French polyethylene catheter with a terminal fine 21-gauge needle. The needle is inserted approximately 3 to 4 mm below the ureteral orifice and is advanced in the submucosal portion of the ureter at the 6 o'clock position (Figure 16–3). The paste is then injected slowly. Afterward, the orifice takes on a volcanic appearance. There appears to be little doubt that the STING procedure is a useful adjunct for treatment of vesicoureteral reflux; however, the use of polytetrafluoroethylene has not been approved in the United States for this purpose and animal experiments have shown migration of polytetrafluoroethylene particles throughout the bladder.[13,14] Investigators are in the process of evaluating other substances including crosslinked collagen, beads, and fat as alternative materials.

Though not a frequent occurrence, ureteroceles can be managed endoscopically with success.[15,16] For those who need immediate management in the neonatal period, endoscopic incision provides a satisfactory method of drainage. Unfortunately, ureteral obstruction has resulted from this technique in many patients; however, a procedure involving a low ureteral incision in a single system described by Rich et al produced reflux in only one of seven patients.[15] With this technique, a 2- to 3-mm low transverse incision is made in the ureterocele with a Bugbee electrode just above the distal junction of the ureterocele with the bladder (Figure 16–4). Incision of the ureterocele at the proper position avoids leaving a flap that might obstruct the bladder outlet and leaves a flap valve in the collapsed ureterocele.

Confirmation of Neoplasia

Cystoscopy in children for neoplasia is a confirmatory procedure rather than a diagnostic or treatment-oriented modality. With rhabdomyosarcoma, the diagnosis usually has been established by its characteristic appearance on radiographic evaluation such as voiding cystourethrogram (VCUG) or computed tomography (CT) scan. Cystoscopy, however, is helpful in determining whether the origin is bladder or prostatic in boys or cystic or vaginal in girls. The extent of

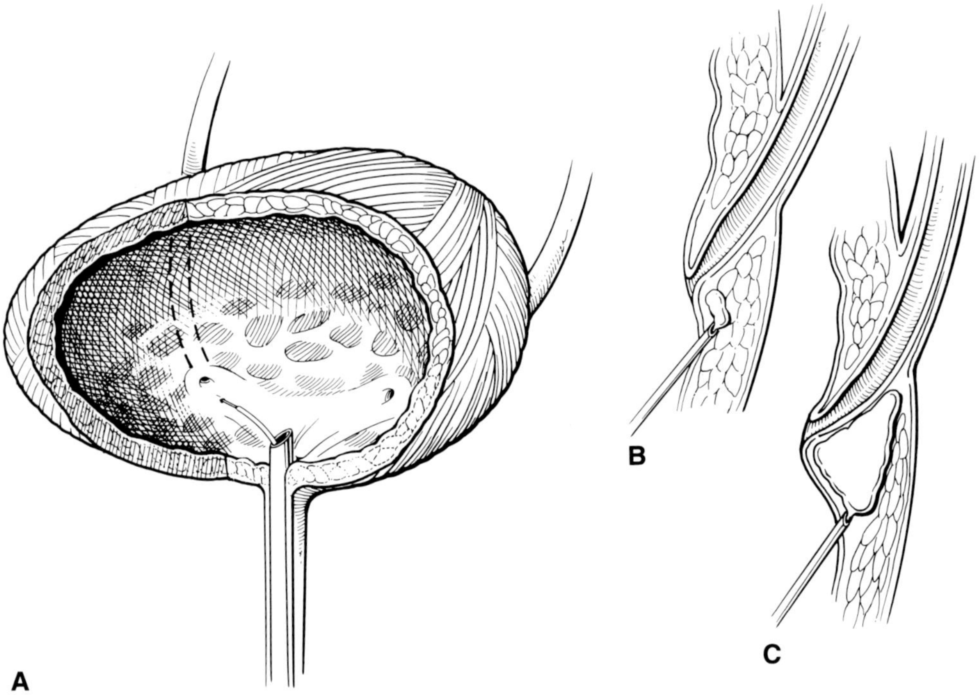

Figure 16–3. In Europe and Ireland, endoscopic subureteral injection of various substances has been used for management of vesicoureteral reflux. One substance is polytetrafluoroethylene (Teflon) paste. Under endoscopic visualization, a fine needle is inserted 3 to 4 mm below the ureteral orifice **(A)** and advanced into the submucosal portion of the ureter at the 6 o'clock position **(B)**. The orifice resembles a volcano following injection of the paste **(C)**.

the tumor can be determined and confirmatory biopsies performed.

With the advent of more aggressive chemotherapeutic regimens, the International Rhabdomyosarcoma Study Group has been very aggressive in trying to treat bladder rhabdomyosarcoma with organ-sparing regimens. Cystoscopy is needed as a second-look procedure to determine effectiveness of treatment. At second-look cystoscopy, the previous sites of tumor are inspected and endoscopic biopsies performed.

Renal parenchymal tumors rarely require cystoscopy as part of the evaluation. Their characteristic appearance on radiologic evaluation render retrograde pyelography and endoscopy of minimal use; however, extravesical lesions arising in the pelvis may impinge on the bladder and can be noted on pelvic radiographs. In those patients, cystoscopy may be helpful in confirming or excluding genitourinary tract involvement.

Evaluation of Cloacal Malformations

The spectrum of anatomic abnormalities in urogenital sinus and cloacal malformations is quite varied. En-

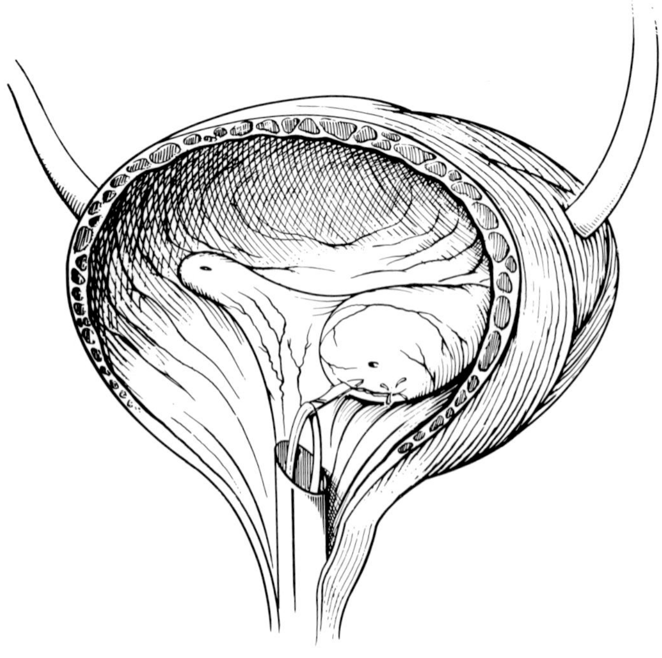

Figure 16–4. Endoscopic management of ureteroceles has been described. A short low transverse incision is made in the ureterocele with a Bugbee electrode just above the distal junction of the ureterocele with the bladder.

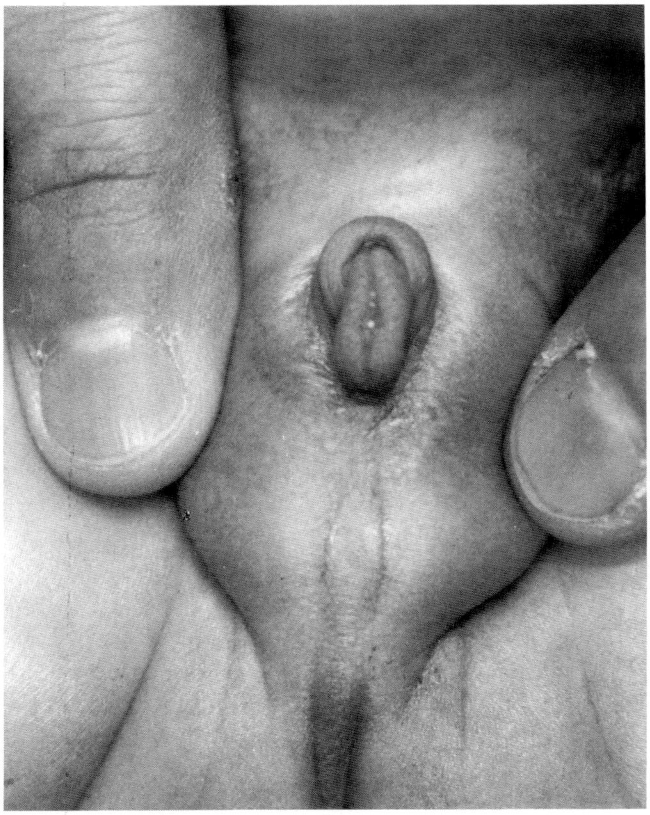

Figure 16–5. Endoscopy serves an important role in the evaluation of children with cloacal malformations. A single perineal opening is shown in this infant.

doscopy serves an important role in the evaluation of these children.[17] Female newborns with severe cloacal malformations present with an abnormal perineum (Figure 16–5). Abdominal distention is common and abdominal radiographs show a large fluid-filled structure in the midabdomen. Most commonly, this pelvic structure is the vagina, but in some cases, the bladder is distended. Ultrasonography is helpful in determining the position of the bladder and the vagina. The bladder is most often small and displaced anteriorly by the large fluid-filled vagina. Catheterization of the urogenital sinus usually results in entry into the vaginal opening. Endoscopy is required in some cases in the neonate for decompression of the bladder and vagina. Cystoscopy is performed, and a 5-French feeding tube is directed into the bladder and vagina separately and secured. Some children require dilation of the vaginal opening to decompress the distended vagina and relieve bladder obstruction. With bladder decompression, intermittent catheterization is not necessary.

Endoscopic evaluation of the cloacal abnormality is invaluable in children prior to reconstruction.[18,19] A definitive look at levels of entry of the vagina, rectum, and bladder into the urogenital sinus is essential before correction is planned. Also, catheters may be directed into the vaginal canal or rectum for contrast studies (Figure 16–6).

URETEROSCOPY

Development of the microlens with small telescopes and endoscopes with working channels has allowed the pediatric urologist to evaluate and treat upper urinary tract anomalies (Table 16–1). This new technology has coincided with development of the laser beam and lithotripsy. With these smaller instruments, stones in the mid- and upper ureter can be manipulated back into the renal pelvis for extracorporeal shockwave lithotripsy. Another option is treatment in situ with either electrohydraulic lithotripsy (EHL) or the pulse dye laser; however, EHL is not possible at present for pediatric patients because of size limitations of the

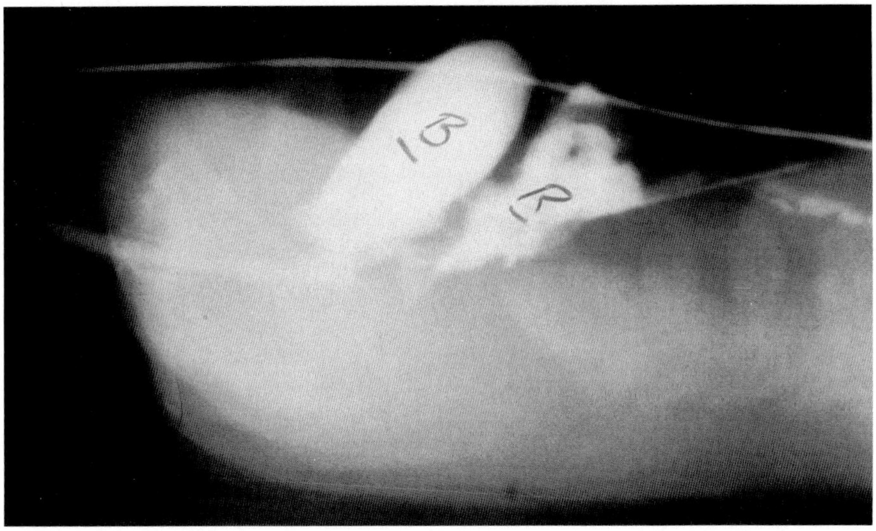

Figure 16–6. For the infant with a cloacal malformation, endoscopic evaluation allows placement of catheters into the vagina or rectum for contrast studies. This contrast study was performed outlining the bladder **(B)** and rectum **(R)**.

TABLE 16–1. AVAILABLE RIGID URETERONEPHROSCOPES[a]

Company	Size of Sheath (Tip) (French)	Length of Endoscope (cm)	Accessory Channel (French)	Lens (degrees)
Storz	11.5	25	4	6
		41	4	6, 70
Olympus	10.5	45	—	0
	11.0	34	3	0
	11.0	45	5	5
Wolf	7.5		3.3	0
	9.5	43	5	5
	11.5	28	6 or 5 and 3	5, 25, 70
Circon/ ACMI	6.9	33/41	3.4 and 2.3	5
	10.0	43	5	5, 90
Candela	7.2	41	2.1 and 2.1	0

[a] The endoscopes listed represent the smallest endoscope available from each manufacturer at the time of publication.

equipment. Moreover, it is important to realize that the use of the EHL is associated with potentially significant complications such as perforation and stricture. The use of the pulse dye laser through the ureteroscope is quite helpful in disintegrating stones that are too large for extraction. The 3-French laser fiber is used to contact the stone directly, and pulsed energy disintegrates the stone. The smaller particles are then either extracted or allowed to pass spontaneously.

The technique of ureteroscopy and passage of the scope is important to prevent complications.[20,21] Cystoscopy is performed initially and a guidewire of appropriate size is passed per ureteral orifice. The wire functions as a guide for possible balloon dilation of the ureter and allows access to the ureter for either placement of a stenting catheter or passage of the scope over the wire. After placement of the wire, the cystoscope is removed and the ureteroscope inserted adjacent to the wire into the bladder. In most children, balloon dilation of the ureter is not necessary to advance the scope into the orifice. Rotation of the scope 180 degrees allows its beak to gently dilate the orifice, thereby facilitating passage into the ureter. The scope is advanced under direct vision up the ureter to the area of concern. Following either diagnostic visualization or stone extraction, the ureteroscope is withdrawn. An external/internal stent, or internal stent alone, may be placed in the ureter depending on the degree of manipulation and subsequent edema. In most cases, use of the flexible ureteroscope has been limited to diagnostic maneuvers. Unfortunately, although the flexible laser fiber and EHL probes are available, the irrigating channel on this scope does not allow a flow rate sufficient for adequate visualization, even with the aid of pumps.

Long-term effects of ureteroscopy in children are unknown at present. Stricture formation and vesicoureteral reflux remain major concerns, but the incidence in small pediatric series remains minimal.[22]

ENDOPYELOTOMY

A new and emerging area in endourology is the management of urinary obstruction.[23] Balloon dilation of stricture disease of the upper urinary system has been well described in adults with varied results.[24,25] Access to the area has been through the conventional bladder route in a retrograde fashion and antegrade by way of a nephrostomy tube. The technique of retrograde endopyelotomy involves passage of a guidewire from the bladder to renal pelvis. For antegrade endopyelotomy, a nephrostomy tube is placed and the tract dilated with 18- to 24-French catheters, depending on the size of the child. A rigid panendoscope is used to visualize the intrarenal collecting system. A guidewire is passed antegrade into the bladder (Figure 16–7). Both wires are insulated with a 5-French angiographic catheter and normal saline is placed 40 cm above the table used for irrigation during the diagnostic phase. Glycine or sorbitol is used during the

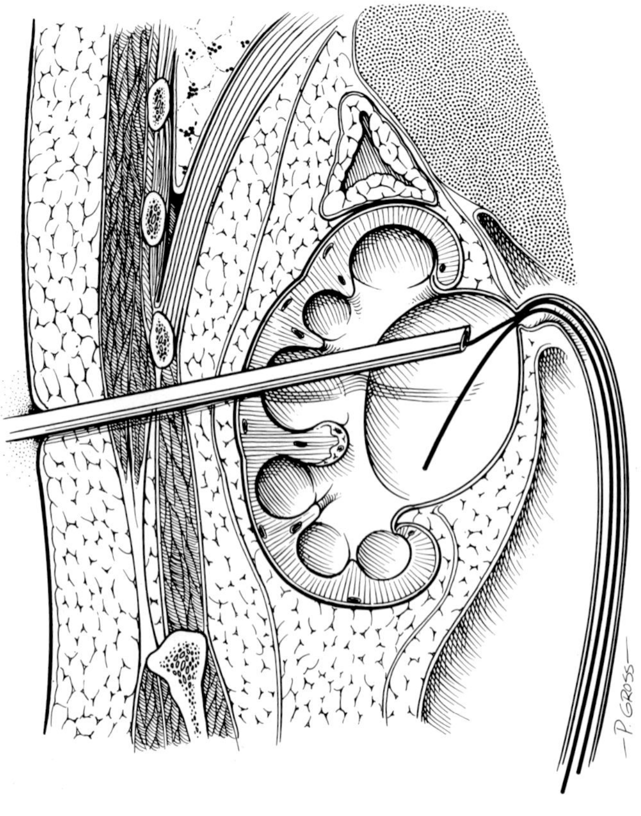

Figure 16–7. For endopyelotomy, guidewires are passed antegrade and retrograde through the ureteropelvic stenosis. Antegrade passage is accomplished using a panendoscope placed through a previously dilated nephrostomy tube tract.

pyelotomy. Endopyelotomy has been carried out using a 3- or 5-French electrocautery probe with the cutting current set at 50 to 100 W. The incision is made in the posterior lateral aspect of the ureteropelvic junction (UPJ) and deepened until fat is seen (Figure 16–8). The incision is then carried at least 1 cm on each side of the strictured area. A 5- or 6-mm balloon is inserted in the antegrade direction and inflated in the area of the incision to ensure the incision is adequate. This is visualized fluoroscopically (Figure 16–9). A ureteral stent is placed and left for 6 weeks. A nephrostomy tube is inserted and left for variable lengths of time. Endopyelotomy has been recommended for use in both primary and secondary ureteropelvic junction obstructions.[22,26] Its success appears most likely in the patient who is postsurgical with an anastomotic stricture secondary to periureteral fibrosis or induration. Its use in primary ureteropelvic junction obstruction has been reported, but long-term evaluation has not been possible.

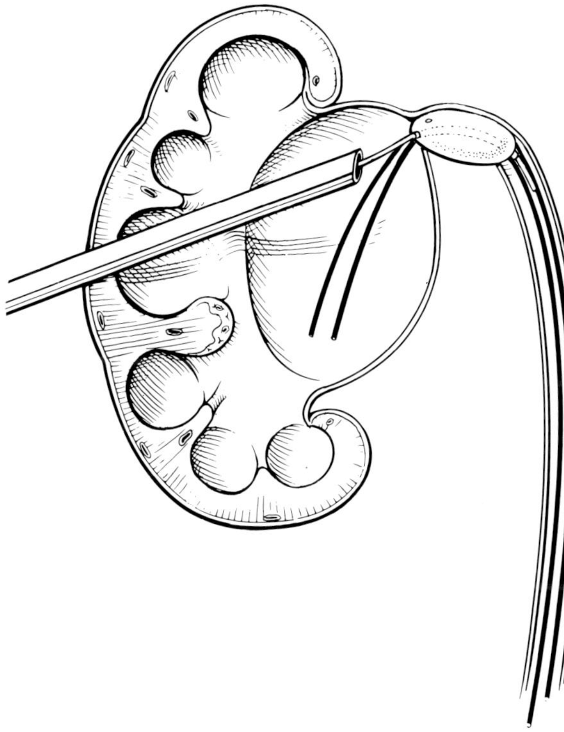

Figure 16–9. A balloon dilator is then inserted in the antegrade direction and inflated under fluoroscopic visualization in the area of the incision to ensure adequate ablation of the stenosis.

SUMMARY

Endoscopy of the genitourinary system in children will continue to change significantly in the coming years. Refinements in radiographic and ultrasonographic technology may alter the indications for endoscopy. Technologic advances will continue to drive our interest and possibly our indications. Ultimately, however, the physician responsible for the patient's care must be the determining force in deciding the proper use of genitourinary endoscopy in children.

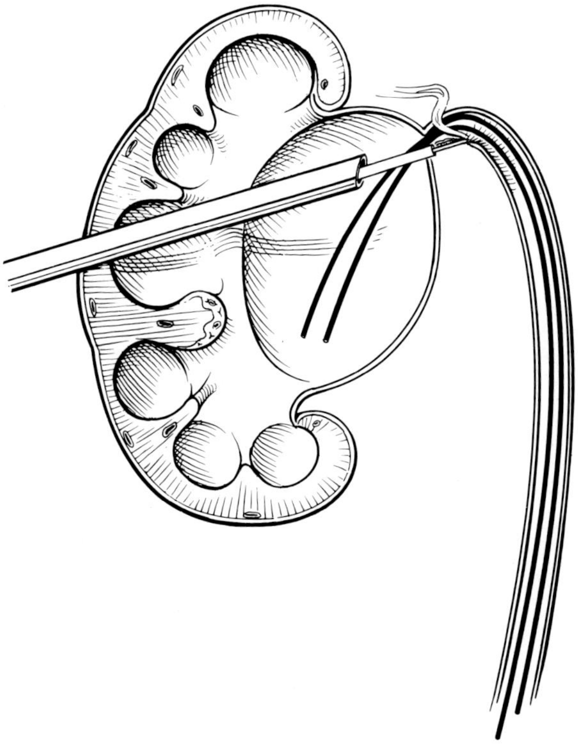

Figure 16–8. Under endoscopic visualization, an incision is made in the posterolateral aspect of the ureteropelvic junction and deepened until fat is seen.

REFERENCES

1. Litvak AS, Morris JA, McRoberts JW. Normal size of the urethral meatus in boys. *J Urol.* 1976;115:736.
2. Johnson DK, Kroovand RL, Perlmutter AD. The changing role of cystoscopy in the pediatric patient. *J Urol.* 1980;123:232.
3. Walther PC, Kaplan GW. Cystoscopy in children: Indications for its use in common urologic problems. *J Urol.* 1980;123:232.
4. Kaplan GW, Brock WA. Idiopathic urethrorrhagia in boys. *J Urol.* 1982;128:1001.
5. Whitaker RH, Keeton JE, Williams DI. Posterior urethral valves: A study of urinary control after operation. *J Urol.* 1972;108:167.
6. Zaontz MR, Firlit CF. Percutaneous antegrade ablation of posterior urethral valves in infants with small caliber urethras: An alternative to urinary diversion. *J Urol.* 1986;136:247.
7. Churchill BM, Krueger RP, Fleisher MH, et al. Compli-

cations of posterior urethral valve surgery and their prevention. *Urol Clin North Am.* 1983;10:519.
8. Scherz HC, Kaplan GW. Etiology, diagnosis and management of urethral strictures in children. *Urol Clin North Am.* 1990;17(2):389.
9. Scherz HC, Kaplan JW, Packer MG, Brock WA. Posthypospadias repair of urethral strictures: A review of 30 cases. *J Urol.* 1988;140:1253.
10. Noe HN. Complications and management of childhood urethral stricture disease. *Urol Clin North Am.* 1983;10: 531.
11. Walker RD. Stricture formation after perineal urethrostomy. Presented at Annual Meeting, Section on Urology, American Academy of Pediatrics, 1972.
12. O'Donnell B, Puri P. Treatment of vesicoureteral reflux by endoscopic injection of Teflon. *Br Med J.* 1984; 289:7.
13. Malizia AA Jr, Woodard JR, Rushton HG, et al. Migration and granulomatous reaction after subureteric injection of Teflon paste in primates. Unpublished data.
14. Malizia AA Jr, Reiman HM, Myers RP, et al. Migration and granulomatous reaction after periurethral injection of Polytef (Teflon). *JAMA.* 1984;251:3277.
15. Rich MA, Keating MA, Snyder HM, et al. Low transurethral incision of single system intravesical ureteroceles in children. *J Urol.* 1990;144:120.
16. Tank ES. Experience with endoscopic incision and open unroofing of ureteroceles. *J Urol.* 1986;136:241.
17. Hendren WH. Urological aspects of cloacal malformations. *J Urol.* 1988;140:1207.
18. Hendren WH. Surgical management of urogenital sinus abnormalities. *J Pediatr Surg.* 1977;12(3):339.
19. Hendren WH. Cloacal malformations. In: *Campbell's Urology*, 1992.
20. Hill DE, Segura JW, Patterson DE, et al. Ureteroscopy in children. *J Urol.* 1990;144:481.
21. Shepherd P, Thomas R, Harmon EP. Urolithiasis in children: Innovations in management. *J Urol.* 1988;140:790.
22. Ball WS Jr, Towbin R, Strife JL, et al. Interventional genitourinary radiology in children: A review of 61 procedures. *AJR* 1986;147(2):791.
23. Kavoussi LR, Meretyk S, Dierks SM, et al. Endopyelotomy for secondary ureteropelvic junction obstruction in children. *J Urol.* 1991;145:345.
24. Brannen GE, Bush WH, Lewis GP. Endopyelotomy for primary repair of ureteropelvic junction obstruction. *J Urol.* 1988;139:29.
25. Clayman RV, Basler JW, Kavoussi L, et al. Ureteronephroscopic endopyelotomy. *J Urol.* 1990;144:246.
26. Towbin RB, Wacksman J, Ball WS. Percutaneous pyeloplasty in children: Experience in three patients. *Radiology.* 1987;163:381.

CHAPTER 17

Fetoscopic Surgery

JAMES M. ESTES • N. SCOTT ADZICK
MICHAEL R. HARRISON

Endoscopic procedures have revolutionized the approach to surgery. Advances in optical equipment and instrumentation have facilitated the application of minimally invasive methods to many surgical specialties. Virtually all surgeons must now broaden their repertoire to include these new endoscopic techniques. This revolutionary surgical approach can also be applied to the fetus.

In utero surgery can salvage fetuses with several life-threatening malformations including congenital diaphragmatic hernia, cystic adenomatoid malformation, obstructive uropathy, and massive sacrococcygeal teratoma.[1] This aggressive approach carries risks to both mother and child, and these risks must be carefully considered. It is imperative that maternal morbidity is minimal, without adverse effects on future pregnancies, and this minimal morbidity has been confirmed by a review of our first 17 patients.[2] Experience, however, also demonstrates that significant fetal morbidity results from postoperative preterm labor. This phenomenon is due to uterine irritability caused by the hysterotomy incision. It is therefore possible that the risks of in utero surgery could be substantially reduced by developing minimally invasive methods for fetal intervention.

Until recently, the development of the fetus was shrouded in mystery and secrecy because there were no modalities to observe this phenomenon. As early as 1954, however, Westin visualized the fetus in situ using a 10-mm "hysteroscope" that was introduced transcervically.[3] In 1972, Valenti described the "endamnioscope," which was a modified cystoscope introduced into the uterine cavity prior to hysterotomy in six patients between 16 and 18 weeks of gestation.[4] Using this technique, he was able to obtain fetal skin biopsies under direct vision.

Techniques rapidly improved such that fetal endoscopy was no longer limited to examinations prior to second-trimester pregnancy terminations. Hobbins and Mahoney extended the applications of *fetoscopy* (a term coined in 1974)[5] to prenatal diagnosis. Their technique involved piercing the abdominal wall fascia and uterus with an outer cannula (2.2 × 2.7 mm) through which was passed a 1.7-mm Dyonics Needlescope. This device contained a straight rod lens and a coaxial fiberoptic bundle for illumination. In a series of 84 patients, they examined the fetus and obtained tissue samples. Seventeen abnormal fetuses were diagnosed and electively terminated while approximately 80% of the remaining pregnancies proceeded to term[6]; however, the small optical channel and limited mobility of the Needlescope severely restricted visualization, as only a small fraction of the fetus could be examined in an average study.[7]

Although fetoscopy produced revolutionary changes in prenatal diagnosis, it played a very limited role in fetal therapy. With the exception of in utero blood transfusion, fetoscopy was used predominantly for diagnosis through tissue sampling and blood aspiration in fetuses between 18 and 23 weeks of gestation.[8] Furthermore, even at experienced centers, this technique carried a fetal loss rate of 5 to 7%.[9] As noninvasive imaging techniques improved, fetoscopy was largely replaced by other methods, chiefly percutaneous umbilical blood sampling (PUBS). PUBS uses high-resolution ultrasound to guide a 20- or 22-gauge needle into the umbilical cord vessels, and pregnancy loss is only 0.5%.[10] Ultrasound-guided needle aspiration also provided a means for fluid aspiration, cyst decompression, and fetal transfusion.

Despite the loss in popularity, technologic advances have facilitated some innovations in fetoscopic therapy. DeVore and co-workers used a neodymium:YAG (Nd:YAG) laser to cut and coagulate fetal lamb tissue under endoscopic visualization.[11] DeLia and colleagues have also used this type of laser to successfully coagulate placental vessels in primates and placental anastomoses in the twin–twin transfusion syndrome.[12] We have extended the application of fetoscopic therapy to include direct surgical manipulation.

DEVELOPMENT OF FETOSCOPIC SURGERY

Ultrasound and fetoscopy have dramatically enhanced prenatal diagnostic capabilities; however, these techniques offer limited potential for in utero fetal intervention. Frustrated by this deficiency, our research group, as part of the Fetal Treatment Center at the University of California, San Francisco, has developed techniques for in utero surgery. Highly selected fetuses with life-threatening malformations including congenital diaphragmatic hernia, cystic adenomatoid malformation, obstructive uropathy, and massive sacrococcygeal teratoma have undergone successful surgical repair by open hysterotomy.[1] Prenatal repair corrects the malformation, which allows further growth to overcome the adverse developmental consequences. For example, correction of diaphragmatic hernia and reduction of herniated viscera in utero prevent pulmonary hypoplasia, which is often fatal in severely affected neonates.[13]

These experiences have shown that the major risk of fetal surgery is preterm labor, which is caused by the large hysterotomy required for fetal exposure. To solve this problem we have combined the minimally invasive attributes of fetoscopy with specialized techniques and instrumentation to provide a safer alternative to open fetal surgery.

FETAL CLEFT LIP

The application of endoscopy to in utero fetal intervention required significant modifications to laparoscopic techniques. Our initial studies were performed in fetal lambs because of their large size and relative resistance to spontaneous abortion following hysterotomy. The initial questions we addressed concerned cannulation methods, types of insufflation media, and fetal tolerance to insufflation.

To explore these issues we developed a model for the endoscopic creation and repair of fetal cleft lip. In these experiments we exposed the ovine uterus by maternal laparotomy. Several 5-mm trocars were placed through a uterine pursestring suture, which served to maintain an airtight seal, and a 5-mm rod lens was passed into the intrauterine space (Figure 17–1). Amniotic fluid was usually too cloudy for adequate visualization so carbon dioxide was used to distend the uterus. The resulting gas-filled pocket afforded excellent fetal visualization and allowed the use of unipolar cautery.

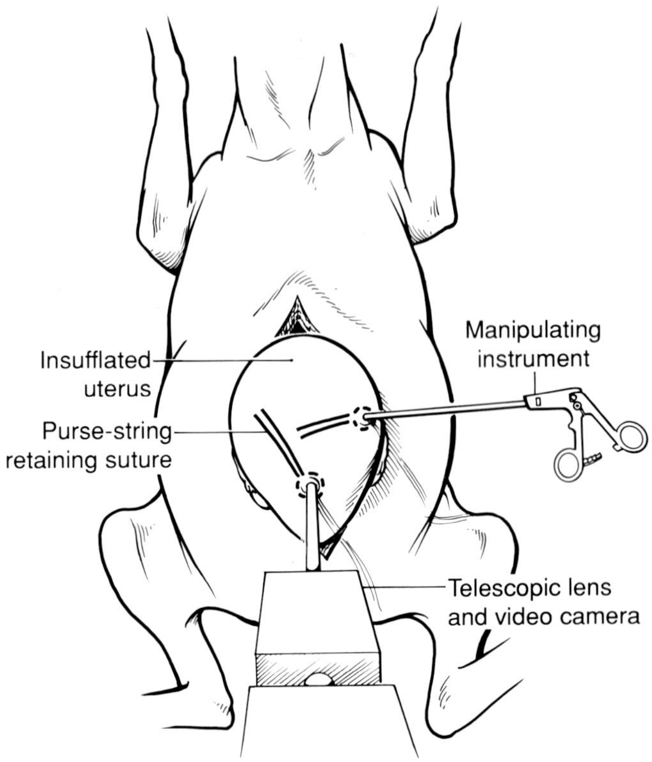

Figure 17–1. Diagram of the ovine uterus exposed by laparotomy. Two 5-mm ports are placed for the camera and operating instruments. Pursestring sutures are used to maintain an airtight seal around the trocars.

These initial experiments were associated with a high incidence of fetal mortality. This mortality was due to impaired umbilical venous flow (normal umbilical venous pressure is 4 to 6 cm H_2O) and was obviated by using insufflation pressures no greater than 5 cm H_2O.

Once the technical problems of uterine cannulation and insufflation were solved, we focused our approach on instrumentation. Conventional laparoscopic instruments have large grasping jaws and awkward scissor grips, which make them unsuitable for precision work in a highly magnified surgical field. Our techniques required the design and manufacture of miniaturized graspers and needleholders that facilitated precise tissue manipulation and suture placement (Figure 17–2). Methods for "microendoscopic" suturing were adapted from existing microsurgical techniques[14] and were practiced in an inanimate trainer model prior to use in animals.[15] Our method of microendoscopic knot tying quickly and reliably produced a secure square knot (Figure 17–3).

These techniques were then applied to chronic animal experiments.[16] Fetal lambs at 80 days of gestation (term = 145 days) were selected because they are

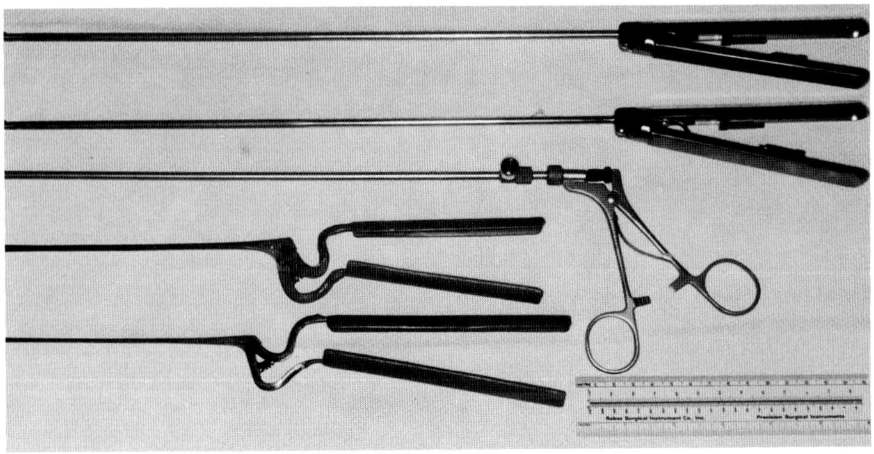

Figure 17–2. Comparison of a standard laparoscopic needle holder (*middle*) with specially designed instruments for microendoscopic surgery (*top and bottom*). Note the modified handles that provide precision action through the full range of rotation. These instruments also have curved grasping tips that facilitate needle driving at various angles.

well developed and also because there is a more favorable amniotic fluid-to-fetal size ratio than later in gestation. The relatively large amount of amniotic fluid facilitated fetal positioning and visualization during the procedure. A simulated cleft lip was created by excising a wedge of tissue incorporating part of the upper lip and alveolar plate (Figure 17–4). Following its creation, the defect was approximated with interrupted 6-0 "pliabilized" nylon sutures (Ethicon, Inc, Somerville, NJ) using the intracorporeal methods previously described. At the end of the procedure, the carbon dioxide was removed and 50 mL of warmed Ringer's lactate containing 1 g of penicillin was instilled.

The procedures were well tolerated and there was no maternal or fetal morbidity. Fourteen days later the fetuses were removed and the lip wounds examined. Gross and histologic analysis revealed no evidence of

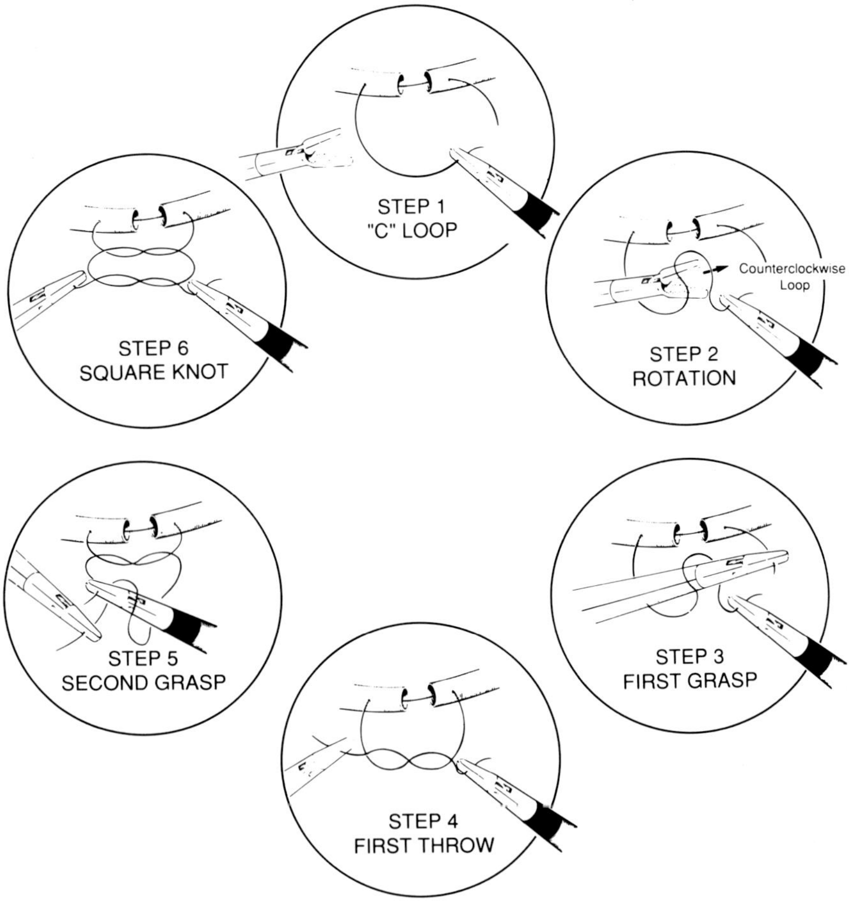

Figure 17–3. Method for intracorporeal knot tying. Step 1 demonstrates creation of the "C" loop. The assisting grasper is placed over the loop, and the suture is wrapped around the instrument in a counterclockwise direction (step 2). The free suture end is grasped (step 3) and pulled through, creating a square first throw (step 4). The procedure is reversed for the second throw (steps 5 and 6) and a square knot is created. (*Reprinted, with permission, from Estes et al.*[15])

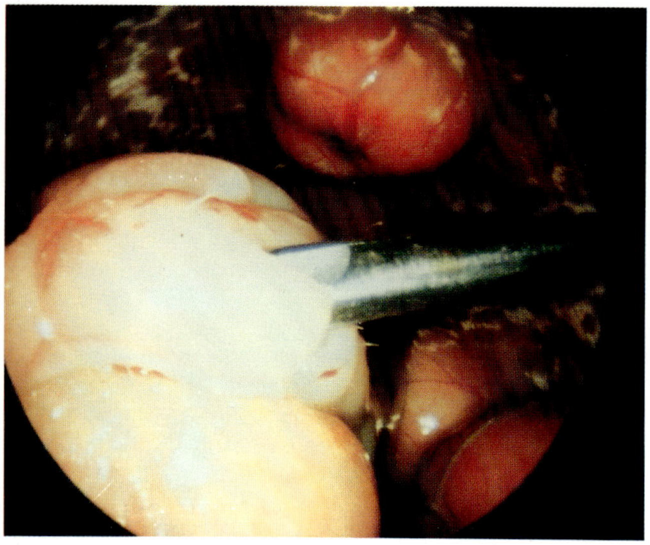

Figure 17–4. Hooked scissors are used to create the full-thickness lip defect. The placental cotyledons are seen attached to the uterine wall in the background.

scarring (Figure 17–5), consistent with previous studies of fetal lip wounds using open surgical techniques.[17]

Because of the less invasive nature of this technique, we hypothesized that fetoscopic surgery could be performed much earlier in gestation than open manipulation. In our experience with fetal lambs, 60 days represents the earliest gestational age that open surgery is tolerated. At this point even minimal surgical manipulation carries a mortality of about 50%, probably because of a marked susceptibility and sensitivity to hypothermia. We performed endoscopic surgery on two 45-day-gestation (first-trimester) lamb fetuses by resecting a large wedge of lip tissue. At this age the fetus is about 6 cm long, so the magnification provided by the 5-mm telescope was essential to the operation. Both fetuses survived and the large lip defect had healed without scar or deformity.[18] These studies clearly demonstrated the feasibility of endoscopic fetal surgery. Although the cleft lip model described here is conceptually simple, it has allowed the development of fundamental techniques for fetoscopic surgery. Further improvements in instrumentation and methods were, however, necessary before we could apply minimally invasive surgery to fetal therapy.

OBSTRUCTIVE UROPATHY

Congenital obstructive uropathy is a common malformation affecting approximately one in every 1000 fetuses.[19] In those severely affected, bilateral hydronephrosis causes early postnatal death as a result of pulmonary hypoplasia and renal failure. Fetal surgery has been successful in treating a few highly selected cases of this anomaly.[20] Ultrasound-guided percutaneous catheter placement is also used to treat this mal-

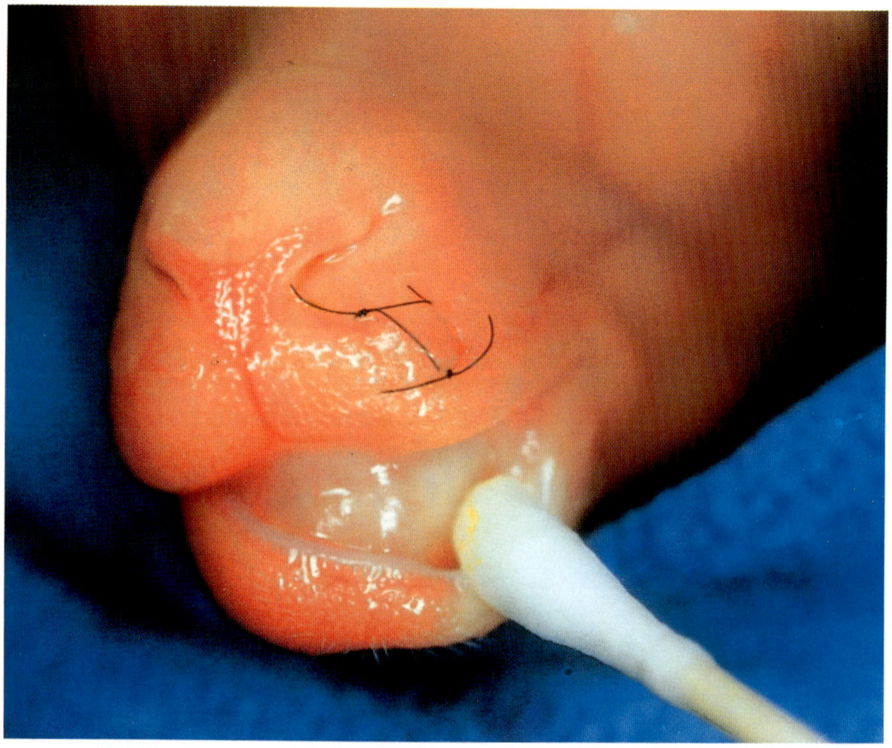

Figure 17–5. Appearance of the lip wound 14 days after endoscopic repair. The wound has healed without visible scar or deformity.

formation in utero, but often fails because of catheter obstruction and migration, thereby limiting this approach to short-term therapy.[21,22] Catheter placement has also resulted in iatrogenic cases of gastroschisis and other fetal injuries.[22,23] These complications were attributed to imprecise needle placement and unsatisfactory fetal visualization.

Hydronephrosis is easily diagnosed in utero. Unilateral hydronephrosis is managed conservatively; bilateral disease can present as a spectrum of severity. Criteria have been developed to assess renal function in utero, and these parameters include urine electrolytes, ultrasonographic appearance of kidneys (presence or absence of dysplastic cysts), and amniotic fluid volume.[24] Several case reports in humans and experimental work in lambs have demonstrated that in utero bladder drainage may restore amniotic fluid volume and prevent progressive renal deterioration and pulmonary hypoplasia, thus providing the scientific rationale for aggressive prenatal treatment.[24,25]

The prenatal management of obstructive uropathy provides an ideal opportunity for innovation. Open fetal surgery can reliably palliate bladder obstruction but it carries high risks because of preterm labor. Moreover, percutaneous methods are unreliable for long-term bladder decompression. Therefore, we have devised endoscopic techniques to treat fetal urinary tract obstruction. The magnified view provided by the endoscope facilitates precise fetal manipulation and minimizes unnecessary injury. The endoscopic approach can also decrease the risks of fetal surgery by causing less uterine trauma and preterm labor.

This procedure was initially developed in fetal lambs.[18] A complete lower urinary obstruction was created by ligation of the urethra and urachus at 80 days of gestation. Seven days later the endoscopic procedure was performed. Two 5-mm trocars were placed for the telescopic lens and operating port. The distended lower abdominal wall was visualized with the umbilical cord and urethral meatus serving as landmarks, and a longitudinal incision was made with unipolar cautery through the skin and fascia of the lower midline abdominal wall. It is crucial to remain in the midline during this procedure to avoid injury to the umbilical arteries, which are adherent to the bladder and course posterolaterally.

The vesicocutaneous fistula is created using a novel expandable wire-mesh stent developed by Schneider U.S. Stent, Inc (Minneapolis, MN). The Wallstent is placed in compressed form on a 7-French catheter (Figure 17–6). When deployed, the device expands and forms a semirigid conduit that maintains the bladder fistula (Figure 17–7). The stent catheter is placed over a guidewire passed into the bladder by transuterine needle localization. The stent is then deployed within the abdominal wall under direct endoscopic vision (Figure 17–8).

This technique was well tolerated and there was no fetal or maternal morbidity. The stent was effective in relieving obstruction in all cases. Examination 7 days later revealed completely decompressed urinary systems in the treated animals and severe megacystis and hydroureters in the controls.

PRIMATE STUDIES

The fetal lamb model was useful for the development of techniques and instrumentation for endoscopic fetal surgery; however, critical examination of this method

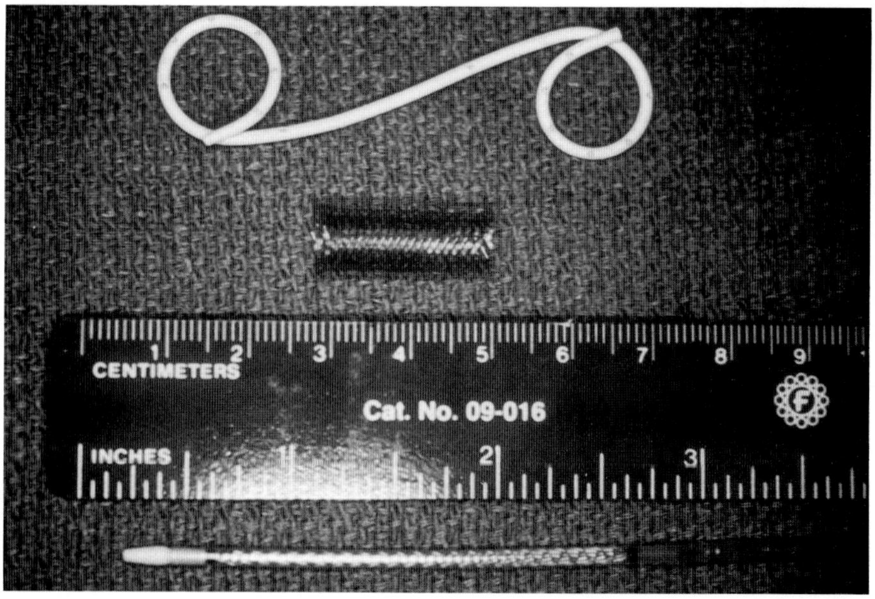

Figure 17–6. Compare the Wallstent (*middle*) with a conventional fetal bladder catheter (*top*). When deployed, the stent measures 8 × 20 mm and provides a significantly larger channel for bladder drainage than the catheter. The wire-mesh design also promotes firm tissue fixation. The stent is also shown in compressed form on the 7-French introducer catheter (*bottom*).

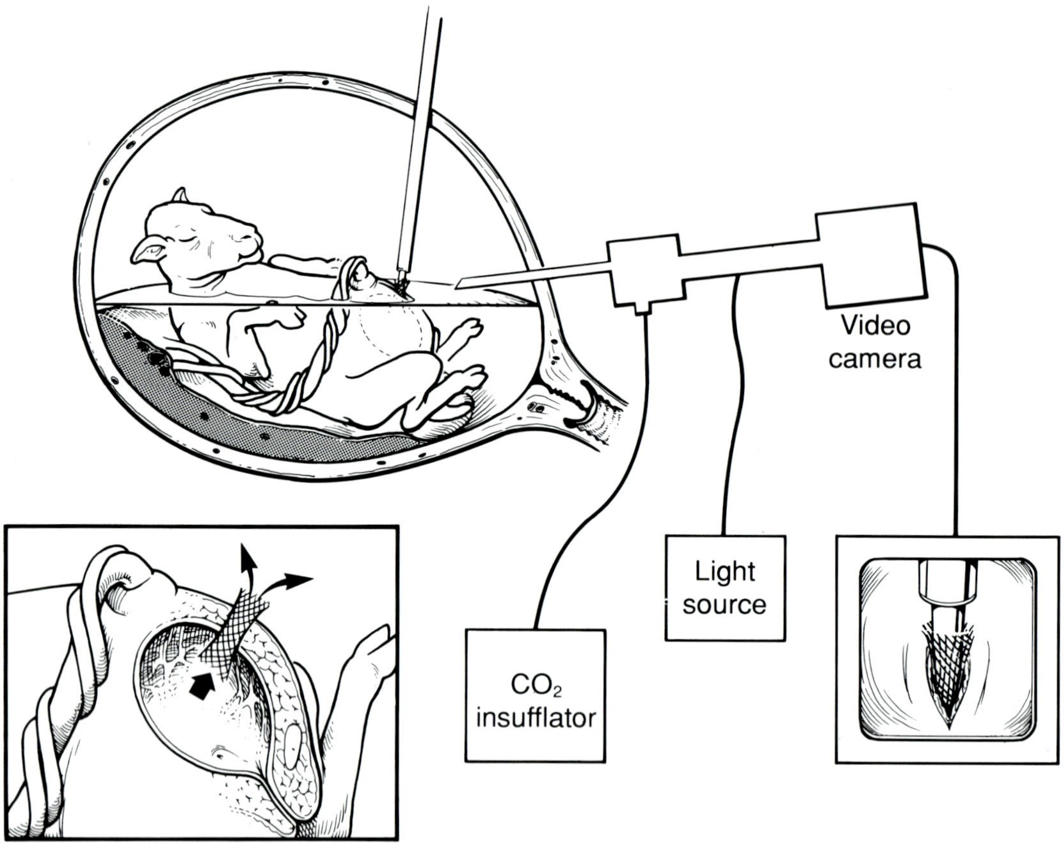

Figure 17–7. Arrangement of the 5-mm lens and stent catheter as seen through the uterus. Insufflation is used to create a gas pocket to facilitate visualization. The stent is deployed within the abdominal wall, thereby decompressing the bladder by creating a large vesicocutaneous fistula (*inset*). (*Reprinted, with permission, from Estes et al.*[18])

requires experimentation in nonhuman primates. The primate uterus is much thicker and more vascular than that of the sheep. It is also much more "irritable" following surgical manipulation and more likely to develop preterm labor. Therefore, to simulate fetoscopic surgery in humans, we chose the rhesus monkey (*Macaca mulatta*) as our next experimental model. We have previously described the general aspects of anesthetic management for fetal surgery in this animal.[26] Several modifications of our fetoscopic techniques were necessary because of the thickness and muscularity of the rhesus uterus.

Intraoperative ultrasound was required to identify fetal position prior to port placement. Using a high-resolution device with color doppler capabilities (Model 128/XP, Acuson Corporation, Mountain View, CA), we identified the placental disks and umbilical cord to prevent injury during port insertion.

The primate uterus presented several new obstacles. The thick muscular wall prohibited port placement using a sharp trocar, as this required excessive force and usually caused dissection of amniotic membranes. Port placement could be accomplished via cut-

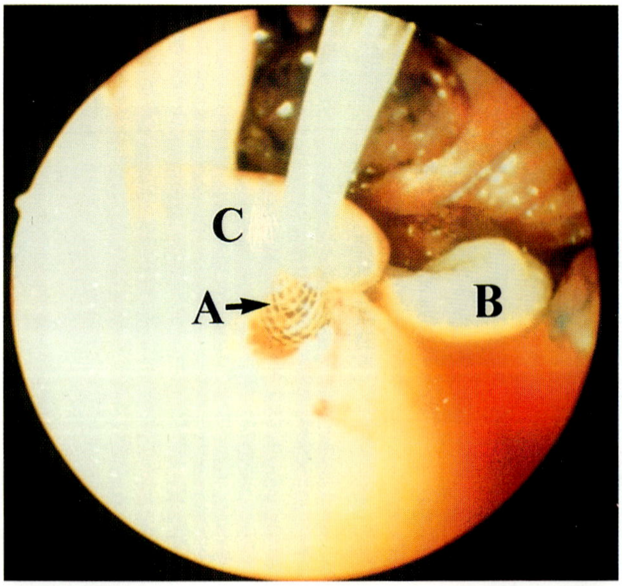

Figure 17–8. Intrauterine view as seen through the endoscope. The Wallstent is deployed within the vesicocutaneous fistula. A = Wallstent. B = Umbilical cord. C = Scrotum. (*Reprinted, with permission, from Estes et al.*[18])

down through the myometrium, thereby exposing the membranes and allowing trocar insertion into the amniotic space under direct vision. This method, however, is unsuitable because it adds significant uterine trauma to a procedure that should be minimally invasive.

A better approach used progressive dilation of the "hysterostomy." The intraamniotic space is localized with a 16-gauge angiocatheter and guidewire. With a series of tapered dilators, the hysterostomy is gradually enlarged to accommodate a 5-mm trocar which is passed over the last dilator. This technique causes little uterine trauma and avoids amniotic membrane dissection.

The second problem was insufflation. As in the fetal lamb, amniotic fluid usually contains particulate debris (vernix caseosum) that scatters light, making it unsatisfactory as a visualization medium. Unlike the sheep, however, the primate uterus is much less compliant and therefore less distensible. We initially tried carbon dioxide insufflation with good results, but because of the smaller working space around the fetus, proper port placement and fetal positioning were critical to the success of the procedure.

An alternative insufflation medium is fluid. We experimented with continuous warmed saline irrigation and found that it provided excellent visualization. There were, however, several disadvantages: small amounts of blood obscured the field, and a second port was required to provide flow rates effective enough to clear shed blood. Also, unipolar cautery was ineffective during saline irrigation, but the use of a Nd:YAG laser or a less ionic medium such as glycine would prevent this problem.

We are presently applying the endoscopic techniques for bladder decompression to the rhesus monkey with the ultimate goal of human applications. Some of the basic problems with uterine cannulation and insufflation have been solved, and studies are now underway to assess the long-term efficacy and safety of this endoscopic technique.

FUTURE OF ENDOSCOPIC FETAL SURGERY

Endoscopic fetal surgery offers considerable promise for the future of antenatal therapy. By decreasing the risks of fetal manipulation, this technique may provide the means to correct certain non-life-threatening malformations in utero such as cleft lip and palate, neural tube defects, and amniotic bands (Table 17–1). We also have the capability to provide chronic vascular access via the placental bed to the sick fetus afflicted with growth retardation or hydrops. In utero repair also offers the potential for scarless fetal wound healing, a remarkable property yet to be clinically exploited.[27] Future research will undoubtedly expand the possibilities and applications of fetoscopic surgery.

TABLE 17–1. MALFORMATIONS AND DISEASES THAT MAY BE CORRECTED IN UTERO BY FETOSCOPIC SURGERY

Cleft lip and palate
Obstructive uropathy
Neural tube defects
Amniotic bands
Syndactyly
Pedunculated sacrococcygeal teratomas
Twin–twin transfusion
Growth retardation (chronic placental catheter placement for intravenous nutrition)

REFERENCES

1. Harrison MR, Adzick NS. The fetus as a patient: Surgical considerations. *Ann Surg.* 1991;213:279.
2. Longaker MT, Golbus MS, Filly RA, et al. Maternal outcome after open fetal surgery. A review of the first 17 cases. *JAMA.* 1991;265:737.
3. Westin B. Hysteroscopy in early pregnancy. *Lancet.* 1954;2:872.
4. Valenti C. Endoamnioscopy and fetal biopsy: A new technique. *Am J Obstet Gynecol.* 1972;114:561.
5. Phillips JM. Fetoscopy: Its genesis and promise. *J Reprod Med.* 1978;21:115.
6. Hobbins JC. Diagnosing with the fetoscope. *Contemp Obstet Gynecol.* 1979;13:143.
7. Benzie RJ, Doran TA. The "fetoscope"—A new clinical tool for prenatal diagnosis. *Am J Obstet Gynecol.* 1975;121:460.
8. Schwartz DB, Zweibel WJ, Donovan D, et al. Fetoscopic visualization in second trimester pregnancies. *Am J Obstet Gynecol.* 1983;145:51.
9. Grannum PA, Copel JA. Invasive fetal procedures. *Radiol Clin North Am.* 1990;28:217.
10. Daffos F, Capella-Pavlovsky M, Forestier F. Fetal blood sampling during pregnancy with the use of a needle guided by ultrasound: A study of 606 consecutive cases. *Am J Obstet Gynecol.* 1985;153:655.
11. DeVore GR, Dixon JA, Hobbins JC. Fetoscope-directed neodymium-YAG laser: A potential tool for fetal surgery. *Am J Obstet Gynecol.* 1983;145:379.
12. DeLia JE, Cukierski MA, Lundergan DK, et al. Neodymium:yttrium–aluminum–garnet laser occlusion of rhesus placental vasculature via fetoscopy. *Am J Obstet Gynecol.* 1989;160:485.
13. Harrison MR, Bressack MA, Churg AM, et al. Correction of congenital diaphragmatic hernia *in utero.* II. Simulated correction permits fetal lung growth with survival at birth. *Surgery.* 1980;88:260.
14. Buncke HJ, Chater NL, Szabo Z. *The Manual of Micro-*

vascular Surgery. San Francisco: Davis and Geck; 1975: 13.

15. Estes JM, Szabo Z, Harrison MR. Techniques for *in utero* endoscopic surgery: A new approach for fetal intervention. *Surg Endosc.* 1992;6:215.
16. Estes JM, Whitby DJ, Lorenz HP, et al. Endoscopic creation and repair of fetal cleft lip. *Plast Reconstr Surg.* 1992;90:743.
17. Longaker MT, Stern M, Lorenz HP, et al. A model for fetal cleft lip repair in lambs. *Plast Reconstr Surg.* 1992;90:750.
18. Estes JM, MacGillivray TE, Hedrick MH, et al. Fetoscopic surgery for the treatment of congenital anomalies. *J Pediatr Surg.* 1992;27:950.
19. Flake AW, Adzick NS, Glick PL, et al. Evaluation of the fetus with hydronephrosis. In: deVere White RW, Palmer JM, eds. *New Techniques in Urology.* Mount Kisco, NY: Futura; 1987:271.
20. Crombleholme TM, Harrison MR, Golbus MS, et al. Fetal intervention in obstructive uropathy: Prognostic indicators and efficacy of intervention. *Am J Obstet Gynecol.* 1990;162:1239.
21. Harrison MR, Golbus MS, Filly RA, et al. Fetal hydronephrosis: Selection and surgical repair. *J Pediatr Surg.* 1987;22:556.
22. Glick PL, Harrison MR, Golbus MS, et al. Management of the fetus with congenital hydronephrosis. II. Prognostic criteria and selection for treatment. *J Pediatr Surg.* 1985;20:376.
23. Manning FA, Harrison MR, Rodeck C. Catheter shunts for fetal hydronephrosis and hydrocephalus. Report of the International Fetal Surgery Registry. *N Engl J Med.* 1986;315:336.
24. Crombleholme TM, Harrison MR, Longaker MT, et al. Prenatal diagnosis and management of bilateral hydronephrosis. *Pediatr Nephrol.* 1988;2:334.
25. Harrison MR, Nakayama DK, Noall R. Correction of congenital hydronephrosis *in utero.* II. Decompression reverses the effects of obstruction on the fetal lung and urinary tract. *J Pediatr Surg.* 1981;17:965.
26. Harrison MR, Anderson J, Rosen MA, et al. Fetal surgery in the primate. I. Anesthetic, surgical, and tocolytic management to maximize fetal–neonatal survival. *J Pediatr Surg.* 1985;17:115.
27. Longaker MT, Adzick NS. The biology of fetal wound healing: A review. *Plast Reconstr Surg.* 1991;87:788.

CHAPTER 18

Anesthetic Management for Endoscopic Procedures

JOSEPH D. TOBIAS

With the recent advances in technique and refinement of equipment,[1,2] the applications of endoscopic procedures in children has continued to increase. Therefore, anesthesiologists are faced with an increasing number of children who require anesthetic care during such procedures. Anesthesia for endoscopy includes considerations for a wide range of procedures including laryngoscopy, bronchoscopy, esophagoscopy, thoracoscopy, and laparoscopy. This chapter attempts to deal with the specific anesthetic implications of these endoscopic procedures in children, including intraoperative anesthetic care and monitoring and the physiologic alterations induced by the endoscopic procedure.

PREOPERATIVE EVALUATION

Prior to formulation of the anesthetic plan, the anesthesiologist must have a thorough understanding of the anticipated procedure. Unlike most other surgical procedures in which the airway is the responsibility solely of the anesthesiologist, endoscopic procedures of the upper airway require that the airway be shared between surgeon and anesthesiologist. Therefore, cooperation and communication are especially important to ensure adequate intraoperative conditions for endoscopy as well as to ensure patient safety.

Regardless of the surgical procedure, anesthetic care should begin with a thorough preoperative history and physical examination. Numerous possible scenarios may be present, from an outpatient, elective procedure on an otherwise healthy patient to emergency laparoscopy to evaluate an acute abdomen in a patient with a severe systemic illness. Therefore, premedication and anesthetic induction will vary according to the clinical status of the patient. The child with an acute abdomen requires rapid-sequence endotracheal intubation to reduce the possibility of aspiration, whereas the child with an anterior mediastinal mass requires careful preoperative assessment prior to any surgical procedure requiring general anesthesia or sedation.[3]

In the healthy outpatient without signs of airway compromise, oral premedication with midazolam (0.5 to 0.75 mg/kg) 15 to 20 minutes prior to the procedure provides excellent relief from anxiety and allows for easy separation from parents. This is generally followed by inhalation induction by mask with halothane and nitrous oxide in oxygen. Additional premedications may include the administration of H_2 antagonists (ranitidine) and metoclopramide, for patients at risk for acid aspiration, and antisialogogues (atropine or glycopyrrolate), to decrease secretions and improve airway visualization. Additionally, the preoperative administration of dexamethasone (0.25 to 0.5 mg/kg) should be considered in patients at risk for upper airway edema resulting from laser therapy or prolonged manipulation of the airway.

Preoperative laboratory evaluation depends on the clinical status of the patient more than the endoscopic procedure itself. The healthy outpatient requires a hematocrit and blood draw for type and screen, whereas a more thorough preoperative evaluation should be pursued in patients with systemic diseases. Although blood loss is generally minimal during endoscopic procedures, it is necessary to remember that a laparoscopy may turn into a laparotomy and a thoracoscopy may turn into a thoracotomy. Therefore, blood (10 to 20 mL/kg packed red blood cells) should be available. Furthermore, adequate venous access should be secured prior to the start of these procedures, as inadvertent injury by the trocar and endoscopic instruments to visceral structures may occur.

Central venous access may occasionally be necessary in children with limited peripheral access but is not routine; however, when it is necessary, internal jugular or subclavian vein cannulation on the side of the thoracoscopy is recommended. This avoids the possibility of bilateral pneumothoraces (the intentional pneumothorax induced on the side of the thoracoscopy and the unintentional pneumothorax as a complication of the venous access procedure). Invasive hemodynamic monitoring of arterial blood pressure is not routinely used unless indicated by the clinical status of the patient. Standard intraoperative monitoring includes continuous electrocardiogram, automated blood pressure cuff, pulse oximetry, esophageal stethoscope, temperature probe, and end-tidal carbon dioxide measurement.

INTRAOPERATIVE CARE

Laryngoscopy

Laryngoscopy and upper airway endoscopy may be performed either as a diagnostic procedure to investigate upper airway pathology or during the use of laser therapy in the treatment of various abnormalities. Regardless of the reason, many of these children may have airway pathology that makes usual induction techniques and airway management difficult. Therefore, the first priority is to determine whether airway access will be adequate to permit intubation. In patients at risk for airway compromise (epiglottitis, foreign body), the necessary equipment for needle cricothyrotomy and jet ventilation should be readily available.[4] Additionally, the surgical team should be ready for surgical cricothyrotomy.

Although several options exist for securing the airway in adults with upper airway pathology (awake intubation, fiberoptic intubation),[5] such procedures are difficult and often impossible in a child who is unable to comprehend the situation. Although anecdotal success has been reported in children with various airway management techniques, including retrograde wire-guided intubation,[6] flexible fiberoptic intubation,[7] and retrograde-assisted fiberoptic tracheal intubation,[8] an inhalation induction with halothane in 100% oxygen is the best option in most children.[9] This allows for maintenance of spontaneous ventilation until direct laryngoscopy and airway visualization can be performed; however, airway compromise may increase and complete obstruction may occur as the induction proceeds with loss of upper airway muscle tone.

Halothane may also be administered in a mixture of oxygen and helium to decrease the density of the inhaled gases and thereby increase air flow past a fixed obstruction.[10,11] Although this can be done only at the expense of lowering the inspired fraction of oxygen, air exchange may significantly increase in patients with partially obstructed airways.

Following mask induction and prior to airway manipulation, airway reflexes may be blunted and the risk of laryngospasm decreased by the administration of intravenous lidocaine (1 to 2 mg/kg) or the application of topical lidocaine (5 mg/kg). Muscle relaxants are avoided until successful intubation is accomplished and the airway secured. The one exception is the administration of succinylcholine (1 to 2 mg/kg intravenously) if laryngospasm occurs during induction and is unresponsive to positive-pressure ventilation.

Following induction, the next decisions involve placement of an endotracheal (ET) tube and mode of ventilation. Advantages of placement of an ET tube during laryngoscopy include airway security, protection of the lower airway from particulate matter produced during upper airway laser procedures, ability to control and monitor the adequacy of ventilation, and ability to administer volatile anesthetic agents such as halothane. Disadvantages of ET tube placement include obscuring the upper airway and risk of combustion during laser use.

The major risk during laser surgery of the airway is ET tube fire, with a reported incidence of 0.5 to 2.0%.[12,13] Several scenarios can result in ET tube ignition including tube ignition by either direct laser illumination, reflected laser ignition, or ignited particles from the upper airway surgical site. Regardless of the cause, if the fire is unrecognized, it may burn through the ET tube and ignite the gas flow, resulting in an airway fire. Minimizing the chance of this complication entails reducing the inspired fraction of oxygen to less than 0.40 (Table 18–1). This can be accomplished by diluting the inspired gases with either air or helium. Although it decreases the inspired oxygen concentration, the use of nitrous oxide does not significantly alter the flammability of the gas flow.[14]

Another measure to limit operative airway fire is the use of ET tubes with limited combustibility. Commonly used tubes are either red rubber or polyvinyl chloride (PVC). Although conflicting reports exist, it is generally agreed that PVC tubes are more combustible than red rubber tubes.[15,16] Further protection may be obtained by wrapping the red rubber tube with metallic tape. Although this will not protect the cuff, it will protect the remainder of the tube. Several studies have attempted to identify the most

TABLE 18–1. AIRWAY FIRE DURING ENDOTRACHEAL LASER SURGERY

- MEASURES THAT MINIMIZE RISK OF OCCURRENCE
  1. Reduce fraction of inspired oxygen to less than 0.40
  2. Use ET tubes with limited combustibility
  3. Wrap ET tube with copper tape
  4. Use ET tube only when necessary

- MANAGEMENT OF AIRWAY FIRE
  1. Discontinue gas flow
  2. Remove present ET tube
  3. Reintubate with new ET tube when fire is extinguished
  4. Perform endoscopy to assess damage
  5. Administer systemic corticosteroids, if severe
  6. Repeat endoscopic assessment in 24 to 48 hours to assess response to therapy

effective tape to protect the tube from inadvertent laser damage.[17,18] The general consensus is that copper tape provides the most ignition protection from all three types of lasers (carbon dioxide, Nd:YAG, and KTP Nd:YAG).

Two additional types of ET tubes have been used during laser surgery: a metal tube and a silicone/aluminum-impregnated tube. Because of size constraints, the former is not commonly used in the pediatric population. The Xomed Lasershield (Xomed-Treace, Jacksonville, FL) tube contains an outer coating impregnated with aluminum–silica powder. It should, however, be remembered that resistance to combustion is only relative and airway fires have been reported even with the Xomed tube.[19]

The risk of airway fire can be reduced if an ET tube is not positioned during laser use. This may be accomplished by several methods. The easiest method is intermittent removal of the tube during laser use. With this technique, the patient is anesthetized with intravenous agents and ventilated with 100% oxygen. The ET tube is removed for brief periods (60 to 90 seconds) while the patient's saturation is monitored by pulse oximetry. The laser surgery is performed during these periods of brief apnea. The tube is then replaced, the patient ventilated, and the procedure repeated as needed.

Jet ventilation may also be used during laser surgery. When this modality is used, the patient is anesthetized with intravenous agents and a catheter is placed above the glottic opening. Alternatively, jet ventilation may be accomplished through a central channel in the laryngoscope or by securing an injection needle to the side of the operating laryngoscope. With either method, the jet is connected to an oxygen source with a driving pressure of 50 psi. Ventilation and oxygenation occur by intermittently opening the system, which allows the pressurized oxygen to pass through the tubing to the patient.

Regardless of the method of ventilation and the type of ET tube employed, morbidity from airway fire can be reduced with a preconceived plan to manage this complication (see Table 18–1). If an airway fire occurs, the gas flow should be discontinued and the patient extubated. The patient should be reintubated with another tube followed by direct inspection of the upper and lower airway to assess the degree of damage. Patients with significant airway trauma should be treated with systemic corticosteroids and their trachea should remain intubated for airway protection. Repeat bronchoscopy is necessary to evaluate the degree of airway damage and assess the appropriate time for endotracheal extubation.

Bronchoscopy

Bronchoscopy may be accomplished using either a flexible or a rigid endoscope. Flexible bronchoscopy is generally performed during spontaneous ventilation with intravenous sedation. Prior to the procedure, intravenous access is obtained and an antisialogogue (glycopyrrolate 0.01 mg/kg) administered. Nasal and upper airway anesthesia is accomplished with topical lidocaine (maximum dose 5 mg/kg), which limits the requirement for intravenous sedation. A combination of benzodiazepines and narcotics is used for sedation. Our current preference is the combination of midazolam (incremental doses of 0.03 to 0.05 mg/kg) and fentanyl (incremental doses of 1 μg/kg). Ketamine (1 mg/kg) may be used as the sole agent in younger patients. Although ketamine may increase secretions, its advantages include the maintenance of protective airway reflexes and ventilatory drive.

Flexible bronchoscopy may also be performed during general anesthesia with ET intubation. In these cases, the bronchoscope is passed through the ET tube and ventilation is maintained around the bronchoscope. This requires higher than usual airway pressures because of the reduction in the cross-sectional area of the ET tube lumen by the bronchoscope. Hand ventilation is generally more efficient than relying on the anesthesia machine ventilator. During this time oxygen saturation is monitored and chest excursions are observed to ensure adequate oxygenation and ventilation. In smaller patients with limited airway access (endotracheal tube size less than 4.5 to 5.0 mm), intermittent apnea may be needed, as ventilation around the bronchoscope may not be possible.

General anesthesia is required for rigid bronchoscopy. Following the intravenous or inhalation induction of general anesthesia (depending on the presence of airway pathology), short-acting muscle relaxants are administered (vecuronium 0.1 mg/kg or atracurium 0.5 mg/kg). Neuromuscular function is monitored and neuromuscular blockade maintained during the procedure because of the risks of bleeding and airway trauma if excessive movement occurs while the rigid bronchoscope is positioned. Although the airway may be instrumented and the trachea intubated prior to rigid examination, this is never done when a foreign body is suspected because of the risks of dislodging the foreign body and impacting it deeper into the airway. Following bronchoscope placement, ventilation is maintained through the side arm attachment. The side-arm attachment has a standard 15-mm adapter that connects to the anesthesia system. In smaller patients, ventilation may be impaired when instruments and the telescope are passed through the rigid bronchoscope. Therefore, it may be necessary to withdraw the telescope intermittently to allow adequate ventilation and oxygenation. During the procedure, anesthesia may be maintained with either intravenous or inhalational agents. Postoperatively, the patient is extubated when awake and transported to the recovery room. Extreme vigilance concerning airway integrity is required, as airway manipulation during bronchoscopy may result in edema, bleeding, or barotrauma.

Esophagoscopy

Esophagoscopy may likewise be performed with either a flexible or a rigid instrument. Intravenous sedation is commonly used for flexible esophagoscopy, whereas general anesthesia and muscle relaxation are required for rigid procedures. The choice of anesthetic induction technique depends on the nature of the patient's problem and clinical condition. Rapid-sequence induction is indicated in patients with a suspected foreign body, as retention of food and aspiration are possible. On the other hand, intravenous or inhalation induction is acceptable for the outpatient who has been NPO for an acceptable period. Some of these patients may have gastroesophageal reflux and preoperative administration of H_2 antagonists may be warranted. Following induction and tracheal intubation, anesthesia is continued with either intravenous or inhalational agents. Muscle relaxation is achieved with short-acting, nondepolarizing agents prior to endoscopy. As with rigid bronchoscopy, neuromuscular function should be monitored closely to ensure adequate relaxation and avoid trauma induced by movement during the procedure.

Thoracoscopy

The anesthetic options for thoracoscopy include local anesthetic infiltration, regional anesthesia, and general anesthesia. Although in adults thoracoscopy is often performed using local infiltration and intravenous sedation,[20] this is not practical in younger children because of their inability to comprehend instructions. In older children or teenagers, intravenous sedation supplemented with local anesthetic infiltration may be an option. Following adequate intravenous sedation, the lateral chest wall and parietal pleura are infiltrated with local anesthetic to provide anesthesia for port placement.

Options for regional anesthesia include thoracic epidural anesthesia and multiple intercostal blocks. As with local infiltration, these techniques are often combined with intravenous sedation. Intercostal blocks performed at the level of the incision and two interspaces above and below will provide analgesia for cannula insertion. Thoracic epidural anesthesia provides cutaneous analgesia and eliminates the need for repeated injections at separate interspaces; however, both these techniques provide only cutaneous analgesia and do not block visceral afferents in the phrenic, vagus, or recurrent laryngeal nerves. Therefore, if regional or local infiltration techniques are employed, it may be necessary to provide visceral analgesia using a stellate ganglion block.[21] In addition, this will block the cough reflex which may occur during manipulation of the pulmonary hilum.

Regional and local anesthetic techniques are beneficial during thoracoscopy as they allow spontaneous ventilation. This mode of ventilation is advantageous because it interferes less with surgical exposure than controlled positive-pressure ventilation. During spontaneous ventilation, lung movement does not obscure the surgical field; however, during controlled ventilation, each positive-pressure breath obscures the surgical field unless some means of one-lung ventilation is used.

In younger children, regional anesthetic techniques are limited by the expertise of the anesthesiologist. Furthermore, these blocks are contraindicated in patients with coagulation disturbances. Dosing of these anesthetics is difficult because of rapid intravascular absorption, especially from the intercostal space.

One additional regional anesthetic technique that may find some application during thoracoscopy is intrapleural analgesia (IPA). Although initially described in adults, this technique has been successfully used in children to provide analgesia following thoracotomy.[22] IPA involves the percutaneous placement of a catheter in the paravertebral space. Somatic analgesia results primarily from multiple intercostal nerve blocks, which occur after the local anesthetic has diffused from the pleural space through the parietal pleura.[23] The advantage of this technique over other regional anesthetic techniques (intercostal or epidural anesthesia) is that IPA may also block visceral affer-

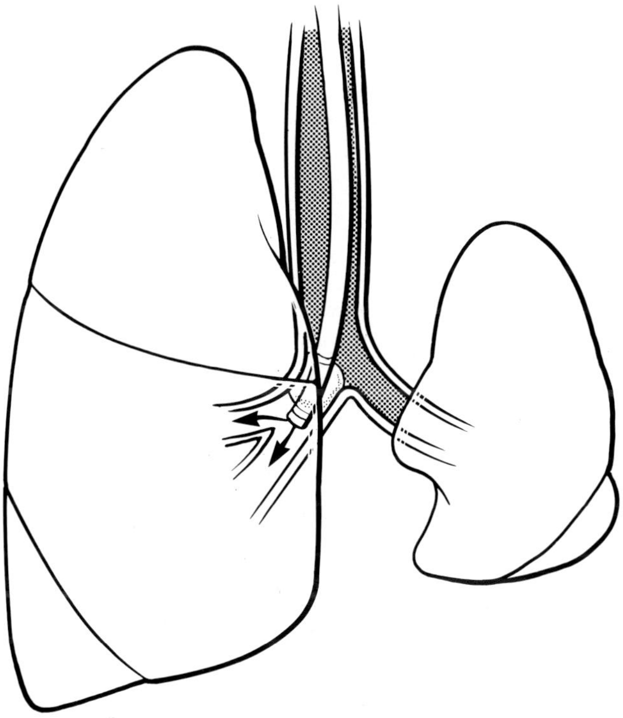

Figure 18–1. The endotracheal tube is positioned in the right mainstem bronchus, which provides ventilation to the right lung only. This can usually be accomplished blindly for right mainstem bronchial intubation, but may require bronchoscopy for placement in the left mainstem bronchus.

ents in the phrenic, vagus, and recurrent laryngeal nerves in addition to the sympathetic chain, thereby providing both cutaneous and visceral analgesia.

Because of the limitations of the regional anesthetic techniques, we prefer general anesthesia in most circumstances. As standard positive-pressure ventilation will interfere with the artificial pneumothorax induced to facilitate the procedure, we use positive-pressure ventilation with one-lung anesthesia. Although commonly used in adult thoracic surgery, one-lung anesthesia is less commonly employed in pediatric anesthesia. In adults, standard double-lumen endotracheal tubes are used to isolate the individual lungs. Because of size limitations, this is possible only in patients greater than 30 to 35 kg.

In smaller patients, two options are available for one-lung anesthesia: selective endobronchial intubation or the use of bronchial blockers. We generally use selective endobronchial intubation. This can be done blindly for right-sided intubation, but usually requires either bronchoscopic guidance or fluoroscopy to ensure left mainstem intubation.[24,25] Following standard anesthetic induction, the patient's trachea is intubated with a cuffed ET tube (one half to one size smaller than usual). The fiberoptic bronchoscope is passed through the ET tube and maneuvered into the mainstem bronchus of the side opposite the surgical pathology. The ET tube is advanced over the bronchoscope. The balloon is inflated so that collateral ventilation of the opposite lung does not occur (Figure 18–1). A standard 3.5-mm (external diameter) fiberoptic bronchoscope will fit through a 5.0-mm or greater endotracheal tube. Following the procedure, the endotracheal tube is withdrawn into the midtracheal position and two-lung ventilation initiated.

If one chooses to use bronchial blockers to occlude the involved bronchus, a Fogarty embolectomy catheter or a standard Swan-Ganz catheter may be used (Figure 18–2). Both of these are also placed using fiberoptic guidance. The Swan-Ganz catheter allows delivery of oxygen to the involved lung through the distal port of the catheter. This may improve oxygenation during one-lung anesthesia.[26] Disadvantages of this technique include difficulty with catheter placement and catheter dislodgement during surgery. The latter may result in obstruction of the tracheal lumen distal to the endotracheal tube. Therefore, when these techniques are used, continuous monitoring of breath sounds and pulmonary compliance is mandatory. In such cases, hand ventilation is recommended to accurately follow compliance during the procedure.

In older patients, a double-lumen endotracheal

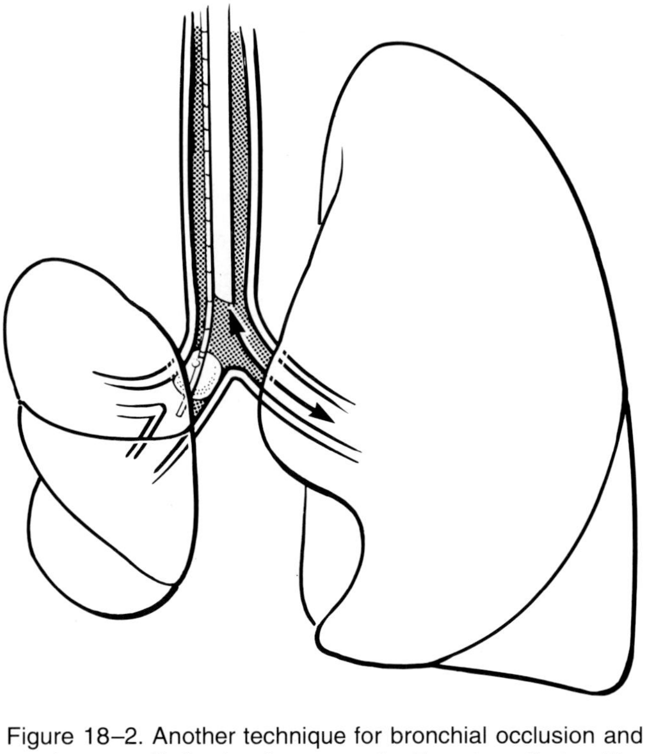

Figure 18–2. Another technique for bronchial occlusion and one-lung ventilation involves use of a Fogarty catheter. The catheter is positioned beside the endotracheal tube and placed in the appropriate mainstem bronchus. The balloon on the catheter is then inflated.

tube may be used for one-lung anesthesia. This technique provides the opportunity to change from one-lung to two-lung ventilation without repositioning the endotracheal tube. Although a 25- or 27-French double-lumen tube may be used in patients weighing 30 to 35 kg, the lumina of these tubes will not accept a 3.5-mm bronchoscope. Therefore, blind placement is necessary without guidance or confirmation by fiberoptic bronchoscopy. In patients greater than 50 kg, standard, left-sided double-lumen tubes (35, 37, 39, and 41 French) may be used. The 3.5-mm bronchoscope will pass through both lumina of these tubes and may be used to facilitate and confirm placement.

Following successful isolation of one lung, anesthesia is maintained with a combination of intravenous and inhalational agents. In the choice of an inhalational agent, isoflurane has the advantage of interfering less with hypoxic pulmonary vasoconstriction (HPV) than halothane or enflurane.[27] These inhalational agents are administered with 100% oxygen and limited to 0.5 to 1.0 minimum alveolar concentration (MAC) to avoid interference with HPV. Anesthesia is supplemented as needed with intravenous narcotics (usually fentanyl 3 to 10 μg/kg) or other intravenous agents (ketamine, benzodiazepines, barbiturates) that have little or no effect on HPV.[28] Intraoperatively, nitrous oxide is avoided because of the risks of expanding an inadvertent venous air embolism (discussed later) or the artificial pneumothorax. This is especially important after evacuation of the pneumothorax at the completion of the procedure.

Positioning includes the standard right or left lateral decubitus position as used for routine thoracotomy. Following induction, an artificial pneumothorax may be created by the surgeon with the injection of 50 to 100 mL of air. This should be performed in the third or fourth interspace, as the hemidiaphragm will move cephalad during one-lung ventilation and needle entry at a lower point may result in hepatic or splenic injury. During this time, cardiorespiratory function should be carefully monitored. The moderate displacement of intrathoracic contents is generally well tolerated in the euvolemic patient with normal cardiac function. Creation of an excessive pneumothorax (either volume or pressure) may lead to decreased venous return and increased afterload, resulting in hypotension. Therefore, frequent monitoring of blood pressure is recommended during this time.

Hypovolemia or abnormal cardiac function may predispose patients to hypotension in response to the alterations in preload and afterload induced by the artificial pneumothorax. Therefore, intravascular deficits should be corrected and cardiovascular function optimized prior to the creation of the artificial pneumothorax. Additionally, invasive monitoring (central venous pressure and arterial line placement) should be considered in such patients.

The second risk during the creation of the artificial pneumothorax is inadvertent injection of air either into an intercostal vessel or into the pulmonary circulation. Careful aspiration and slow injection are necessary to ensure that this catastrophic event does not occur. The consequences and clinical manifestations of air embolism are dependent on several factors: volume of air, rate of entrainment, use of nitrous oxide, and general cardiorespiratory status of the patient. Small volumes of air are removed by the pulmonary vasculature and excreted. When the rate of entrainment exceeds the rate of excretion, pulmonary artery pressures rise and cardiac output falls.[29]

Treatment of this catastrophic event is directed primarily at early detection and prevention (Table 18–2). Detection techniques can be separated into those that detect venous air embolism prior to clinical signs (precordial doppler, end-tidal nitrogen, end-tidal carbon dioxide, and pulmonary artery pressure monitoring) and those that monitor the clinical sequelae (decreased cardiac output, central venous pressure, oxygen saturation).[30] Precordial doppler and end-tidal nitrogen monitoring are extremely sensitive measures and will detect as little as 0.5 mL of air.[31] As these techniques are non-invasive and easily applied to most patients, their use is recommended. More invasive techniques such as pulmonary artery pressure monitoring and central venous pressure monitoring add little to the ability to detect this unlikely event. Moreover, they are relatively nonspecific and provide little warning.

Management includes notifying the surgeon to stop the injection and then restoring intravascular volume and administering inotropic agents to treat the cardiovascular sequelae. If these measures are not successful in restoring cardiovascular stability, the patient should be placed supine. This maneuver promotes venous return and allows more effective external cardiac massage in extreme cases.

Although such catastrophic events are possible, the artificial pneumothorax is usually well tolerated. Following the creation of the artificial pneumothorax,

TABLE 18–2. MANAGEMENT OF AIR EMBOLUS

Early detection
Use precordial doppler
Monitor end-tidal nitrogen
Treatment
Stop injection
Restore intravascular volume
Administer inotropic drugs for cardiovascular sequelae
Place in supine position or Trendelenburg position
Perform external cardiac massage in extreme cases

one-lung ventilation is maintained throughout the surgical procedure. At the completion of the procedure, the pneumothorax is evacuated and two-lung ventilation reinstituted. Auscultation is performed to ensure reinflation of the collapsed lung. Residual neuromuscular blockade is reversed and the patient is extubated when awake. Postoperative analgesia can generally be achieved with oral narcotics and many patients are discharged home the same day.

Laparoscopy

As with thoracoscopy, the options for anesthesia during laparoscopy include local, regional, and general anesthetic techniques.[23,32] Anesthetic induction techniques and agents should be based on the clinical status of the patient. It should be kept in mind that laparoscopy in children is frequently used to evaluate possible appendicitis and other intraabdominal processes, so that these patients should be considered to have a full stomach. Therefore, preoperative H_2 antagonists and metoclopramide followed by rapid-sequence intubation may be indicated.

Although general anesthesia is most commonly used, local anesthesia with intravenous sedation is an option for the healthy, fasted, adult patient [33]; however, laparoscopy in children is done almost exclusively with general anesthesia. Although laparoscopy can be performed with general anesthesia by mask in the low-risk adult patient, ET intubation with controlled ventilation is the anesthetic of choice for the majority of children. This is important as the risk of hypoxemia during spontaneous ventilation is greater in children. The greater likelihood of hypoxemia is the result of a decreased functional residual capacity (FRC) compared with adults. FRC is further reduced by Trendelenburg position, insufflation of the abdomen with carbon dioxide or fluid during the procedure, and administration of volatile anesthetic agents. This combination further reduces the limited FRC of the pediatric patient, resulting in ventilation–perfusion inequalities and hypoxemia during spontaneous ventilation.

Following induction, anesthesia is maintained with inhalational agents (isoflurane or halothane) supplemented with intravenous narcotics. We prefer to avoid the use of nitrous oxide, as the risk of air embolism exists during this procedure with the instillation of carbon dioxide into the peritoneal cavity.[34] Although the risk of air embolism is small and the physiologic consequences lessened by the use of carbon dioxide rather than air, general anesthesia can easily be maintained without nitrous oxide. Additionally, a high inspired concentration of oxygen is recommended especially for the younger patient, who is at risk for hypoxemia during this procedure because of the previously mentioned factors that decrease FRC. In those situations in which 100% oxygen is contraindicated or not required, an air/oxygen mixture can be delivered.

Routine monitoring including the use of end-tidal carbon dioxide should be adequate to detect air embolism, and more sophisticated devices including precordial doppler and measurement of end-tidal nitrogen do not appear necessary. Furthermore, because of the rare occurrence of air embolism during this procedure, the prophylactic placement of a multiorifice central venous catheter for air aspiration does not seem warranted.

Aside from the risk of air embolism, the major physiologic effects of the intraperitoneal insufflation of carbon dioxide relate to the absorption of carbon dioxide by the peritoneum and the cardiopulmonary changes from the increased intraabdominal pressure (Table 18–3). Ventilation may need to be increased 10 to 20% to maintain normocarbia. This is accomplished by monitoring end-tidal carbon dioxide and making appropriate adjustments in respiratory rate. The increased ventilatory demands related to carbon dioxide absorption by the peritoneum combined with the respiratory depressant effects of volatile anesthetic agents may result in significant hypercarbia if ventilation is not controlled.

Significant physiologic effects may occur with increases in intraabdominal pressure. These effects are reduced by monitoring intraabdominal pressure during carbon dioxide insufflation and limiting it to less than 20 mm Hg. Cardiovascular changes including de-

TABLE 18–3. PHYSIOLOGIC EFFECTS OF INTRAABDOMINAL CARBON DIOXIDE INSUFFLATION

Effect	Management
1. Absorption of carbon dioxide and hypercarbia	1. Increase ventilation
2. Increased intraabdominal pressure	
a. Diminished preload	2a. Replace preoperative fluid deficits and ongoing fluid losses
b. Bradycardia	b. Administer atropine and glycopyrrolate
c. Need for increased airway pressure to maintain tidal volume	c. Increase pressure limits on ventilator to achieve adequate tidal volume
d. Decreased functional residual capacity	d. Increase positive end expiratory pressure

creased blood pressure may occur as a result of diminished venous return and preload. Such changes are well tolerated in the euvolemic patient, but may be exaggerated in the volume-depleted patient. Preoperative and intraoperative fluid administration should be used to maintain normovolemia by replacing preoperative deficits in addition to ongoing losses. Additionally, the intraperitoneal insufflation of carbon dioxide may occasionally lead to bradycardia through vagal reflexes. Preoperative or intraoperative administration of anticholinergic agents (atropine, glycopyrrolate) prevents this occurrence.

Increased intraabdominal pressure can also have significant pulmonary effects. In addition to its effects on FRC, increased intraabdominal pressure requires an increase in airway pressure to maintain tidal volume. Monitoring of exhaled tidal volume is necessary to prevent hypoventilation, as many pediatric ventilators are pressure, not volume, cycled. If this is the case, pressure limits should be increased to maintain tidal volume. In addition, positive end expiratory pressure (PEEP) may be needed to offset the detrimental effects of increased intraabdominal pressure on FRC. The judicious use of PEEP will also improve compliance and deliver an appropriate tidal volume with acceptable mean airway pressures.

Occasionally, fluid is instilled into the peritoneal cavity to create an "artificial ascites" to improve surgical exposure. An isotonic solution such as lactated Ringer's or Plasmalyte should be used, as this fluid may be absorbed by the peritoneum. Hypotonic fluids such as half-normal saline or hypertonic fluids such as normal saline may result in electrolyte disturbances. Although the amount of fluid absorbed is limited, significant amounts of fluid may be absorbed in children with peritonitis.

At the completion of the procedure, residual neuromuscular blockade is reversed and the patient is extubated. Postoperative analgesia is provided by a combination of intravenous and oral narcotics according to the needs of the patient.

REFERENCES

1. Ryckman FC, Rodgers BM. Thoracoscopy for intrathoracic neoplasia in children. *J Pediatr Surg.* 1982;17:521.
2. Rodgers BM, Talbert JL. Thoracoscopy for diagnosis of intrathoracic lesions in children. *J Pediatr Surg.* 1976;11:703.
3. Pullerits J, Holzman R. Anaesthesia for patients with mediastinal masses. *Can J Anaesth.* 1989;36:681.
4. Spoerel WE, Narayanan PD, Singh NP. Transtracheal ventilation. *Br J Anaesth.* 1971;43:932.
5. Donlon JV. Anesthetic management of patients with compromised airways. *Anesth Rev.* 1980;7:22.
6. Borland LM, Swan DM, Leff S. Difficult pediatric endotracheal intubation: A new approach to the retrograde technique. *Anesthesiology.* 1981;55:577.
7. Rucker RW, Silva WJ, Worcester CC. Fiberoptic bronchoscopic nasotracheal intubation in children. *Chest.* 1979;76:56.
8. Audenaert SM, Montgomery CL, Stone B, Akins R, Lock RL. Retrograde-assisted fiberoptic tracheal intubation in children with difficult airways. *Anesth Analg.* 1991;73:660.
9. Oh TG, Motoyama EK. Comparison of nasotracheal intubation and tracheostomy in the management of acute epiglottitis. *Anesthesiology.* 1977;46:214.
10. Mizrahi S, Yaari Y, Lugassy G, Cotev S. Major airway obstruction relieved by helium/oxygen breathing. *Crit Care Med.* 1986;14:986.
11. Skrinskas GJ, Hyland RH, Hutcheon MA. Using helium–oxygen mixtures in the management of acute upper airway obstruction. *Can Med Assoc J.* 1983;128:555.
12. Snow JC, Norton ML, Salvja TS, Estanislao AF. Fire hazard during CO_2 laser microsurgery on the larynx and trachea. *Anesth Analg.* 1976;55:146.
13. Hermens JM, Bennett MJ, Hirshman CA. Anesthesia for laser surgery. *Anesth Analg.* 1983;62:218.
14. Wolf GL, Simpson JI. Flammability of endotracheal tubes in oxygen and nitrous oxide enriched atmospheres. *Anesthesiology.* 1987;67:236.
15. Ossoff RH, Duncavage JA, Eisenman TS, Karlan MS. Comparison of tracheal damage from laser-ignited endotracheal tube fires. *Ann Otol Rhinol Laryngol.* 1983;92:333.
16. Rampil IJ: Anesthetic considerations for laser surgery. *Anesth Analg.* 1992;74:424.
17. Sosis MB. Evaluation of five metallic tapes for protection of endotracheal tubes during CO_2 laser surgery. *Anesth Analg.* 1989;68:392.
18. Sosis M, Dillon F. What is the safest foil tape for endotracheal tube protection during Nd-YAG laser surgery? A comparative study. *Anesthesiology.* 1990;72:553.
19. Laser-resistant endotracheal tubes and wraps. *Health Devices.* 1990;19:112.
20. Morton JR, Guinn GA. Thoracoscopy using local anesthesia. *Am J Surg.* 1971;122:696.
21. Parris WCV, Reddy BC, White HW, McGrath DM. Stellate ganglion blocks in pediatric patients. *Anesth Analg.* 1991;72:552.
22. Tobias JD, Martin LD, Oakes L, Rao B, Wetzel RC. Postoperative analgesia following thoracotomy in children: Intrapleural catheters. *J Pediatr Surg.* In press.
23. Riegler FX, Vadeboncouer TR, Pelligrino DA. An animal model of interpleural analgesia. *Anesthesiology.* 1989;71:744.
24. Watson CB, Bowe EA, Burk W. One lung anesthesia for pediatric surgery: A new use for the fiberoptic bronchoscope. *Anesthesiology.* 1982;56:314.
25. Rao CC, Krishna G, Grosfeld JL, Weber TR. One lung pediatric anesthesia. *Anesth Analg.* 1981;60:450.
26. Dalens B, Labbe A, Haberer JP. Selective endobronchial blocking versus selective intubation (letter). *Anesthesiology.* 1982;57:555.

27. Benumof JL, Augustine SD, Gibbons JA. Halothane and isoflurane only slightly impair arterial oxygenation during one-lung ventilation in patients undergoing thoracotomy. *Anesthesiology.* 1987;67:910.
28. Benumof JL, Wahrenbrock EA. Local effects of anesthetics on regional hypoxic pulmonary vasoconstriction. *Anesthesiology.* 1975;43:525.
29. Verstappen FTJ, Bernards JA, Kreuzer F. Effects of pulmonary gas embolism on circulation and respiration in the dog. *Pflueger's Arch.* 1977;368:89.
30. Brechner VL, Bethune R. Recent advances in monitoring pulmonary air embolism. *Anesth Analg.* 1971;50:255.
31. Maroon JF, Albin MS. Air embolism diagnosed by doppler ultrasound. *Anesth Analg.* 1974;53:399.
32. Bridenbaugh LD. Regional anaesthesia for outpatient surgery—A summary of 12 years' experience. *Can Anaesth Soc J.* 1983;30:548.
33. Wheeless CR Jr. Outpatient laparoscope sterilization under local anesthesia. *Obstet Gynecol.* 1972;39:767.
34. Munsen ES, Merrick HC. Effect of nitrous oxide on venous air embolism. *Anesthesiology.* 1966;27:783.

CHAPTER 19

Future Applications in Children

GEORGE W. HOLCOMB III

In the preceding chapters, new endoscopic techniques have been described for children. Laparoscopic and thoracoscopic procedures have proliferated over a very short period and it is unknown what the future holds for these methods. It is, however, very likely that these procedures will survive and other improvements and applications will be developed.

At this time, several other laparoscopic procedures either are in the developmental stage or have been used in a small number of patients. Included in this group are laparoscopic liver biopsy, laparoscopic Meckel's diverticulectomy, laparoscopy for insertion of peritoneal dialysis catheters, laparoscopy for assistance with insertion of ventriculoperitoneal shunts, and laparoscopic splenectomy. Laparoscopic intestinal resection has been performed in a relatively large series of adult patients and may develop application for children.

LAPAROSCOPIC LIVER BIOPSY

Open liver biopsies are often required for diagnostic purposes. Following diagnostic laparoscopy through an umbilical incision, the liver is easily identified and several areas are sampled percutaneously under laparoscopic visualization. The advantages of this technique are the ability to identify specific sites within the liver for biopsy and the ability to evaluate bleeding following the biopsy. Control of hemorrhage with cauterization can be accomplished, if needed, through a 5 mm cannula which can be placed at the site of introduction of the percutaneous needle.

LAPAROSCOPIC MECKEL'S DIVERTICULECTOMY

Diverticulectomy can be performed using the laparoscopic technique. Following diagnostic laparoscopy through a 5-mm umbilical port, a 12-mm incision is made in the left lower quadrant and a 5-mm incision in the right inguinal crease (Figure 19–1). Through the 5-mm site, the diverticulum is grasped and elevated. By use of an endostapler inserted through the 12-mm cannula, the diverticulum is stapled and excised (Figure 19–2). The specimen can then be extracted through the 12-mm site.

Whether this procedure will be safer and more advantageous than a small right midabdominal incision is not evident at this time. It can, however, be performed and has been reported.[1]

LAPAROSCOPY FOR PERITONEAL DIALYSIS CATHETERS

Laparoscopy can be employed for assistance with insertion of peritoneal dialysis catheters and offers some advantages over an open technique. Either a 9.5-French, 31-cm-long or 15.0-French, 42-cm-long silicone catheter (Cook, Bloomington, IN) can be inserted through a site in the midabdominal wall using the Seldinger technique. Initially, diagnostic laparoscopy is performed through a 5-mm umbilical cannula and a site is selected for insertion of the catheter. A needle is inserted in an oblique fashion followed by insertion of the guidewire, which is positioned in the pelvis under direct visualization.

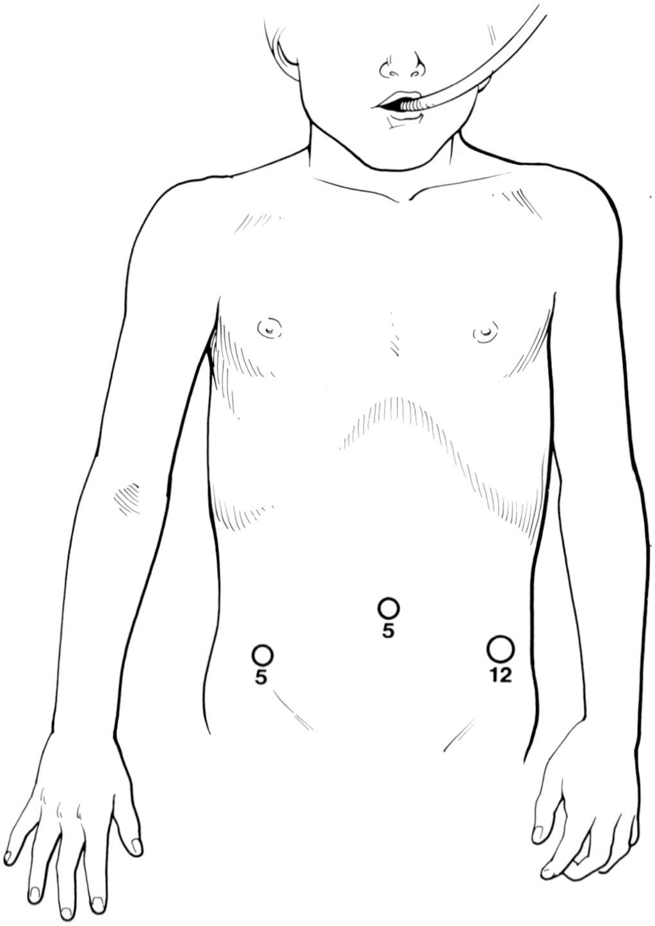

Figure 19–1. For laparoscopic Meckel's diverticulectomy, a three-port technique similar to laparoscopic appendectomy is used. The endostapler is inserted through the left lower quadrant port and the Meckel's diverticulum is elevated with a grasping forceps placed through the 5-mm right lower quadrant port.

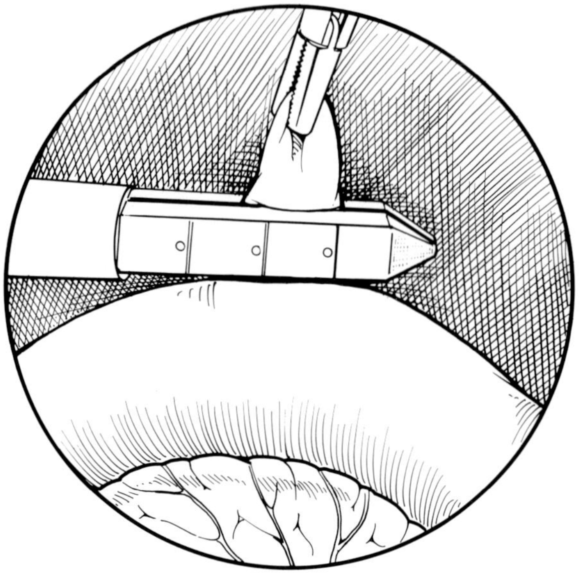

Figure 19–2. The endostapler being placed across the base of the Meckel's diverticulum.

Dilator and sheath are then inserted over the guidewire, guidewire and dilator are removed, and the catheter is placed through the sheath and directed into the pelvis under visualization (Figure 19–3). The sheath is then peeled away and the catheter is secured at the skin.

Advantages of the laparoscopic approach include the avoidance of peritoneal closure with resultant leak at the site of catheter insertion and decreased operating time. Moreover, with abdominal insufflation, the bowel is displaced posteriorly; thus the needle can be inserted without concern for intestinal injury. With this technique, the only closure required is the 5-mm umbilical incision. This procedure has been performed at Children's Hospital–Vanderbilt University Medical Center (CH-VUMC) without complications in two children.

LAPAROSCOPY FOR ASSISTANCE WITH VENTRICULOPERITONEAL SHUNTS

In a fashion similar to that for the previously mentioned peritoneal dialysis catheters, laparoscopic assistance is available for ventriculoperitoneal (VP) shunts. Again, following diagnostic laparoscopy, and after the tubing has been tunneled from its cranial insertion, a site is selected for entry into the abdominal cavity. With the Seldinger technique and equipment similar to that used for peritoneal dialysis catheters, the shunt tube is threaded through a sheath that is then peeled away following placement of the tube in a dependent position. Though laparoscopic assistance may not be needed on each occasion, it can be employed in selected cases. This has been performed in a patient with a large abdominal pseudocyst. Moreover, the lining of the pseudocyst was resected laparoscopically. It has also been used in four other children at CH-VUMC. In two children, the retained intraabdominal portion of a previously placed ventriculoperitoneal shunt was removed from the abdominal cavity.

LAPAROSCOPIC SPLENECTOMY

Laparoscopic splenectomy has been described by Tulman and colleagues and has been performed on a limited basis[2,3]; however, it may attract surgeons in the

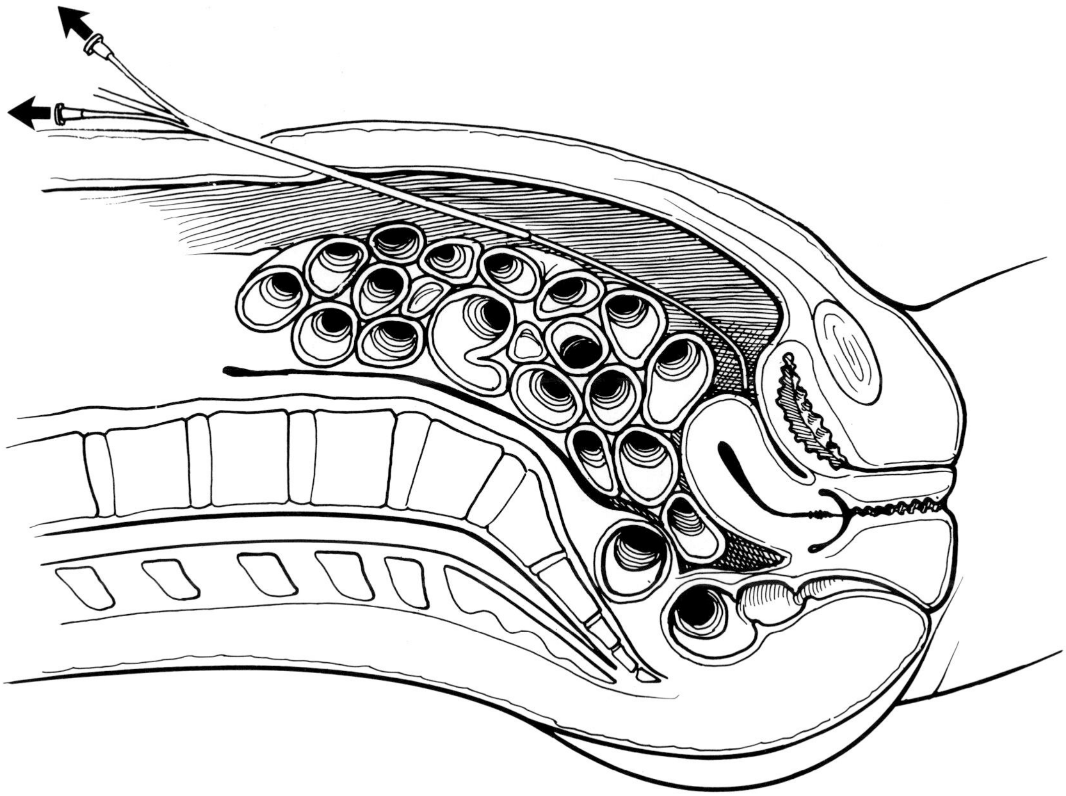

Figure 19–3. For laparoscopic assistance with insertion of peritoneal catheters, the Seldinger technique is employed. In this diagram, the catheter has been placed through a sheath and directed into the pelvis, and the sheath is being peeled away.

future if the procedure can be performed safely. The ideal candidate would be a child with idiopathic thrombocytopenia purpura (ITP), as the spleen should be small. In addition, it may be possible to combine laparoscopic splenectomy with staging laparoscopy and node biopsy for Hodgkin's disease.

Following establishment of an adequate pneumoperitoneum, a 10-mm trocar and cannula are inserted through the umbilicus for video laparoscopy. A 5-mm port is then placed halfway between the umbilicus and xiphoid and 12-mm ports are placed in the left midclavicular and anterior axillary lines at the level of the umbilicus (Figure 19–4).

Initially, the short gastric vessels are divided. Next the splenocolic ligament is dissected and divided, allowing a probe to be passed posteriorly to the spleen which lifts the hilum anteriorly (Figure 19–5). The hilar vessels are then identified and exposed, which enables placement of endovascular clips and ligatures for vascular control (Figure 19–6). The splenic artery and vein are divided, with the vessels secured by clips and extracorporeal ligatures. In an alternative technique, the endostapler is used for ligation and division of the splenic hilum. Hemostasis is very important during the procedure and all maneuvers should be performed very cautiously. Following division of all the ligaments as well as vascular attachments, the spleen is freed and introduced into a sterile bag. The open portion of the bag is exteriorized through the 12-mm incision in the anterior axillary position. Either a morcellator or a finger is used for splenic fracture, which will enable piecemeal removal. Following complete extraction of the splenic tissue, the peritoneal cavity is inspected, all cannulas are removed, and the incisions are closed.

Should it be necessary to remove the spleen intact, either the anterior axillary line or midclavicular incision may be enlarged and the intact spleen easily removed. This usually requires only a 2.5- to 3.0-cm incision if the spleen is small.

The major disadvantage of the laparoscopic approach for splenectomy is the expertise and time required. The procedure will probably require 4 to 5 hours because of the necessity for cautiously dividing the vessels in the splenic hilum; however, the patients can leave the hospital as early as the next day and, on

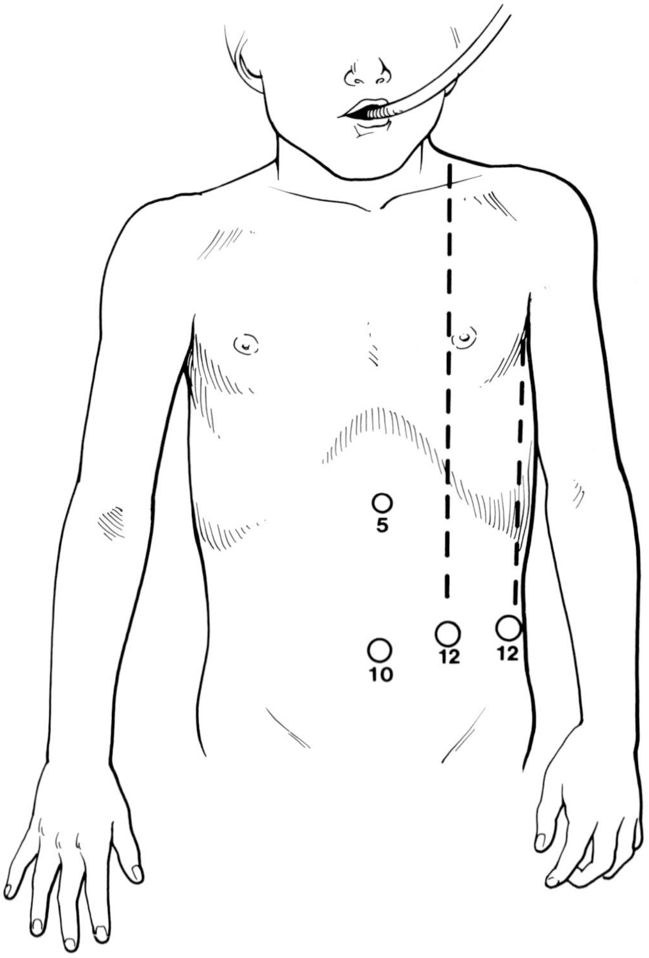

Figure 19–4. For laparoscopic splenectomy, at least four ports are needed and should be placed as shown.

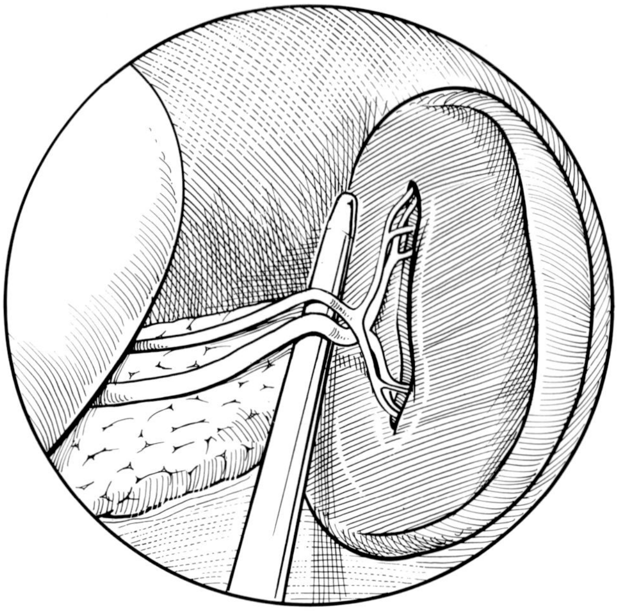

Figure 19–5. Following division of the short gastric vessels and exposure of the splenic hilum, a probe is passed posteriorly to the spleen which elevates the hilum for improved exposure.

the basis of very limited experience, appear to have much less discomfort compared with an open procedure.[3]

As mentioned earlier, laparoscopic splenectomy can be combined with lymph node sampling and liver biopsy for staging of Hodgkin's disease. This has been described in a single child without complication.[3]

INTESTINAL RESECTION

In the future, intestinal resection may be a procedure performed laparoscopically by experienced pediatric surgical endoscopists. Experience with laparoscopic colectomy has already been described in adult patients.[4] In this report of 51 laparoscopic colectomies, 7 cases (14%) were converted to facilitated procedures and 4 cases (8%) were converted to an open laparotomy. Four patients (8%) developed complications but none were related specifically to the laparoscopic approach.

Potential application of laparoscopic intestinal resection to pediatric patients would involve such diseases as Crohn's disease, ulcerative colitis and, possi-

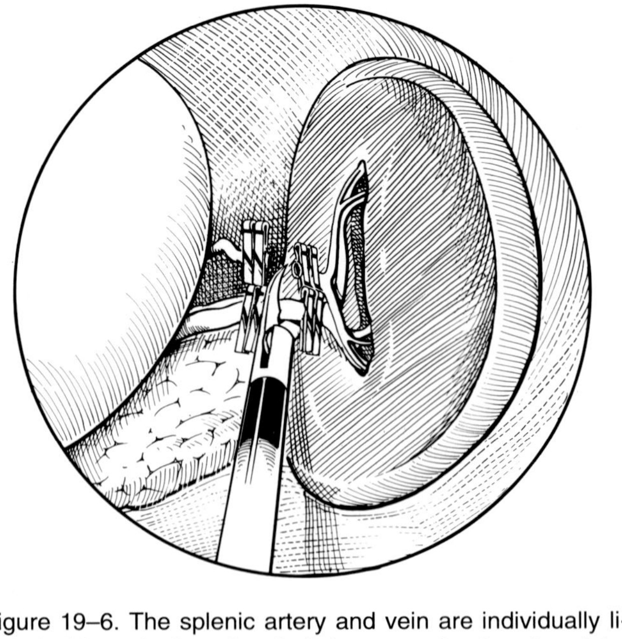

Figure 19–6. The splenic artery and vein are individually ligated with endoclips. Surgical ties may also be placed for added security. In an alternative technique, the endostapler is used across the splenic hilum.

bly, Hirschsprung's disease. A laparoscopic small bowel resection or colonic resection might be applicable to a child with segmental Crohn's disease. With respect to ulcerative colitis, perhaps a two-stage approach would be more beneficial than the very long, time-consuming, single operative approach now used by some surgeons. At the first stage, the colon could be removed laparoscopically, with the colonic mesentery controlled by endoclips or ligatures. The rectum would be divided with an endostapler and the specimen removed through the site of the ileostomy. The advantage of this two-stage approach would be that the patient could be discharged on the first or second day postoperatively following the laparoscopic colectomy and would return at a later date for the endorectal pull-through procedure. With this approach, a low transverse incision could be used at the second stage, and the postoperative ileus, it is hoped, would be decreased as compared with the postoperative ileus resulting from the long single-stage operative approach now used in some centers. Whether or not Hirschsprung's disease will lend itself to laparoscopic management is debatable. There is, however, at least one report of a laparoscopic Soavé procedure and a laparoscopic Duhamel procedure (T. Lobe and K. Georgeson, personal communication, 1993).

The actual technique for laparoscopic intestinal resection in children will vary depending on the size of the patient and the specific part of the intestine to be removed. In general, four or five ports will probably be needed, with control of the mesentery of the resected bowel being accomplished with the endostapler or endoclips. Division at the two ends of the specimen can be accomplished with the endostapler, and the two ends to be anastomosed can be delivered through one of the 10-mm incisions and an extracorporeal anastomosis performed. An intracorporeal anastomosis is possible but is technically difficult and will probably lead to anastomotic complications early in one's experience. It would seem easier to externalize the intestinal segments and perform an extracorporeal anastomosis, which should be much safer in children.

TUMOR MANAGEMENT

What the future holds for endoscopic assistance for tumor management is unknown; however, quite likely, laparoscopy and thoracoscopy will begin to play an important role in diagnostic evaluation of children with tumors. For instance, laparoscopy to evaluate resectability of tumors may be beneficial to the pediatric surgeon and laparoscopy to diagnose the extent of tumors such as pelvic rhabdomyosarcoma and germ cell tumors may also be helpful.

As far as endoscopic management of tumors, thoracoscopic wedge resections for metastatic tumors such as osteosarcoma may prevent the need for repeated thoracotomies for this purpose. In addition, pelvic lymph node dissections may be useful for certain tumors, such as paratesticular rhabdomyosarcoma, that may need retroperitoneal node dissection for staging. Laparoscopy for liver biopsy may also be helpful when hepatic lesions are noted on imaging studies in patients with known tumors.

SUMMARY

As can be seen from the present and preceding chapters, numerous different operative procedures can be performed laparoscopically or with laparoscopic assistance. Most of these procedures have advantages over their open counterparts, primarily in terms of smaller incisions, less discomfort, and, usually, shorter hospitalization. It is, however, extremely important to ensure that the safety of the patient is not compromised. If laparoscopic procedures can be performed with additional benefits to patients and with the same morbidity as open operations, then the laparoscopic route should be preferable. With that in mind, it will be important for pediatric surgeons to learn some laparoscopic techniques to offer these advantages to their patients. By the time this book is published, many of these techniques may already be accepted as the standard of care for children. Others may have been discarded for lack of advantage over the open technique. Only through experience can we determine which techniques should be applied and which should be abandoned.

REFERENCES

1. Huang CS, Lin LH. Laparoscopic Meckel's diverticulum in infants: Report of three cases. Submitted for publication.
2. Tulman S, Reynhout J. Laparoscopic splenectomy (video). Presented at the Society of American Gastrointestinal Endoscopic Surgeons (SAGES) 1992 Scientific Session, April 11–12, Washington, DC.
3. Tulman S, Holcomb GW III, Karamanoukian HL, Reynhout J. Pediatric laparoscopic splenectomy. *J Pediatr Surg.* 1993;28:689.
4. Phillips EH, Franklin M, Carroll BJ, et al. Laparoscopic colectomy. *Ann Surg.* 1992;216:703.

Index

Page numbers followed by *f* refer to figures and by *t* to tables.